ESSENTIALS OF
ORAL PATHOLOGY AND ORAL MEDICINE

For Churchill Livingstone:

Publisher: Michael Parkinson
Project Editors: Ninette Premdas, Janice Urquhart
Copy Editor: Rosaline Crum
Design Direction: Erik Bigland
Project Controller: Kay Hunston

ESSENTIALS OF ORAL PATHOLOGY AND ORAL MEDICINE

R. A. Cawson MD BDS FDS RCPS(Glas) FRCPath

Emeritus Professor of Oral Medicine and Pathology,
University of London, Department of Surgery,
United Medical and Dental Schools, of Guy's
and St Thomas's Hospitals and Visiting Professor
in Oral Pathology, Baylor Dental College, Dallas,
Texas and Eastman Dental Institute, London

E. W. Odell BDS FDS RCS MSc PhD MRCPath

Senior Lecturer and Honorary Consultant, United Medical and Dental Schools,
Guy's and St Thomas's Hospitals, London

SIXTH EDITION

CHURCHILL
LIVINGSTONE

EDINBURGH LONDON NEW YORK PHILADELPHIA SAN FRANCISCO SYDNEY TORONTO 1998

CHURCHILL LIVINGSTONE
A Division of Harcourt Brace and Company Limited

© Longman Group UK Limited 1991
Assigned to Pearson Professional 1995
This edition © Harcourt Brace and Company Limited 1998

⧨ is a registered trade mark of Harcourt Brace and Company Limited

First edition 1962
Second edition 1968
Third edition 1978
Fourth edition 1984
Fifth edition 1991
Sixth edition 1998

Standard Edition ISBN 0 443 05348 0

International Student Edition ISBN 0 443 06121 1

Formerly published as *Essentials of Dental Surgery and Pathology*

British Library of Cataloguing in Publication Data
A catalogue record for this book is available from the British Library.

Library of Congress Cataloging in Publication Data
A catalog record for this book is available from the Library of Congress.

Medical knowledge is constantly changing. As new information becomes
available, changes in treatment, procedures, equipment and the use of
drugs become necessary. The authors and the publishers have, as far as it is
possible, taken care to ensure that the information given in this text is
accurate and up to date. However, readers are strongly advised to confirm
that the information, especially with regard to drug usage, complies with
current legislation and standards of practice.

The
publisher's
policy is to use
**paper manufactured
from sustainable forests**

Produced by Addison Wesley Longman China Limited, Hong Kong
GCC/01

Preface

This book was originally written to cover as much as possible of the contents of the final degree examination in Dental Surgery. At the time this was an entirely new approach, but times have of course changed and this book has been repeatedly updated accordingly. Substantial advances have been made in investigative measures, such as imaging techniques and immunohistochemistry, and in the understanding in particular, of many mucosal diseases and neoplasms. Not merely has knowledge advanced but there is also the healthy trend for the subjects of Oral Pathology and Oral Medicine to unite. Combined departments are being formed both here and in the United States, and with the growing financial pressures on Universities, such moves are likely to continue.

Moreover, for the reader, it is far more satisfactory and informative to learn not merely the pathology of oral disease but also its clinical manifestations and any medical implications. Clinicopathological correlations have therefore been emphasised, as have been the principles of management.

Another problem is that of the growing number of medically-compromised patients who are attending for dental treatment. This is due to such factors as an ageing population, the advent of new diseases such as AIDS, and the problems of modern medical treatment such as the increasing use of immunosuppressive and cytotoxic drugs. Some of these patients, such as those with AIDS, will have oral disease related to their underlying condition. Others require only routine dentistry, but their medical condition may require it to be modified to varying degrees. There has therefore been a trend to set up Units for the care of these special needs patients, and of instituting higher degrees in this subject.

The term 'special needs' is open to various interpretations but typically includes such considerations as management of patients who are medically compromised or who have physical or mental handicaps, such that their care requires more than general practice can usually provide. Considerable attention (within the constraints of the space available) has therefore been given, in Section 3 of this book, to the nature and management of such conditions.

Quite apart from the professional responsibilities of dentists towards their patients, it has unfortunately to be accepted that this is an age of increasing litigation. Dentists must therefore know much more about medical conditions that can affect the management of their patients than was acceptable only a few years ago, if they are to avoid the anxiety and loss of time engendered by medico-legal claims.

For this edition the Publishers have made a generous allowance of colour pictures which should make the recognition of histopathology material and mucosal lesions considerably easier.

London, 1997   R. A. C.
                                                                 E. W. O.

Contents

Principles of investigation and diagnosis

The principles of patient investigation and diagnosis are summarised in Table 1.1.

Table 1.1   Principles of investigation and diagnosis

- A detailed history
- Clinical examination
    Extraoral
    Intraoral
- Special investigations (as appropriate)
    Radiography or other imaging techniques
    Biopsy for histopathology (including immunofluorescence,
        immunocytochemistry, electron microscopy, molecular
        biological tests)
    Specimen for microbial culture
    Haematological or biochemical tests

Taking a history

History-taking needs to be tailored to suit the individual patient but it is sometimes difficult to get a clear idea of the complaint. Many patients are nervous, some are inarticulate, others are confused.

Rapport is critical for eliciting useful information. Initial questions should allow patients to speak at some length and to gain confidence. It is usually best to start with an 'open' question. Medical jargon should be avoided: even regular hospital attenders who appear to understand medical terminology may use it wrongly and cause misunderstanding. Leading questions, which suggest a particular answer, should be avoided because patients often feel compelled to agree with the clinician.

Type of question	Example
Open	Tell me about the pain?
Closed	What does the pain feel like?
Leading	Does the pain feel like an electric shock?

It is sometimes difficult to avoid interrupting patients when trying to structure the history for the records. Structure can only be given after the patient has had time to give the information. Constant note-taking while patients are speaking is undesirable.

Questioning technique is most critical when eliciting any relevant social or psychological history or dealing with embarrassing medical conditions. It may be appropriate to delay asking such questions until after rapport has been gained. Some patients do not consider medical questions to be the concern of the dentist and it is important to give reasons for such questions when necessary (Table 1.2).

During history-taking, the mental and emotional state of the patient should be assessed. This may have a bearing on psychosomatic disease and will also suggest what the patient expects

Type of question	Advantages	Disadvantages
Open	Allows patients to use their own words and summarise their view of the problem	Clinicians must listen carefully and avoid interruptions to extract the relevant information
	Allows patients to partly direct the history-taking, gives them confidence and quickly generates rapport	Patients tend to decide what information is relevant
Closed	Elicits specific information quickly Useful to fill gaps in the information given in response to open questions	Patients may infer that the clinician is not really interested in their problem if only closed questions are asked
	Prevents vague patients from rambling away from the complaint	Important information may be lost if not specifically requested
		Restricts the patient's opportunities to talk

to gain from the consultation and treatment. If the patient's expectations are unreasonable it is important to try to modify them during the consultation, otherwise no treatment may be satisfactory.

Table 1.2 Essential principles of history-taking technique

- Introduce yourself and greet the patient by name
- Put patients at their ease
- Start with an open question
- Mix open and closed questions
- Avoid leading questions
- Avoid jargon
- Explain the need for specific questions
- Assess the patient's mental state
- Assess the patient's expectations from treatment

Demographic details

The age, gender, ethnic group and occupation of the patient should be noted. Such information is occasionally critical. For instance, an elderly woman with arthritis and a dry mouth is likely to have Sjögren's syndrome (Ch. 18), but a young man with a parotid swelling due to similar lymphoproliferation is far more likely to have HIV infection (Ch. 24). Some diseases such as oral submucous fibrosis (Ch. 11) have a restricted ethnic distribution.

History of the present complaint

Frequently a complaint, such as toothache, suggests the diagnosis. In many cases a detailed history (Table 1.3) is required and sometimes, as in aphthous ulceration, the diagnosis can be made on the history before examination or investigation.

Table 1.3 History of the present complaint

- Record the description of the complaint *in the patient's own* words
- Elicit the exact meaning of those words
- Record the duration and the time course of any changes in symptoms or signs
- Include any relevant facts in the patient's medical history
- Note any temporal relationship between them and the present complaint
- Consider any previous treatments and their effectiveness

If earlier treatment has been ineffective, the diagnosis should be reconsidered. Many patients' lives have been shortened by having malignant tumours treated with repeated courses of antibiotics.

Pain is completely subjective and when physical signs are absent special care must be taken to detail all its features

(Table 1.4). Especially important are features suggesting a dental cause. A fractured tooth or cusp, dentinal hypersensitivity or occlusal pain are easily misdiagnosed.

Table 1.4 Taking a pain history

Characteristic	Informative features
Type	Ache, tenderness, dull pain, throbbing, stabbing, electric shock. These terms are of limited use and the constancy of pain is more useful
Severity	Mild — managed with mild analgesics (e.g. aspirin/paracetamol) Moderate — unresponsive to mild analgesics Severe — disturbs sleep
Duration	Time since onset. Duration of pain or attacks
Nature	Continuous, in attacks or paroxysmal. If not continuous, is pain present between attacks?
Initiating factors	Any potential initiating factors. Association with dental treatment or lack of it is especially important in eliminating dental causes
Exacerbating and relieving factors	Record all and note especially hot and cold sensitivity or pain on eating which suggest a dental cause
Localisation	The patient should map out the distribution of pain if possible. Is it well or poorly defined?
Referral	Try to determine whether the pain could be referred

Factors triggering different causes of pain are discussed in detail in Chapter 34.

The medical history

A medical history is important as it aids the diagnosis of oral manifestations of systemic disease. It also ensures that medical conditions and medication which affect dental or surgical treatment are identified.

To ensure that nothing significant is forgotten, a printed questionnaire for patients to complete is valuable and saves time. It also helps to avoid medicolegal problems by providing a written record that the patient's medical background has been considered. The questions in Table 1.5 are the minimum that should be asked.

Medical warning cards may indicate that the patient is, for example, a haemophiliac, on long-term corticosteroid therapy or allergic to penicillin. It is also worthwhile to leave a final section open for patients to supply any other information that they think might be relevant.

A questionnaire does *not* constitute a medical history and the information must be checked verbally, verified and augmented as necessary. It is important to assess whether the patient's reading ability and understanding are sufficient to provide valid answers to the questionnaire.

A detailed drug history is essential. Drugs can have oral

Table 1.5 A basic medical questionnaire

A Anaemia or Allergies?
B Bleeding tendencies?
C Cardiorespiratory complaints?
D Drug treatment?
E Endocrine disorders?
F Fits or faints?
G Gastrointestinal complaints?
H Hospital admission or attendance?
I Infections including HIV/AIDS?
J Jaundice or other liver disease?
K Kidney disease?
L Likelihood of, or existing pregnancy?
M Medical warning card being carried?

effects or complicate dental management in important ways (Chs 13 and 35).

The medical history should also include questions on consumption of alcohol and tobacco. In some ethnic groups, enquiry should be made concerning habits such as betel quid (pan) or smokeless tobacco use.

The dental history

A dental history and examination is obviously essential for the diagnosis of dental pain or to exclude teeth as cause of symptoms in the head and neck region.

Symptoms of toothache are very variable and may masquerade as a variety of conditions from trivial to sinister. The relationship between symptoms and any dental treatment, or lack of it, should be noted.

The family and social history

Whenever a symptom or sign suggests an inherited disorder, such as haemophilia, the family history should be elicited. Ideally, this is recorded as a pedigree diagram noting the proband (presenting case) and all family members for at least three generations. Even when no familial disease is suspected, questions about other family members often usefully lead naturally into questions about home circumstances, relatives and social history which can be revealing if psychosomatic factors are suspected.

Clinical examination — extraoral

First, *look* at the patient, before looking into the patient's mouth. Anaemia, thyroid disease, long-term corticosteroid treatment, parotid swellings or significantly enlarged cervical nodes are a few conditions that can affect the facial appearance.

The parotid glands, temporomandibular joints (for clicks, crepitus or deviation), cervical and submandibular lymph nodes and thyroid gland should be palpated. Lymphadenopathy (Ch. 26) is a common manifestation of infection but may also

signify malignancy — the cervical lymph nodes are often the first affected by lymphomas. Note the character (site, shape, size, surface texture and consistency) of any enlargement. Press on the maxilla and frontal bone over the sinuses to elicit tenderness if sinusitis is suspected.

Oral examination

Examination of the oral cavity can only be performed adequately with good light, mirrors and compressed air or other means of drying the teeth. If viscid saliva prevents visualisation of the tissues and teeth a rinse with sodium bicarbonate mouthwash will help.

Soft tissues

The soft tissues of the mouth should usually be inspected first. Examination should be systematic to include all areas of the mouth. Care should be taken that mirrors or retractors do not obscure lesions. To ensure complete examination of the lateral tongue and posterior floor of mouth the tongue must be held in gauze and gently extended from side to side.

Abnormal-looking areas of mucosa should be palpated for scarring or induration indicating previous ulceration, inflammation or malignancy. Examination should include deeper tissues accessible to palpation, including the submandibular glands.

If lesions extend close to the gingiva the gingival crevice or pockets should be probed for any communication. Mucosal nodules, especially those on the gingiva or alveolar mucosa, which suggest sinus openings should be probed to identify any sinus or fistula. Check the openings of the salivary ducts while expressing saliva by gentle pressure. Check that saliva flows freely and equally from all glands and is clear in colour. Do not mistake anatomical variations (Table 1.6) for lesions.

After examination of the oral mucosa try to visualise the oropharynx and tonsils.

Teeth

As a minimum, the standing teeth, with a summary of their periodontal health, caries and restorative state, should be recorded. Tooth wear should be checked for 'parafunction'. Dental examination should be thorough both for the patient's sake and for medicolegal reasons. When dental pain is a possibility, full charting, assessment of mobility and percussion of teeth are necessary and further dental investigations will probably be required.

Testing vitality of teeth

The vitality of teeth must be checked if they appear to be causing symptoms. It is also essential to determine the vitality of teeth in the region of cysts and other radiolucent lesions in the

Table 1.6 Some anatomical variants and normal structures often misdiagnosed as lesions

Structure	Description
Fordyce's spots	Sebaceous glands lying superficially in the mucosa are visible as white or cream-coloured spots up to 0.5 mm across. Usually labial mucosa and buccal mucosa. Occasionally prominent and very numerous (see Fig. 15.4)
Lingual tonsils	Enlarge with viral infection and occasionally noted by patients. Sometimes large or ectopic and then mistaken for disease (Figs 1.1 and 1.2)
Circumvallate papillae	Readily identifiable but sometimes prominent and misinterpreted by patients or health care workers
Retrocuspid papilla	Firm pink nodule 0.5–4 mm diameter on the attached gingiva lingual to the lower canine and lateral incisor, usually bilateral but sometimes unilateral. Prominent in children but regress with age
Dorsal tongue fur	Furring of the dorsal tongue mucosa is very variable and is heavier when the diet is soft. Even light furring is regarded as pathological by many patients. When pigmented black by bacteria the condition is called black hairy tongue (Ch. 14)
Leukoedema	A milky-white translucent whitening of the oral mucosa which disappears or fades on stretching. Commoner in black races (Ch. 15)
Tori	Exostoses in the midline of the palate or in the lingual alveolus in the premolar region are termed tori (Ch. 9)

Fig. 1.2 Section showing the nodular surface and lymphoid follicles in a foliate papilla.

jaws at presentation. The information may be essential for diagnosis.

To be absolutely certain, several methods may have to be used. Checking hot and cold sensitivity and electric pulp testing are relatively easily performed (Table 1.7).

Table 1.7 Precautions for electric pulp testing

- Isolate individual teeth with a small portion of rubber dam if necessary
- Always record electric pulp test values in the notes — a progressive change in reading over time may indicate declining vitality
- If results remain uncertain, cut a test cavity or remove suspect restorations without local anaesthetic
- Poorly localised pulp pain from teeth of dubious vitality can be difficult to ascribe to an individual tooth. In such circumstances a diagnostic local anaesthetic injection on a suspect tooth may stop the pain and indicate its source
- Other sources of referred pain may sometimes be identified by the same means

Unfortunately it may not be apparent that a pulp test result is misleading. Care must always be taken to avoid causes of false-positive or false-negative results (Table 1.8).

Medical examination

If the history suggests, or examination reveals, any condition beyond the scope of the dentist's experience or clinical knowledge, referral for specialist medical examination may be necessary. In practice it is usual for some investigation to be performed first. The dentist should be capable of performing simple medical examinations of the head and neck. Examination of the skin of the face, hair, scalp and neck may reveal unexpected foci of infection to account for cervical lymphadenopathy or even malignant neoplasms. The eye can readily be inspected for conjunctivitis or signs of mucous membrane pemphigoid, anaemia or jaundice. Examination of the hands

Fig. 1.1 Large foliate papilla on the side of the tongue which may be mistaken for a lesion.

Table 1.8 Possible causes of misleading electric pulp test results

Problem	Causes to consider
Pulp bypassed by electric current	Electrical contact with next tooth by touching amalgam restorations
	Electrical contact with gingival margin by amalgam restoration or saliva film
Electrical insulation of the pulp	Large composite or non-conducting restorations
Falsely low reading	Incompletely formed root apex
Partially vital pulps	Multiple canals
No check on validity of results	No normal teeth for comparison
Patient fails to report accurately	Failure to differentiate pulpal from soft tissue sensation

Fig. 1.3 Hands with taut shiny pale skin on the tapering fingers, a result of Raynaud's phenomenon, in this case in systemic sclerosis.

may also reveal relevant information (Table 1.9). Dentists should be able to examine cranial nerve function but more extensive medical examination by dentists is usually done in hospital.

Table 1.9 Useful diagnostic information from examination of the hands

Site	Signs
Flexor surface of wrist	Rash (or history of rash) consisting of purplish papules suggests lichen planus, especially if itchy
Finger morphology	Clubbing may be associated with chronic respiratory and cardiac conditions (including infective endocarditis) and sometimes remote malignancy
	Joint changes may suggest rheumatoid arthritis (joint swelling, ulnar drift) or osteoarthritis (Heberden's nodules)
Abnormal nails	Koilonychia suggests long-standing anaemia Hypoplastic nails may be associated with several inherited epithelial disorders of oral significance, including ectodermal dysplasia and dyskeratosis congenita
Skin of fingers	May be thin, shiny and white in Raynaud's phenomenon (periodic ischaemia resulting from exposure to cold) — often associated with autoimmune conditions particularly systemic sclerosis (Fig. 1.3) or Sjögren's syndrome
	Note any tobacco staining. Is the degree commensurate with the patient's reported tobacco use?
Palmar–plantar keratosis	Associated with several syndromes including Papillon–Lefèvre syndrome (includes juvenile periodontitis)

Making a clinical differential diagnosis and investigation plan

The diagnosis and appropriate treatment may be obvious from the history and examination. More frequently there are various possible diagnoses and a clinical differential diagnosis and plan of investigation should be worked out. Possible diagnoses should be recorded in order of probability, based on their prevalence and likelihood of causing the symptoms and signs. Even if only one diagnosis seems appropriate it is worthwhile noting the next most likely possibility and any other causes which should be excluded. This ensures that all appropriate investigations are remembered and reduces the possibility of the patient having to return for further investigations. Drawing up such a written differential diagnosis helps even experienced clinicians to organise their thoughts. The list also forms the basis on which special investigations are selected. Precise diagnosis may depend on histological findings so that a preliminary generic diagnosis, such as 'benign neoplasm' or 'odontogenic tumour', often has to be made.

Special investigations

Innumerable types of investigation are possible, and it may be difficult to refrain from asking for every conceivable investigation in the anxiety not to miss something unsuspected and to avoid medicolegal complications. Though it may be tempting to explore every possibility, however remote, this approach may prove counterproductive in that it can produce a plethora of reports that confuse rather than inform. Laboratory staff soon also become aware of, and become less than helpful towards, those who overburden them.

Special investigations should only be requested to answer specific questions about a possible diagnosis, not as a routine. Some investigations have a high specificity and sensitivity for particular diseases, but few investigations provide a specific diagnosis. A few diseases, such as mumps, may be diagnosed on the basis of a single test, but others, such as Sjögren's syndrome, may require many tests. Therefore, the usefulness of each investigation must be borne in mind when interpreting the results.

Table 1.10 Imaging techniques for lesions of the head and neck

Technique	Advantages	Disadvantages
Conventional radiography	Simple, widely available, many common lesions may be identified with a high degree of accuracy Panoramic radiographs can show unsuspected lesions	Difficult to interpret in some areas of the jaws because of the complex anatomy X-ray dose unavoidable Little information about soft-tissue lesions
Computerised tomography	Provides tomographic (sectional) images of high clarity in any plane without superimposition Very useful where complex anatomy hinders interpretation of plain radiographs	Expensive and not always available Higher X-ray dose than plain radiographs Radiopaque dental restorations cause artefactual shadows which can obscure part of the image Less information on soft-tissue lesions than MRI
Use of contrast media with plain radiography or computerised tomography	Useful for outlining the extent of duct systems (e.g. the salivary gland ducts in sialography), hollow lesions such as cysts or blood vessels (arteriography) Can be used to outline lesions in soft tissues	Requires more expertise than plain radiography
Magnetic resonance imaging	No X-ray dose Produces clear tomograms without superimposition Particularly good for soft-tissue lesions	Expensive and limited availability Does not image bone
Ultrasound	No X-ray dose Shows soft tissue masses and cysts well Useful for salivary gland cysts and stones and to detect lesions in the thyroid gland and neck	Requires expertise in interpretation Overlying bone obscures soft-tissue lesions
Technetium scan	Provides an assessment of function in each salivary gland Can be used if sialography is not possible	Equipment not always available Radiation dose

Imaging

The most informative imaging techniques in the head and neck are radiography and computerised tomography (CT), magnetic resonance imaging (MRI) and ultrasound. Their advantages and disadvantages are shown in Table 1.10.

Plain radiography is widely available but the value of additional techniques should be understood (Table 1.11). Even simple manoeuvres such as introducing a gutta percha point or probe into a sinus to trace its origins may provide critical information. It is also advisable to request a formal radiologist's report on radiographic films whenever the radiographic features appear unusual or beyond the experience of the clinician.

Histopathology

Value and limitations

Removal of a biopsy specimen for histopathological examination is the mainstay of diagnosis for diseases of the mucosa, soft tissues and bone. In the few conditions in which a biopsy is

Table 1.11 Requirements for useful radiographic information

- Always take bite-wings when dental pain is suspected. Small carious lesions may be missed in periapical films and poorly localised pain may originate in the opposing arch
- When imaging bony swellings always take two views at right angles
- Panoramic tomograms cannot provide high definition of bony lesions. Only a cross-section of the lesion is in the focal trough and if the bone is greatly expanded only a small portion will be in focus. For more information, oblique lateral views of the mandible or oblique occlusal films should be taken
- Radiography of soft tissues is occasionally useful, for instance to detect a foreign body or calcification in lymph nodes

not helpful, it may still be valuable to exclude other possible causes (Table 1.12).

As with all other investigations, biopsy must address a specific question. For instance, recurrent aphthae lack specific microscopic features and biopsy is rarely justified. Conversely, a major aphtha may mimic a carcinoma which only microscopy will exclude.

Table 1.12   Possible reasons for failures of histological diagnosis

- Specimen poorly fixed or damaged during removal (Figs 1.4 and 1.5)
- Specimen is unrepresentative of the lesion or too small
- Plane of histological section does not include critical features
- The condition does not have diagnostic histological features, e.g. aphthous ulcers
- The histological features have several possible causes, e.g. granulomas (Ch. 28 and 29)
- The histological features are difficult to interpret, e.g. malignant tumours may be so poorly differentiated that their type cannot be determined
- Inflammation may mask the correct diagnosis

Fig. 1.4   An artefactual polyp produced by grasping normal mucosa with forceps to steady it during biopsy.

Fig. 1.5   Stringy artefact. This appearance is due to breakage of cells and their nuclei when the specimen is stretched or crushed. It is particularly common in lymphoma and some types of carcinoma.

Biopsy

Biopsy is the removal and examination of a part or the whole of a lesion. There are several types of biopsy technique (Table 1.13). The most important is surgical biopsy. The only important contraindication is incisional biopsy of parotid gland tumours. The most common type (pleomorphic adenoma) has an unusual tendency to seed its cells and recur in the incision wound. Such tumours should therefore be examined microscopically only *after* excision with a margin of surrounding normal tissue.

Table 1.13   Types of biopsy

- Surgical biopsy (incisional or excisional)
  Fixed specimen for paraffin blocks
  Frozen sections
- Fine needle aspiration biopsy
- Thick needle/core biopsy

Surgical biopsy

Incisional biopsy (removal of part of a lesion) is used to determine the diagnosis before treatment. Excisional biopsy (removal of the whole lesion such as a mucocele) is used to confirm a clinical diagnosis. It is a simple procedure but certain precautions must be observed (Table 1.14).

Table 1.14   Essential biopsy principles

- Choose most suspicious area, e.g. red area when premalignancy is suspected
- Avoid ulcers sloughs or necrotic areas
- Give regional or local anaesthetic — *not* into the lesion
- Include normal tissue margin
- Specimen should preferably be at least 1×0.6 cm by 2 mm deep
- Specimen edges should be vertical not bevelled
- Pass a suture through the specimen to control it and prevent it being swallowed or aspirated by the suction
- For large lesions, several areas may need to be sampled
- Include every fragment for histological examination
- Label specimen bottle with patient's name and clinical details
- Suture and control any bleeding
- Warn patient of possible soreness afterwards. Give an analgesic
- Check the report is consistent with the clinical diagnosis and investigations
- Discuss with pathologist or repeat biopsy if diagnosis is unclear or not understood

Occasionally general anaesthesia is required for children or problem patients. For those that gag, a short-acting benzodiazepine is usually effective. The request form should contain all the clinical information used to reach the clinical diagnosis. The purpose is to ensure an accurate diagnosis — not (as some clinicians seem to think) to see if the pathologist can guess it without the relevant information. If appropriate, give the vitality of teeth associated with the lesion.

Frozen sections

Frozen section technique allows a stained slide to be examined within 10 minutes of taking the specimen but has some limitations (Table 1.15). The tissue is sent fresh to the laboratory to be quickly frozen, preferably to about −70°C by, for example, immersion in liquid nitrogen or dry ice. A section is then cut on a refrigerated microtome and stained. The theatre suite often includes equipment for frozen sections to speed the process even further.

Table 1.15   Advantages and limitations of frozen sections

- Can establish, at operation, whether or not a tumour is malignant and whether excision needs to be extended
- Can confirm, at operation, that excision margins are free of tumour
- Appearances differ from those in fixed material
- Freezing artefacts due to poor technique can distort the cellular picture
- Definitive diagnosis sometimes impossible

Frozen sections can only be justified if the rapidity of the result will make an immediate difference to the operation in progress. If a rapid diagnosis is required in other circumstances, alternative techniques such as fine needle aspiration biopsy may be used.

Fine needle aspiration (FNA) biopsy (Table 1.16)

Even if not completely conclusive, the information from fine needle aspiration is often sufficient to distinguish benign from malignant neoplasms, to initiate treatment, or to indicate a need for further investigations. Needle/core biopsy is an alternative.

Table 1.16   Principles and uses of fine needle aspiration biopsy

- A 21 gauge needle is inserted into the lesion and cells aspirated and smeared on a slide
- Rapid and usually effective aid to diagnosis of swellings in lymph nodes and parotid tumours especially
- Cells can be fixed, stained and examined within minutes
- Valuable when surgical biopsy could spread tumour cells (e.g. pleomorphic adenomas)
- For deep lesions ultrasound or radiological guidance may be used to ensure that the needle enters the lesion
- No significant complications
- Small size of the needle avoids damage to vital structures in the head and neck
- Disadvantages
  - Experience required for interpretation
  - Small specimen may be unrepresentative
  - Definitive diagnosis not always possible

Needle/core biopsy (Table 1.17)

Table 1.17   Advantages and limitations of needle/core biopsy

- Needle up to 2 mm diameter used to remove a core of tissue
- Specimen processed as for a surgical biopsy
- Larger sample than FNA preserves tissue architecture in the specimen
- Definitive diagnosis more likely than with FNA
- Risk of seeding some types of neoplasms into the tissues
- Risk of damaging adjacent anatomical structures
- Useful for inaccessible tumours, e.g. in the pharynx
- Less used in the head and neck now that FNA is more widely available

---

Exfoliative cytology

Exfoliative cytology is examination of cells scraped from the surface of a lesion or occasionally of material in aspirates of a cyst (Table 1.18). Biopsy is always more reliable and can be so readily carried out in the mouth that it is mandatory when cancer or premalignancy is suspected. Exfoliative cytology samples only surface cells and provides no information on deeper tissues.

Table 1.18   Uses and limitations of exfoliative cytology

- Quick, easy
- Local anaesthetic not required
- Special techniques such as immunostaining can be applied
- Most useful for detecting virally-damaged cells, acantholytic cells of pemphigus or candidal hyphae
- Unreliable for diagnosing cancer. Frequent false-positive or false-negative results

---

Laboratory procedures

Although a clinician does not need to understand the details of laboratory procedures, it is necessary to understand the principles to enable the optimal results to be obtained.

Fixation

Important precautions are as follows (Table 1.19).

In the absence of proper fixative it is better to delay the biopsy and obtain the correct solution. Specimens placed in alcohols, saline or other materials commonly available in dental surgeries are frequently useless for diagnosis.

Special types of fixative are required for electron microscopy and for urgent specimens. Whenever microbiological culture is required the specimen should be sent fresh to the laboratory or a separate specimen should be taken because fixation will kill any microorganisms.

Table 1.19 Essential points about specimen fixation

- Fixation is necessary to prevent autolysis and destruction of microscopic features of the specimen
- The usual, routine fixative is 10% formal saline (formaldehyde solution in normal saline or a neutral pH buffer)
- Fixation must be complete before the specimen can be processed
- Fixative must diffuse into the specimen — a slow process
- Small surgical specimens fix overnight but large specimens take 24 hours or longer
- The centre of large specimens can autolyse before being fixed but the pathologist can incise them to allow fixative to penetrate
- Chemical reaction with the tissue causes the fixative to become weaker as fixation proceeds. Therefore specimens should generally be put in at least 10 times their own volume of fixative

Tissue processing

The fixed tissue is dehydrated by immersion in a series of solvents, and impregnated with paraffin wax. The wax block is mounted on a microtome and sections, usually 4 μm thick, are cut and mounted on glass microscope slides for staining. It takes 24–48 hours to fix, process, section and stain a specimen before the pathologist can report on it.

Some common stains used for microscopy

The combination of haematoxylin and eosin (H & E) is the most common routine histological stain. Haematoxylin is a blue-black basic dye, eosin is a red acid dye. Their typical staining patterns are shown in Table 1.20.

Table 1.20 Example of haematoxylin and eosin staining of various tissues

Eosin (red)	Haematoxylin (blue)
Cytoplasm of most cells* Keratin	Nuclei (DNA and RNA)
Muscle cytoplasm	Mucopolysaccharide-rich ground substance
Bone (decalcified only) Collagen	Reversal lines in decalcified bone

*The cytoplasm of some cells (as in some salivary gland tumours) is intensely eosinophilic. In others such as plasma cells it is basophilic or intermediate (amphophilic).

Periodic acid–Schiff (PAS) stain is probably the second most frequently used stain. It stains carbohydrates and mucinous substances pink. This is useful to identify salivary and other mucins, glycogen and candidal hyphae in sections. Silver staining is also useful for identifying fungi in sections but Gram-staining is quicker and more useful for smears.

Silver stains also stain reticulin fibres black.

Decalcified and ground (undecalcified) sections

Specimens containing bone and teeth need to be softened by decalcifying in acid to enable a thin section to be cut. This delays the diagnosis by days or weeks according to the size of the specimen.

Decalcification must be avoided if examination of dental enamel is required, for instance to aid diagnosis of amelogenesis imperfecta, because the heavily mineralised enamel is almost completely dissolved. In such cases a ground section is prepared by sawing and grinding using special saws and abrasives.

Immunofluorescent and immunohistochemical staining

Immunostaining methods make use of the highly specific binding between antibodies and antigens to stain specific molecules within the tissues. Fresh (unfixed) tissue is sometimes required.

Immunostaining has revolutionised histological diagnosis and has made some more complex techniques such as electron microscopy almost redundant. It is time-consuming and must be meticulously carried out with adequate controls to avoid both false-positive and false-negative results.

The main circumstances where diagnosis depends on immunostaining are shown in Table 1.21.

Antibodies, often monoclonal, can be purchased. They react with the target molecule and the combination is labelled, either by being coupled to a fluorescein or an enzyme such as peroxi-

Table 1.21 Important uses of immunostaining techniques

Disease	Molecule detected	Significance
Pemphigus	Autoantibody bound to the epithelial prickle cells	Indicates pemphigus
Pemphigoid	Autoantibody and/or complement C3 bound to the basement membrane	Indicates pemphigoid
Suspected lymphoma	κ and λ light chains of immunoglobulin expressed by B lymphocytes or plasma cells	Normal inflammatory infiltrates contain B lymphocytes secreting antibody with both κ and λ light chains. If all cells in an infiltrate express only one type of light chain the infiltrate is monoclonal and therefore neoplastic
Lymphoma	Cell surface markers specific for T or B lymphocytes	Indicate whether a lymphoma is of B or T cell origin
Undifferentiated malignant neoplasms	Intermediate filaments (components of the cytoskeleton), including keratins (in epithelial cells), vimentin (in mesenchymal tissues) or desmin (in muscle)	Indicate the type of tumour in an undifferentiated malignancy

dase. The antibody is incubated on the section where it binds specifically to the target molecule. Surplus reagent is washed off and any binding (a positive reaction) is visible by its fluorescence in an ultraviolet light microscope or by reacting the enzyme with synthetic substrate to produce a coloured product (Figs 1.6–1.8).

Molecular biological tests

Molecular biological diagnostic tests have revolutionised diagnosis, particularly in screening for and identification of genetic abnormalities and rapid identification of bacteria and viruses. Some malignant neoplasms have characteristic genetic abnormalities, mostly chromosomal translocations, which can be detected by cytogenetics, polymerase chain reaction (PCR) or fluorescent in situ hybridisation. Molecular techniques are also the method of choice for the diagnosis of some lymphomas which cannot be accurately categorised by routine histological methods.

Identification of many bacteria and viruses is now often undertaken using PCR. In this test the clinical sample is solubilised and the nucleic acids hybridised with complementary probes which are specific for known pathogens. If the pathogen is present in the sample PCR will copy the nucleic acid repeatedly until enough is synthesised to be seen in an electrophoresis gel (Fig. 1.9). If no pathogen is present no nucleic acid is synthesised. Identification of mycobacteria is a good example of the value of this type of test. Previously, identification of

mycobacterial infection required approximately 6 weeks to culture the sample. PCR can be performed in 48 hours, is more sensitive and differentiates different types of mycobacteria with a high degree of precision. This test is therefore ideal for investigation of enlarged lymph nodes in the neck. A more recent application of PCR, to detect micrometastases of tumours, is potentially also of enormous value.

Such methods have yet to become widespread in dentistry, even in hospital specialties. However, when confronted with a difficult diagnosis it is sensible to discuss the case with the pathologist or microbiologist before biopsy, to ensure that appropriate samples are available for these specialised tests.

Haematology, clinical chemistry and serology

Blood investigations are clearly essential for the diagnosis of diseases such as leukaemias, myelomas or leukopenias which have oral manifestations, or for defects of haemostasis which can greatly affect management. Blood investigations are also helpful in the diagnosis of other conditions such as some infections, and sore tongues or recurrent aphthae which are sometimes associated with anaemia.

There are many different types of haematological examinations but, despite the frequent use of the term 'routine blood test', no test should ever be requested as a routine, only to answer a specific question (Table 1.22) The request form should always be completed with sufficient clinical detail to

Fig. 1.6 Method and application of direct immunofluorescence. Example: Diagnosis of pemphigus and pemphigoid. Aim: To detect the site of the IgG autoantibody already bound to the tissues in a biopsy.

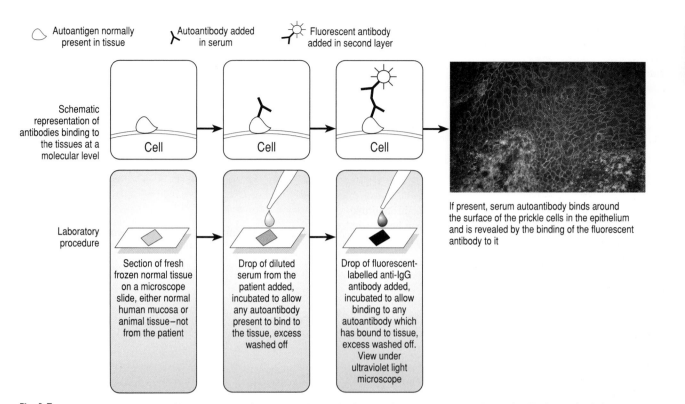

Fig. 1.7 Method and application of indirect immunofluorescence. Example: Control of treatment for pemphigus. Aim: To detect circulating autoantibody in the serum of patients with pemphigus.

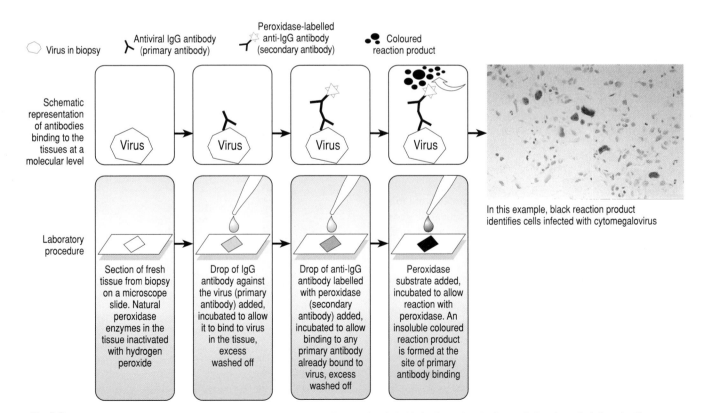

Fig. 1.8 Method and application of immunocytochemistry. Example: Diagnosis of viral infection. Aim: To detect viral antigens in infected cells.

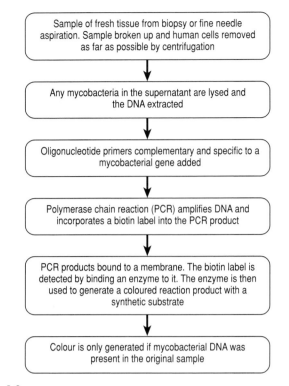

Fig. 1.9 Example application for the technique of polymerase chain reaction. Identification of mycobacterial infection.

allow the haematologist or clinical chemist to check that the appropriate tests have been ordered and to allow the interpretation of the results. It is important to include details of any drug treatment on blood test request forms. Always put the blood into the appropriate tube because some anticoagulants are incompatible with certain tests. A haematologist will not be impressed with a request for assessment of clotting function on a specimen of coagulated blood.

Microbiology

Despite the fact that the most common oral diseases are infective, microbiology is surprisingly rarely of practical diagnostic value in dentistry (Table 1.23). Direct Gram-stained smears will quickly confirm the diagnosis of thrush or acute ulcerative gingivitis, and H & E-stained smears can show the distorted, virally infected epithelial cells in herpetic infections more easily than microbiological tests for the organisms themselves.

A key microbiological investigation is culture and sensitivity of pus organisms. Whenever pus is obtained from a soft tissue or bone infection it should be sent for culture and determination of antibiotic sensitivity of the causative microbes. Those of osteomyelitis, cellulitis, acute parotitis, deep mycoses (frequently mistaken for tumours) or other severe infections need to be identified if appropriate antimicrobial treatment is to be given. However, such treatment has usually to be started empirically without this information but the sensitivity test may dictate a change.

Table 1.22 Types of blood test useful in oral diagnosis (see also Appendix 1.1)

Test	Main uses
'Full blood picture' usually includes erythrocyte number, size and haemoglobin indices and differential white cell count	Anaemia and the effects of sideropenia and vitamin B_{12} deficiency associated with several common oral disorders. Leukaemias
Blood film	Leukaemias, infectious mononucleosis, anaemias
Erythrocyte sedimentation rate	Raised in systemic inflammatory and autoimmune disorders. Particularly important in giant cell arteritis and Wegener's granulomatosis
Serum iron and total iron binding capacity	Iron deficiency associated with several common oral disorders
Serum ferritin	A more sensitive indicator of body stores of iron than serum iron and total iron-binding capacity but not available in all laboratories
Folate level	Folic acid deficiency is sometimes associated with recurrent aphthous ulceration and recurrent candidosis
Vitamin B_{12} level	Vitamin B_{12} deficiency is sometimes associated with recurrent aphthous ulceration and recurrent candidosis
Autoantibodies (e.g. rheumatoid factor, antinuclear factor, DNA binding antibodies, SS-A, SS-B)	Raised in autoimmune diseases. Specific autoantibody levels suggest certain diseases
Viral antibody titres (e.g. herpes simplex, varicella zoster, mumps virus)	A rising titre of specific antibody indicates active infection by the virus
Paul–Bunnell or monospot test	Infectious mononucleosis
Syphilis serology	Syphilis
Complement tests	Occasionally useful in diagnosis of SLE or familial angio-oedema
Serum angiotensin-converting enzyme	Sarcoidosis
Serum calcium, phosphate, and parathormone levels	Paget's disease and hyperparathyroidism
HIV test	HIV infection (testing only possible under particular circumstances)
Serum alkaline phosphatase	Raised in conditions with increased bone turnover, e.g. Paget's disease and hyperparathyroidism. Lowered in hypophosphatasia

Practical point Always take a sample of pus for culture and antibiotic sensitivity from bone and soft tissue infections **before** giving an antibiotic

Viral identification is rarely required for oral diseases as many oral viral infections are clinically typical and indicate the causative virus. A smear alone may show the nuclear changes of herpetic infection in epithelial cells from the margins of mucosal ulcers. A more sensitive and almost as rapid result may be obtained by sending a swab for virus detection using ELISA (enzyme-linked immunosorbent assay).

Table 1.23 Microbiological tests useful in oral diagnosis

Test	Main uses
Culture and antibiotic sensitivity	Detect unusual pathogens, e.g. actinomycosis in soft tissue infection. Antibiotic sensitivity for all infections, particularly osteomyelitis and acute facial soft-tissue infection
Smear for candida	Candidosis
Viral culture or antigen screen	Viral culture identifies many viruses but requires considerable time. Screening for viral antigens is faster but of more limited diagnostic value

Other clinical tests

Several simple clinical tests may be valuable in diagnosis of oral disease. Urine tests are valuable for the diagnosis of diabetes (suggested by repeated candidal or periodontal infection), autoimmune conditions which damage the kidneys, for instance Wegener's granulomatosis, and for the detection of Bence Jones protein in myeloma.

Taking the patient's temperature is an easily forgotten investigation. The temperature should be noted whenever bone or soft tissue infections are suspected. It helps distinguish facial inflammatory oedema from cellulitis and indicates systemic effects of infections and the need for more aggressive treatment.

Practical point Always take the temperature of any patient with a swollen face, enlarged lymph nodes, malaise or other symptom or sign which might indicate infection

Interpreting special investigations and making a diagnosis and treatment plan

The history, examination and results of special investigations should provide the basis for a diagnosis and treatment plan. Check that the results of each investigation are compatible with the preliminary diagnosis and do not indicate any need to avoid a particular treatment.

If a result appears at odds with other information, take into account the normal variation, perhaps with age or diurnal variation, and consider the possibility of false-positive and false-negative results. A common cause of unusual blood test results is a delay in taking blood samples to the laboratory.

Further advice and specialised tests may be appropriate.

General medical, ear, nose and throat, neurological and psychiatric referral are among the specialties to whom patients may be referred. In referrals, it is important to state whether the dentist is requesting the medical specialist to exclude a condition and refer the patient back, or to take over investigation. If the latter, it is essential that dental causes have been completely eliminated as the source of the problem.

Finally, ensure that the patient's notes include a complete record of the consultation and investigation results. This must be correctly dated, legible, limited to relevant facts and include a clear complaint history, list of clinical findings, test results and plan of treatment organised in a suitable form for quick reappraisal. It must be signed by the clinician and, in addition, the name should be printed below if the signature is anything less than perfectly legible. It should be possible for another person to continue to investigate or treat the patient without difficulty on the basis of the clinical record.

Practical point Good clinical record-keeping is essential for good patient management as well as for medicolegal reasons

Photography or computerised video imaging is a very valuable adjunct to the clinical record. Pictures are especially useful in monitoring lesions which may vary in the course of a long follow-up, for instance white patches. It is useful to include teeth or a scale in the frame to allow accurate assessment of small changes in size. Photographs may also be helpful in explaining to patients about their condition and to show the effects of treatment.

SUGGESTED FURTHER READING

Arends M J, Bird C C 1992 Recombinant DNA technology and its diagnostic applications. Histopathology 21:303–313

Ghossein R A, Rosai J 1996 Polymerase chain reaction in the detection of micrometastases and circulating tumor cells. Cancer 78:10–16

Heatley M K 1996 Cytokeratins and cytokeratin staining in diagnostic histopathology. Histopathology 28:479–483

Kabala J, Goddard P, Cook P 1992 Magnetic resonance imaging of extracranial head and neck tumours. Br J Radiol 65:375–383

Komoroski R A, Pappas A, Hough A 1992 Nuclear magnetic resonance imaging in pathology I. Principles and general aspects. Hum Pathol 22:1077–1084

Layton S, Korsen J 1994 Informed consent in oral and maxillofacial surgery: a study of the value of written warnings. Br J Oral Maxillofac Surg 32:34–36

Minden N J, Fast T B 1994 Evaluation of health history forms used in U.S. dental schools. Oral Surg Oral Med Oral Pathol 77:105–109

Nathan A W, Havard C W H 1979 The face in diagnosis. Br J Hosp Med 21:104–111

O'Connor N 1995 Laboratory diagnosis in haematology. Medicine UK 23:489–494

Stanley M W 1995 False-positive diagnosis in exfoliative cytology (editorial). Am J Clin Pathol Editorial 104:117–119

Thibodeau E A, Rossomondo K J 1992 Survey of the medical history questionnaire. Oral Surg Oral Med Oral Pathol 74:400–403

Whaites E 1996 *Essentials of dental radiography and radiology*, 2nd edn. Churchill Livingstone, Edinburgh

Normal haematological values

Red cells

Haemoglobin	Males 13–17 g/dl. Females 11.5–16 g/dl
Haematocrit (packed cell volume – PCV)	Males 40–50 l/l. Females 34–47 l/l
Mean corpuscular volume (MCV)	78–98 fl
Mean corpuscular haemoglobin concentration (MCHC)	30–35 g/dl
Red cell count	Males 4–6×10^{12}l. Females 4–5×10^{12}l
Erythrocyte sedimentation rate (ESR)	0–15 mm/h

White cells

Total count	4–10×10^{9}/l
Neutrophils	2–7.5×10^{9}/l
Lymphocytes	1–3×10^{9}/l
Monocytes	0.15–0.8×10^{9}/l
Eosinophils	0.05–0.4×10^{9}/l
Platelets	150–400×10^{9}/l

Note. These are average values and may vary slightly between laboratories. Also, approximately 5% of normal persons have values outside the figures quoted above.

HARD-TISSUE PATHOLOGY

Disorders of development of the teeth and related tissues

Development of an ideal dentition depends on many factors (Table 2.1).

Table 2.1   Requirements for development of an ideal dentition

- Formation of a full complement of teeth
- Normal structural development of the dental tissues
- Eruption of each group of teeth at the appropriate time into an adequate space
- Eruption of teeth into correct relationship with their opposite numbers

---

Significant structural defects of teeth are uncommon but disorders of occlusion due to irregularities of the teeth in the arch or abnormal relationship of the arches to each other are so common that their treatment has become a specialty in its own right. The main groups of disorders affecting development of the dentition are summarised in Table 2.2.

Table 2.2   Disorders of development of the teeth

- Abnormalities in number
    Anodontia or hypodontia
    Additional teeth (hyperdontia)
- Disorders of eruption
- Defects of structure
    Enamel defects
    Dentine defects
- Developmental anomalies of several dental tissues
    Odontomas

ABNORMALITIES IN THE NUMBER OF TEETH

Isolated hypodontia or anodontia

Failure of development of one or two teeth is relatively common and often hereditary. The teeth most frequently missing are third molars, second premolars or maxillary second incisors (Fig. 2.1). Absence of third molars can be a disadvantage if first or second molars, or both, have been lost. The absence of lower

Fig. 2.1   Congenital absence of lateral incisors with spacing of the anterior teeth.

premolars worsens malocclusion if there is already disparity between an underdeveloped mandible and a normal upper arch. Otherwise absence of these teeth may have little or no noticeable effect.

Absence of lateral incisors can sometimes be conspicuous because the large, pointed canines erupt in the front of the mouth beside the central incisors. It is usually impossible to prevent the canine from erupting into this empty space, even if the patient is seen early. It is also very difficult to make room between the centrals and canines by orthodontic means to replace the laterals. An attempt has often therefore to be made to disguise the shape of the canines.

Total failure of development of a complete dentition (anodontia) is exceedingly rare. If the permanent dentition fails to form, the deciduous dentition is retained for many years, but when these deciduous teeth become excessively worn or too much damaged by caries then they must be replaced by dentures.

Hypodontia or anodontia with systemic defects

Anhidrotic (hereditary) ectodermal dysplasia

The main features are summarised in Table 2.3. In severe cases no teeth form. More often, most of the deciduous teeth form but there are few or no permanent teeth. The teeth are usually peg-shaped or conical (Fig. 2.2).

Table 2.3 **Major features of anhidrotic ectodermal dyplasia**

- Usually a sex-linked recessive trait
- Hypodontia
- Hypotrichosis (scanty hair)
- Anhidrosis (inability to sweat)

Fig. 2.2 Anhidrotic ectodermal dysplasia showing two conical teeth, the only teeth present.

Fig. 2.3 The same case showing typical fine and scanty hair and loss of support for the facial soft tissues.

Fig. 2.4 A paramolar or buccally placed supernumerary molar tooth.

When there is anodontia, the alveolar process, without teeth to support, fails to develop and has too little bone to support implants. The profile then resembles that of an elderly person because of the gross loss of vertical dimension. The hair is fine and sparse (Fig. 2.3), particularly in the tonsural region. The skin is smooth, shiny and dry due to absence of sweat glands. Heat is therefore poorly tolerated. The fingernails are usually also defective. All that can be done to improve the patient's appearance and mastication is to fit dentures, which are usually well tolerated by children.

Other conditions associated with hypodontia

There are many rare syndromes where hypodontia is a feature, but the only common one is Down's syndrome (Ch. 33). One or more third molars are absent in over 90% of these patients, while absence of individual teeth scattered about the arch is also common. Anodontia is rare. Palatal clefts may be associated.

Additional teeth: hyperdontia

Additional teeth are relatively common. They are usually of simple conical shape (*supernumerary teeth*) but less frequently resemble teeth of the normal series (*supplemental teeth*). These are the result of excessive but organised growth of the dental lamina of unknown cause.

Supernumerary teeth. Conical or more seriously malformed additional teeth most frequently form in the incisor or molar region (Fig. 2.4) and, very occasionally, in the midline (mesiodens).

Fig. 2.5 Malocclusion resulting from the eruption of a midline tuberculate supernumerary and two supplemental premolars.

Supplemental teeth. Occasionally an additional maxillary incisor, premolar (Fig. 2.5) or, rarely, a fourth molar develops.

Effects and treatment

Additional teeth usually erupt in abnormal positions, labial or buccal to the arch, and create stagnation areas. Alternatively a supernumerary tooth may prevent a normal tooth from erupting. These additional teeth should usually be extracted.

Syndromes associated with hyperdontia

These syndromes are all rare but probably the best known is cleidocranial dysplasia (Ch. 10) where many additional teeth develop but fail to erupt.

DISORDERS OF ERUPTION

Eruption of deciduous teeth starts at about 6 months, usually with the appearance of the lower incisors, and is complete by about 2 years. Mass failure of eruption is very rare. More often eruption of a single tooth is prevented by local obstruction. In the permanent dentition, delay in eruption of a tooth or, more frequently, too early loss of a deciduous predecessor tends to cause irregularities because movement of adjacent teeth closes the available space.

Delayed eruption associated with skeletal disorders

Metabolic diseases particularly *cretinism* and *rickets* are now uncommon causes of delayed eruption of teeth. *Cleidocranial dysplasia*, has been mentioned earlier. In severe *hereditary gingival fibromatosis*, eruption may apparently fail merely because the teeth are buried in the excessive fibrous gingival tissue and only their tips show in the mouth (*pseudoanodontia*). In *cherubism* (Ch. 10) several teeth may be displaced by the proliferat-

ing connective tissue masses containing giant cells and are prevented from erupting.

Local factors affecting eruption of deciduous teeth

Having no predecessors, deciduous teeth usually erupt unobstructed. Occasionally an eruption cyst may overlie a tooth but is unlikely to block eruption.

Local factors affecting eruption of permanent teeth

A permanent tooth may be prevented from erupting or may be misplaced by various causes (Table 2.4). Treatment depends on the circumstances, but room may be made for the unerupted tooth by orthodontic means or extractions. A retained deciduous tooth should be extracted if radiographs show a normal permanent successor. If a buried tooth partially erupts and becomes infected, it may have to be removed: mandibular third molars are the main source of this complication.

Table 2.4 Local causes of failure of eruption of permanent teeth

- Loss of space
- Abnormal position of the crypt
- Overcrowding
- Supernumerary and supplemental teeth
- Displacement in a dentigerous cyst
- Retention of a deciduous predecessor

Changes affecting buried teeth

Teeth may occasionally remain buried in the jaws for many years without complications. The roots of these teeth may undergo varying degrees of hypercementosis or resorption; alternatively they may become enveloped in dentigerous cysts, as in cleidocranial dysplasia for example.

DEFECTS OF STRUCTURE: HYPOPLASIA AND HYPOCALCIFICATION

Minor structural defects of the teeth, such as pitting or discolouration, or, occasionally, more serious defects may be markers of past disease, but only rarely is the disease still active. Hypoplasia of the teeth is not an important contributory cause of dental caries; indeed, hypoplasia due to fluorosis is associated with enhanced resistance. The main clinical problem is usually cosmetic improvement.

Defects of deciduous teeth

Calcification of deciduous teeth begins about the fourth month of intrauterine life. Disturbances of metabolism or infections that affect the fetus at this early stage without causing abortion are rare. Defective structure of the deciduous teeth is therefore uncommon, but, in a few places, such as parts of India, where the fluoride content of the water is excessively high, the deciduous teeth may be mottled. The deciduous teeth may be discoloured by abnormal pigments circulating in the blood. Severe neonatal jaundice may cause the teeth to become yellow, or there may be bands of greenish discolouration. In congenital porphyria, a rare disorder of haemoglobin metabolism, the teeth are red or purple. Tetracycline given during dental development is the main cause of permanent discolouration.

Defects of permanent teeth

Single permanent teeth may be malformed as a result of local causes such as periapical infection of a predecessor (Turner teeth, Fig. 2.6) or damage by intubation, for instance (Fig. 2.7); or multiple teeth may be malformed in systemic diseases, as summarised in Table 2.5.

Fig. 2.6 Turner tooth, a hypoplastic tooth resulting from periapical infection, usually of the deciduous predecessor.

Fig. 2.7 Localised dental disturbance caused by prolonged intubation during tooth development. The upper left central incisor shows enamel pitting incisally and the upper right central incisor is deformed and has failed to erupt.

Table 2.5 Important causes of multiple malformed permanent teeth

Genetic
Amelogenesis imperfecta
   Hereditary enamel hypoplasia
   Hereditary enamel hypocalcification
   Hypomaturation defects
Dentinogenesis imperfecta
Shell teeth
Dentinal dysplasia
Regional odontodysplasia
Multisystem disorders with associated dental defects

Infective
Congenital syphilis

Metabolic
Childhood infections, rickets, hypoparathyroidism

Drugs
Tetracycline pigmentation
Cytotoxic chemotherapy

Fluorosis

Other acquired developmental anomalies
Fetal alcohol syndrome

Amelogenesis imperfecta

Genetic factors act with variable severity throughout the whole duration of amelogenesis. Characteristically therefore, all teeth are affected and defects involve the whole enamel, or are randomly distributed in it. By contrast, exogenous factors affecting enamel formation (with the important exception of fluorosis) tend to act for a relatively brief period and produce defects related to that period of enamel formation.

Hereditary enamel hypoplasia

The main defect is in formation of the matrix. The enamel is randomly pitted, grooved or very thin, but hard and translucent (Fig. 2.8). The defects tend to become stained, but the teeth are not especially susceptible to caries unless the enamel is scanty and easily damaged.

The main patterns of inheritance are autosomal dominant and recessive and (a genetic rarity) a sex-linked dominant type. In the last there is almost complete failure of enamel formation in affected males, while in females the enamel is vertically ridged (Figs 2.9–2.11). Occasionally cases are difficult to classify (Fig. 2.12).

Hereditary enamel hypocalcification

Enamel matrix is formed in normal quantity but poorly calcified. When newly erupted, the enamel is normal in thickness and form, but weak and opaque or chalky in appearance.

The teeth tend to become stained and relatively rapidly worn away. The upper incisors develop a shouldered form due to the chipping away of the thin, soft enamel of the incisal edge (Fig. 2.13). There are dominant and recessive patterns of inheritance.

Fig. 2.8   Amelogenesis imperfecta, hypoplastic type.

Fig. 2.9   Close-up of X-linked hypoplastic type amelogenesis imperfecta. These teeth from an affected female show the typical vertical ridged pattern of normal and abnormal enamel as a result of Lyonisation.

Fig. 2.10   Amelogenesis imperfecta X-linked hypoplastic form in a male. This premolar has a cap of enamel so thin that the shape of the tooth is virtually that of the dentine core.

Hypomaturation defects

The enamel is of normal form on eruption but opaque, white to brownish-yellow. The teeth appear similar to those with mottled fluoride defects (Figs. 2.14 and 2.15). However, they are soft and vulnerable to attrition but not as severely as the hypocalcified type.

Fig. 2.11   Amelogenesis imperfecta X-linked hypoplastic type in a male showing a thin translucent layer of defective enamel on the dentine surface.

Fig. 2.12   Amelogenesis imperfecta, indeterminate type. Some cases, such as this, are difficult to classify but are clearly inherited, as shown by their long family history.

Fig. 2.13   Amelogenesis imperfecta, hypocalcified type. The soft chalky enamel was virtually of normal thickness and form but has chipped away during mastication.

Fig. 2.14 Amelogenesis imperfecta, hypomaturation type. Tooth morphology is normal but there are opaque white and discoloured patches.

Fig. 2.16 Dentinogenesis imperfecta showing the translucent appearance of the teeth which are of normal morphology.

Fig. 2.15 Amelogenesis imperfecta, one of the several hypomaturation types. In this form there are opaque white flecks and patches affecting the occlusal half of the tooth surface.

Fig. 2.17 Dentinogenesis imperfecta makes the teeth vulnerable to attrition and abrasion because the enamel chips away from defective dentine.

There are several variants of hypomaturation defects, such as a more severe X-linked pattern and hypomaturation combined with hypoplasia.

Dentinogenesis (odontogenesis) imperfecta

This uncommon defect of collagen formation is transmitted as an autosomal dominant trait. The gene is closely related to that of osteogenesis imperfecta (Ch. 10), particularly type IV. The dentine is soft and has an abnormally high water content.

Clinical features

The enamel appears normal but uniformly brownish or purplish and abnormally translucent (Fig. 2.16). The form of the teeth is essentially normal, but the crowns of the molars tend to be bulbous and the roots are usually short. Enamel is weakly attached and tends to chip away from the dentine abnormally easily. In severe cases the teeth become rapidly worn down to the gingivae (Fig. 2.17). Early fitting of full dentures then becomes inevitable, as the relatively soft dentine and short roots make crowning impractical.

In some patients only a few teeth are severely affected, while the remainder appear normal. Radiographically the main features are obliterated pulp chambers and stunted roots.

Pathology

The earliest formed dentine under the amelodentinal junction usually appears normal. The deeper tissue is more defective, tubules become few, calcification is incomplete and the matrix is imperfectly formed. The pulp chamber becomes obliterated early and odontoblasts degenerate, but cellular inclusions in the dentine are common (Fig. 2.18). Scalloping of the amelodentinal junction is sometimes absent. The enamel tends to split from the dentine, but is otherwise normal in typical cases.

Shell teeth

This rare anomaly is so called because only a thin shell of hard dental tissue surrounds overlarge pulp chambers. Shell teeth appear to be a variant of dentinogenesis imperfecta in that there is normal, but thin, mantle dentine which covers irregular dentine (Fig. 2.19). The pulp lacks a normal odontoblast layer and consists of coarse connective tissue which becomes incorporated into the deep surface of the dentine.

Dentinal dysplasia ('rootless' teeth)

In dentinal dysplasia, the roots are very short and conical. The pulp chambers are obliterated by multiple nodules of poorly

Fig. 2.18 Microscopic appearance of dentinogenesis imperfecta showing the grossly disorganised tubular structure with inclusions of pulp in the dentine and obliteration of the pulp cavity.

Fig. 2.19 Shell tooth. In this severe form of dentinogenesis imperfecta only a thin mantle of dentine is formed and no root develops.

organised dentine containing sheaves of tubules. Inevitably, these teeth tend to be lost early in life.

Regional odontodysplasia (ghost teeth)

This is a localised disorder of development affecting a group of teeth. It is recognisable at the time of eruption of the deciduous teeth (2–4 years) or of the permanent teeth (7–11 years).

Maxillary teeth are involved more than twice as frequently as mandibular. They are both malformed and poorly calcified. The enamel is thin, grossly hypoplastic and hypomineralised; it is surrounded by irregular calcifications formed in the reduced enamel epithelium. The dentine is thin and, despite a disproportionately thick zone of predentine, the pulp chamber is abnormally large (Figs 2.20 and 2.21). In radiographs,

Fig. 2.20 Lateral incisor in regional odontodysplasia. Both enamel and dentine are deformed and there is calcification of the reduced enamel epithelium.

Fig. 2.21 Regional odontodysplasia showing dysplastic dentine with a disorganised tubule structure, an irregular enamel space and mineralised enamel epithelium.

ghost teeth appear crumpled and abnormally radiolucent (Fig. 2.22).

These defects are too severe to repair and early tooth loss is inevitable.

Multisystem disorders affecting the teeth

Ehlers–Danlos (floppy joint) syndromes

This group of collagen disorders is characterised (in varying

Fig. 2.22 Radiographic appearance of regional odontodysplasia. On one side of the midline the deciduous incisors have poor root formation with thin radicular dentine and enamel. A poorly organised spotty calcification is present at the site of the permanent successors.

Fig. 2.23 Multiple pulp stones in a case of Ehlers–Danlos syndrome.

degree) by hypermobile joints, loose hyperextensible skin, fragile oral mucosa and, in type VIII, early onset periodontitis.

The main dental abnormalities are small teeth with short roots and multiple pulp stones (Fig. 2.23).

Gardner's syndrome (familial adenomatous polyposis)

Gardner's syndrome is characterised by multiple osteomas, especially of the jaws (Ch. 9), colonic polyps and skin tumours. The majority of patients have dental abnormalities. These include impacted teeth other than third molars, supernumerary or missing teeth and abnormal root formation.

The colonic polyps have an almost 100% frequency of malignant change, and the mortality is high. The dental abnormalities can be detected in childhood or adolescence and recognition of this syndrome may be life-saving by suggesting the need for colectomy.

Epidermolysis bullosa

Epidermolysis bullosa is a blistering disease of skin and

mucosae (Ch. 13). Dental abnormalities include fine or coarse pitting defects, or thin and uneven enamel which may also lack prismatic structure. The amelodentinal junction may be smooth. Dental defects vary in the different subtypes of the disease but are most frequent in the autosomal recessive, scarring type of epidermolysis bullosa in which there may be delayed, or failure of, eruption.

Infection

Congenital syphilis

Prenatal syphilis, the result of maternal infection, can cause a characteristic dental deformity, described by Hutchinson in 1858.

If the fetus becomes infected at a very early stage, abortion follows. Infants born with stigmata of congenital syphilis result from later fetal infection, and the permanent teeth are affected. The characteristic defects are usually seen in the upper central incisors.

The incisors (Hutchinson's incisors) are small, barrel-shaped, and taper towards the tip (Fig. 2.24). The incisal edge sometimes shows a crescentic notch or deep fissure which forms before eruption and can be seen radiographically. An anterior open bite is also characteristic. The first molars may be dome-shaped (Moon's molars) or may have a rough pitted occlusal surface with compressed nodules instead of cusps (mulberry molars). These defects are now largely of historical interest.

Pathology

The effects are due to infection of the dental follicle by *Treponema pallidum*. The postulated consequences are chronic inflammation, fibrosis of the tooth sac, compression of the developing tooth and distortion of the ameloblast layer. *T. pallidum* causes proliferation of the odontogenic epithelium which bulges into the dentine papilla causing the characteristic central notch.

Metabolic disturbances

General disturbances of metabolism affecting the development

Fig. 2.24 Congenital syphilis; Hutchinson's teeth. The characteristics are the notched incisal edge and the peg shape tapering from neck to tip.

of the teeth may be caused by the childhood fevers or severe infantile gastroenteritis.

Unlike inherited forms of hypoplasia, only a restricted area of enamel is defective, corresponding to the state of development at the time of the metabolic disturbance. Measles with severe secondary bacterial infection was the most common cause of this limited type of dental defect, but such defects have become uncommon because of more effective treatment.

Clinically, the typical effect is one or more rows of horizontally disposed pits or grooves across the crown of the incisors. These are usually in the incisal third, suggesting that the disorder had its effect during the first year or two of life, when such infections are most dangerous (Fig. 2.25).

Rickets can cause hypocalcification of the teeth but only if unusually severe.

Early-onset idiopathic hypoparathyroidism is rare. Ectodermal effects are associated. The teeth may therefore be hypoplastic with ridged enamel, short blunt roots and persistently open apices (Fig. 2.26). The nails may be defective and there may be complete absence of hair. Patients with early onset idiopathic hypoparathyroidism may later develop other endocrine deficiencies (polyendocrinopathy syndrome) but chronic candidosis may be the first sign (Ch. 15).

Hypophosphatasia. This rare genetic disorder can have severe skeletal effects as a result of failure of development of mature bone. There may also be failure of cementum formation causing loosening or early loss of teeth (Fig. 2.27).

Drugs

Tetracycline pigmentation

Tetracycline is taken up by calcifying tissues, and the band of tetracycline-stained bone or tooth substance fluoresces bright yellow under ultraviolet light.

The teeth become stained only when tetracycline is given during their development, and it can cross the placenta to stain the developing teeth of the fetus. More frequently, permanent teeth are stained by tetracycline given during infancy.

Fig. 2.26 Teeth in childhood hypoparathyroidism with short blunt roots, open apices and large pulp chambers.

Fig. 2.27 Tooth in hypophosphatasia showing the enlarged pulp chamber and absence of cementum.

Tetracycline is deposited along the incremental lines of the dentine and, to lesser extent, of the enamel.

The more prolonged the course of treatment the broader the band of stain and the deeper the discolouration. The teeth are at first bright yellow, but become a dirty brown or grey (Figs 2.28 and 2.29). The stain is permanent, and when the permanent incisors are affected the ugly appearance can only be disguised. When the history is vague the brownish colour of tetracycline-stained teeth must be distinguished from dentinogenesis imperfecta. In dentinogenesis imperfecta the teeth are obviously more translucent than normal and, in many cases, chipping of the enamel from the dentine can be seen. In tetracycline-induced defects the enamel is not abnormally translucent and is firmly attached to dentine. In very severe cases, intact teeth may fluoresce under ultraviolet light. Otherwise the diagnosis can only be confirmed after a tooth has been extracted. In an undecalcified section the yellow fluorescence of the tetracycline deposited along the incremental lines can be easily seen (Fig. 2.30).

It is no longer necessary to give tetracycline during dental development. There are equally effective alternatives and it

Fig. 2.25 Chronological hypoplasia due to metabolic upset. Unlike the hereditary types of amelogenesis imperfecta, defects are linear and thought to correspond to a short period of amelogenesis disturbed by a concurrent severe illness.

Fig. 2.28 Tetracycline staining. Note the chronological distribution of the dark-brown intrinsic stain.

Fig. 2.29 Tetracycline pigmentation showing the pale yellow discolouration in the newly erupted lower incisors. The typical dark brown stain seen in the upper deciduous incisors develops slowly after eruption.

should be avoided from approximately the fourth month to the 12th year of childhood. Nevertheless, tetracycline pigmentation is still seen.

Cytotoxic chemotherapy

Increasing numbers of children are surviving malignant disease, particularly acute leukaemia, as a result of cytotoxic chemotherapy.

Among survivors, teeth developing during treatment may have short roots, hypoplasia of the crowns and enamel defects. Microscopically, incremental lines may be more prominent, corresponding with the period of chemotherapy, but in extreme cases tooth formation may be aborted.

Fluorosis

Mottled enamel is the most frequently seen and most reliable sign of excess fluoride in the drinking water. It has distinctive features (Table 2.6).

Clinical features

Mottling ranges from paper-white patches to opaque, brown,

Fig. 2.30 Teeth with bands of tetracycline stain. On the left, viewed in transmitted light, the stain appears as brown bands corresponding to the mineralising front in enamel and dentine during administration of each course. On the right, ultraviolet illumination confirms the presence of tetracycline, which is fluorescent, as the cause.

Table 2.6 Distinctive features of dental fluorosis

- Mottling is endemic in areas where fluorides in the drinking water exceed about 2 parts per million, i.e. it has a geographical distribution
- Neighbouring communities with fluoride-free water do not suffer from the disorder
- Only those who have lived in a high-fluoride area during dental development show mottling. The defect is not acquired by older visitors to the area
- Permanent teeth are affected; mottling of deciduous teeth is rare
- Mottled teeth are less susceptible to caries than normal teeth from low-fluoride areas
- A typical effect is paper-white enamel opacities
- Brown staining of these patches may be acquired after eruption

---

pitted and brittle enamel. Clinically, it may be difficult to distinguish fluorotic defects from amelogenesis imperfecta when the degree of exposure to fluoride is unknown (Fig. 2.31).

There is considerable individual variation in the effects of fluorides. A few patients acquire mottling after exposure to relatively low concentrations, while others exposed to higher concentrations appear unaffected.

Changes due to mottling are graded as shown in Table 2.7.

Table 2.7 Grading of mottled enamel

- *Very mild*. Small paper-white areas involve less than 25% of surface
- *Mild*. Opaque areas involve up to 50% surface
- *Moderate*. The whole of the enamel surface may be affected with paper-white or brownish areas or both (Fig. 2.32).
- *Severe*. The enamel is grossly defective, opaque, pitted, stained brown and brittle (Fig. 2.33).

Fig. 2.31 Fluoride mottling. In this case, from an area of endemic fluorosis, there is generalised opaque white mottling with patchy enamel hypoplasia. Note the resemblance to the hypomaturation type of amelogenesis imperfecta.

Fig. 2.33 Fluorosis. Severe effects from an area of endemic fluorosis. Closer view showing irregular depressions caused by hypoplasia and white opaque flecks and patches.

Pathology

Fluoride combines to form calcium fluorapatite in place of part of the hydroxyapatite. Damage to ameloblasts, leading to defective matrix formation, is seen only when the concentrations of fluorides are exceptionally high. At intermediate levels (2–6 p.p.m.) the matrix is normal in structure and quantity. The form of the tooth is unaffected, but there are patches of incomplete calcification beneath the surface layer. These appear as opacities because of high organic and water content. Where there are high concentrations of fluorides (over 6 p.p.m.) the enamel is pitted and brittle, with severe and widespread staining. Deciduous teeth are rarely mottled because excess fluoride is taken up by the maternal skeleton. However, when fluoride levels are excessively high (over 8 p.p.m.), as in parts of India, mottling of deciduous teeth may be seen.

With severe mottling of the enamel, other effects of excessive fluoride intake, especially sclerosis of the skeleton, may develop. Radiographically, increased density of the skeleton may be seen in areas where the fluoride content of the water exceeds 8 p.p.m.

The severity of defects in relation to fluoride concentrations is shown in Table 2.8 and its relationship to caries prevalence in Figure 2.34. Mild dental fluorosis is not readily distinguishable from non-fluoride defects and non-specific defects are more common in areas where the water contains less than 1 p.p.m. of fluorine.

Fig. 2.32 Fluorosis. Severe effects from an area of endemic fluorosis. Irregular patchy discolouration.

Table 2.8 Effects on enamel of increasing fluoride levels

Fluoride concentration (p.p.m.)	Effects	Clinical appearance
Less than 0.5	Very mild or mild defects in up to 6% of patients	Inconspicuous
0.5–1.5	At the upper limit, 22% show very mild defects	
2.5	Very mild or mild defects in over 50%; nearly 10% show apparent 'moderate' or 'severe' defects	Noticeable
4.5	Nearly all patients affected in some degree; 46% have 'moderate' and 18% 'severe' defects	Disfiguring
6.0 and above	All patients affected; 50% severely disfiguring	

Other acquired developmental anomalies

Dilaceration

Trauma to a developing tooth can cause the root to form at an angle to the normal axis of the tooth — a rare deformity known as dilaceration. The sudden disturbance to odontogenesis may cause the formation of highly irregular dentine in the coronal part of the pulp chamber but the angulated root may consist of normal tubular dentine. The hook-shaped tooth is likely to be difficult to extract (Figs 2.35 and 2.36).

Fetal alcohol syndrome

Maternal alcoholism may cause developmental defects in the fetus. The eyes typically slant laterally, the lower half of the face is elongated and there is mental deficiency. Dental development may be delayed and there may be enamel defects such

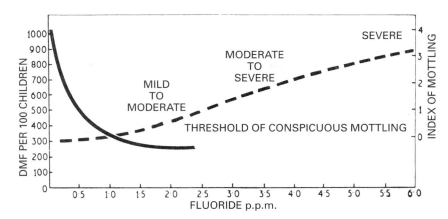

Fig. 2.34 Caries prevalence and mottling. The general relationship between the prevalence of caries (continuous line) and the severity of mottling (broken line) in persons continuously exposed to various levels of fluoride in the water during dental development. The optimum level of fluoride can be seen to be about 1 part per million. Higher concentrations of fluoride cause increasing incidence and severity of mottling without a comparable improvement in resistance to caries. The index of mottling is obtained by giving an arbitrary value for each degree of mottling and relating the numbers of patients with each grade to the total number examined.

Fig. 2.35 A dilacerated upper central incisor. There has been an abrupt change in the direction of root growth after approximately one-third of the root was formed.

as mottled opacities in the enamel near the incisal margins but elsewhere abnormal enamel translucency.

Treatment of hypoplastic defects

Hypoplastic teeth can only be disguised by restorative procedures such as veneers or jacket crowns. The latter should be delayed until adult life. The young pulp is large, is easily damaged during preparation of the tooth, and injuries are more frequent than in older persons.

ODONTOMAS

Odontomas result from aberrant development of the dental lamina. The most minor examples, though they are not usually

Fig. 2.36 Another dilacerated tooth showing, in addition to the deflected root, a change in enamel contour and disorganised coronal dentine formed after the causative trauma.

called odontomas, are slight malformations such as an exaggerated cingulum or extra roots or cusps on otherwise normal teeth. All gradations exist between these anomalies and composite odontomas where the dental tissues have developed in a completely irregular and haphazard manner, bearing no resemblance to a tooth and occasionally forming a large mass (Ch. 8).

Dens invaginatus is an exaggeration of the process of formation of a cingular pit. Dentine and enamel-forming tissue invaginate the whole length of a tooth to appear radiographically as a 'tooth within a tooth' (*dens in dente*, Fig. 2.37). Food debris lodges in the cavity to cause caries which rapidly penetrates the distorted pulp chamber. Extension of this process causes the formation of an invaginated odontome (Fig. 2.38).

Geminated teeth are most common in the maxillary incisor region. The pulp chambers may be entirely separate, joined in the middle of the tooth, or branched, with the pulp chambers of separated crowns sharing a common root canal. The crowns may be entirely separate or divided only by a shallow groove. The roots may be single or double.

These malformed teeth usually need to be removed before they obstruct the eruption of other teeth or become infected, or for cosmetic reasons.

Enamel pearls are uncommon, minor abnormalities, which are formed on otherwise normal teeth by displaced ameloblasts below the amelocemental junction. Enamel pearls may consist of only a nodule of enamel attached to the dentine, or may have a core of dentine containing a horn of the pulp. The pearls are usually round, a few millimetres in diameter, and often form at the bifurcation of upper permanent molars (Fig. 2.39 and 2.40). They may cause a stagnation area at the gingival margin, but, if they contain pulp, this will be exposed when the pearl is removed.

GENETIC DISORDERS OF THE JAWS

Important developmental defects of the jaws are summarised in Table 2.9 and discussed more fully in subsequent chapters.

Fig. 2.37 Dens in dente or mild invaginated odontome. In this radiograph the enamel-lined invagination and its communication with the exterior at the incisal tip are clearly seen. The pulp is compressed to the periphery.

Fig. 2.38 An invaginated odontome in a lateral incisor, sectioned vertically. The central cavity communicates with the exterior through an invagination in the cusp tip.

Hereditary prognathism

Historically, hereditary prognathism is best known in the Spanish branch of the Hapsburg royal family. The defect is seen in striking form in contemporaneous portraits and persisted for 300 years.

CLEFTS OF THE LIP AND PALATE

Clefts can form in the lip or palate alone or in both (Figs 2.41 and 2.42). The aetiology is unknown but there is a genetic component in approximately 40% of cases. The risk of having such defects is greatly increased if one, and particularly if both, of the parents are affected.

Cleft lip (with or without a palatal cleft) is more common in males, while cleft palate alone is approximately twice as common in females. The incidence of cleft lip is about 1 per 1000 live births, while that of isolated palatal clefts is about 1 per 2000 live births. In terms of relative frequencies, cleft lips form about 22%, combined defects of lip and palate form about 58% and isolated palatal clefts form about 20% of this group of defects. The reasons for the variations in the sites of clefts is that the lip and anterior palate (the primary palate) develop before the hard and soft palates (the secondary palate). Fusion of the secondary palate is from behind forwards. Isolated cleft lip is therefore the result of an early developmental disorder, while isolated cleft palate results from influences acting later, after the primary palate has closed. By contrast, a prolonged disorder of development can prevent both primary and secondary palates from closing and leaves a severe combined defect.

Developmental disorders associated with clefting

In Down's syndrome, cleft lip or palate is present in approximately 1 in 200 patients (Ch. 33). In the less common trisomy

Fig. 2.39 An enamel pearl. A rounded nodule of ectopic enamel is seen in the usual position for these malformations, at the bifurcation of the roots of a molar.

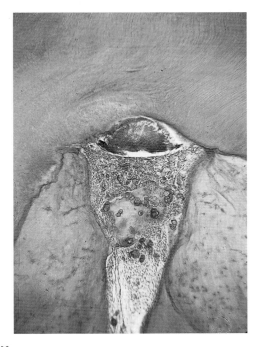

Fig. 2.40 Histological appearance of an enamel pearl showing a small isolated zone of enamel matrix on the root dentine.

13 (Patau's syndrome), cleft lip or palate, or both, is present in up to 70% of cases, but multiple defects of the brain and other organs lead to early death. Clefts are also a feature of many other genetic craniofacial syndromes.

Classification

The main types of cleft lip are summarised in Table 2.10. In the worst cases there is complete separation of the anterior palate, which projects forward with the centre section of the lip and is attached only by the nasal septum.

Associated defects

1. *Local*. Teeth in the region of the defect are typically absent or malformed.
2. *Systemic*. Major congenital defects, particularly heart disease, limb defects, spina bifida or mental defects, are associated

Table 2.9 Developmental defects of the jaws

- Hereditary prognathism
- Clefts of the palate and/or lip
- Craniofacial anomalies
- Cleidocranial dysplasia (Ch. 10)
- Cherubism (Ch. 10)
- Gorlin–Goltz syndrome (Ch. 7)
- Gardner's syndrome (Ch. 9)
- Osteogenesis imperfecta (Ch. 10)

Fig. 2.41 Cleft palate. A broad midline defect is present.

Fig. 2.42 Cleft lip and palate. Complete unilateral cleft of palate, alveolar bone and lip joining the oral and nasal cavities.

Table 2.10 Clefts of lip and/or palate

- Cleft lip
  Unilateral (usually on the left side), with or without an anterior alveolar ridge cleft
  Bilateral, with or without alveolar ridge clefts, complete or incomplete
- Palatal clefts
  Bifid uvula
  Soft palate only
  Both hard and soft palate
- Combined lip and palatal defects
  Unilateral, complete or incomplete
  Cleft palate with bilateral cleft lip, complete or incomplete

in about 50% of these patients and can seriously affect their management. This is particularly so in the case of Down's syndrome.

Management

Important considerations are summarised in Table 2.11. Repair of these clefts has traditionally been carried out at 15–18 months after birth. Nevertheless, early operation can severely inhibit growth, both by damaging the delicate growing tissues and, particularly, by consequent scarring. Severe malocclusion can result, and reoperation may be necessary to lessen the deformity (Fig. 2.43).

However, observation of untreated clefts has shown that the growth potential of these tissues is virtually normal. In some centres, therefore, a soft palate cleft is repaired early but hard palate repair is delayed until 8–9 years after temporary closure with an obturator. The results are good facial growth and occlusion, but speech may be impaired to some degree.

Submucous cleft palate

Submucous clefts are an abnormality of the attachment of the muscles of the soft palate beneath an intact mucosa. They are present in approximately 1 in 1200 births but frequently missed. The chief effects are slowness in feeding and nasal regurgitation. Middle ear infections and speech defects result from the defective muscle attachments as frequently as in those with overt clefts. Symptoms are absent in only 10% of cases.

Clinically, a submucous cleft is visible as a translucent area along the midline of the soft palate and frequently a bifid uvula.

On palpation, a notched posterior nasal spine may be felt. The diagnosis can be confirmed by imaging techniques, such as videofluoroscopy. Operation to repair the muscle attachments is

Table 2.11 Important aspects of management of clefts

- Provision for feeding in infancy when palatal clefts are severe
- Prevention of collapse of the two halves of the maxilla
- Measures to counteract speech defects
- Cosmetic repair of cleft lips

Fig. 2.43 Collapsed maxilla resulting from traditional surgical repair of cleft palate. Scarring and growth disturbance produce a distorted narrow maxilla. (Figures 2.41–2.43 by kind permission of Mrs E Horrocks.)

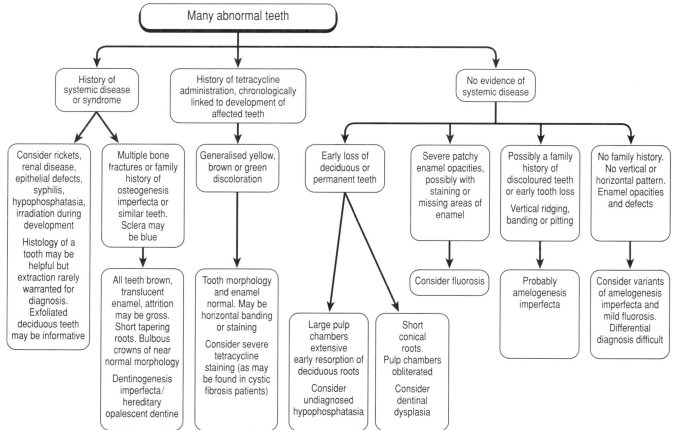

Summary 2.1 Differential diagnosis of developmental defects of the teeth.

usually delayed for about 2.5 years to enable the degree of the defect to be assessed.

DEVELOPMENTAL DEFECTS OF THE ORAL SOFT TISSUES

These defects (Table 2.12) are discussed in more detail in later chapters.

Table 2.12   Important developmental defects of oral soft tissues

• The gingivae and periodontium (Ch. 5)
    Hereditary gingival fibromatosis
    Ehlers–Danlos syndrome type VIII
• The oral mucosa (Ch. 15)
    White sponge naevus
    Epidermolysis bullosa
    Ehlers–Danlos syndrome

OTHER GENETIC DISEASES RELEVANT TO DENTISTRY

There are many rare hereditary disorders which can affect the mouth or jaws, but, from the practical clinical viewpoint, haemophilia is the most important (Ch. 23).

SUGGESTED FURTHER READING

Aine L, Mäki M, Collin P et al 1990 Dental enamel defects in celiac disease. J Oral Pathol Med 19:241–245

Aldred M J 1992 Unusual dentinal changes in dentinogenesis imperfecta associated with osteogenesis imperfecta. A case report. Oral Surg Oral Med Oral Pathol 73:461–464

Bhat M, Nelson K B, Cummins S K, Grether J K 1992 Prevalence of developmental enamel defects in children with cerebral palsy. J Oral Pathol Med 21:241–244

Chapple I L C 1993 Hypophosphatasia: dental aspects and mode of inheritance. J Clin Periodontol 20:615–622

Crawford P J M, Aldred M J 1989 Regional odontodysplasia: a bibliography. J Oral Pathol Med 18:251–263

Fanibunda K B, Soames J V 1996 Odontodysplasia, gingival manifestations, and accompanying abnormalities. Oral Surg Oral Med Oral Pathol Oral Radiol Endod 81:84–88

Mäki M, Aine L, Lipsanen V et al 1991 Dental enamel defects in first-degree relatives of coeliac disease patients. Lancet 337:763–764

Markus A F, Smith W P, Delaire J 1993 Primary closure of cleft palate: a functional approach. Br J Oral Maxillofac Surg 31:71–77

Precious D S, Delaire J 1993 Clinical observations of cleft lip and palate. Oral Surg Oral Med Oral Pathol 75:141–151

Van der Wal J E, Rittersma J, Baart J A, van der Waal I 1993 Odontodysplasia: report of three cases. Int J Oral Maxillofac Surg 22:356–358

Wolff G, Wienker T F, Sander H 1993 On the genetics of mandibular prognathism: analysis of large European noble families. J Med Genet 30:112–116

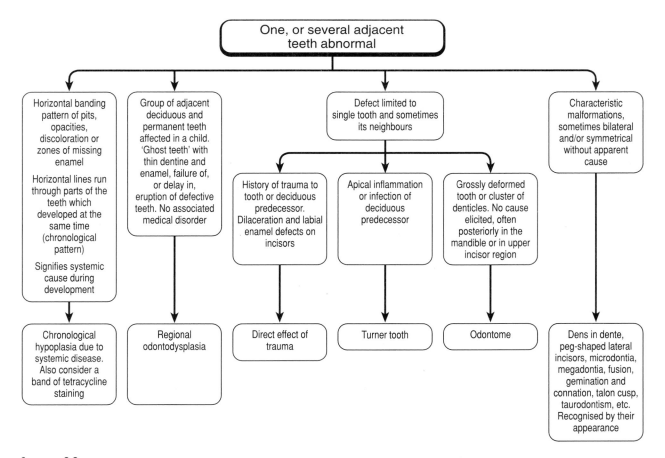

Summary 2.2   Differential diagnosis of developmental and acquired abnormalities of one or a group of teeth.

Dental caries

> *For sweetness and decay are of one root and sweetness ever riots to decay.*
>
> Author, regrettably, unknown

Dental caries is a progressive bacterial damage to teeth exposed to the saliva and initiated by acid production in bacterial plaque. The effect of untreated caries is to break down enamel and dentine, and open the way for bacteria to infect the pulp. The ultimate consequences are inflammation of the pulp and, later, of the periapical tissues. Acute pulpitis and periodontitis caused in this way are the most common causes of toothache. Infection can spread from the periapical region to the jaw and beyond. This is rare in Britain, but people in other countries occasionally die as a result (Ch. 6).

Caries is one of the most common of all diseases and still a major cause of loss of teeth.

AETIOLOGY

In 1890, W. D. Miller showed that lesions similar to dental caries could be produced by incubating teeth in saliva when carbohydrates were added. Miller proposed that caries could result from decalcification caused by bacterial acid production followed by invasion and destruction of any remaining tissue. His basic hypothesis has been upheld, even though the infective nature of the disease was not confirmed until 1954 when Orland and his associates showed that caries did not develop in germ-free animals. However, dental caries develops only in the presence of several interacting variables (Fig. 3.1 and Table 3.1).

BACTERIOLOGY

Germ-free animals do not develop dental caries when fed a sucrose-rich diet which causes caries in animals with a normal oral flora. Substantial evidence indicates that certain streptococci are essential for the initiation of dental caries, particularly of smooth (interstitial) surfaces. These are viridans streptococ-

Possible interventions
Reduce intake cariogenic sugars
(primarily sucrose, glucose and fructose)

Possible interventions
Reduce *Strep. mutans* numbers by:
- reduction in sugar intake
- active or passive immunisation

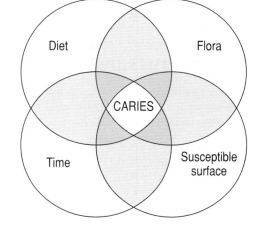

Possible interventions
Avoid frequent sucrose intake ('snacking')
Stimulate salivary flow and sugar clearance

Possible interventions
Water and other types of fluoridation
Prevention during post-eruptive
   maturation
Fissure sealing
Remineralising solutions
Properly contoured restorations

Fig. 3.1   The four major factors in the aetiology of dental caries.

Table 3.1   Essential requirements for development of dental caries

1. Cariogenic bacteria
2. Bacterial plaque
3. Stagnation areas
4. Fermentable bacterial substrate (sugar)
5. Susceptible tooth surfaces
6. Time for the process to develop

ci, which are a heterogeneous group including *Streptococcus mutans*, *S. sobrinus*, *S. salivarius*, *S. mitior* and *S. sanguis*.

Viridans streptococci vary in their ability to attach to different types of tissues, their ability to ferment sugars, particularly sucrose, and the concentrations of acid thus produced. They also differ in the types of polysaccharides that they form.

Certain strains of *S. mutans* are strongly acidogenic and, at low pH, with freely available sucrose, also store an intracellular, glycogen-like, reserve polysaccharide. When the supply of substrate dries up, this reserve is metabolised to sugars which continue acid production for a time. Drastic reduction in dietary sucrose intake is followed by virtual elimination of *S. mutans* from plaque and reduces or abolishes caries activity. When sucrose becomes freely available again, *S. mutans* rapidly recolonises the plaque.

S. mutans is a major component of plaque in human mouths, particularly in persons with a high dietary sucrose intake and high caries activity (Fig. 3.2). *S. mutans* isolated from such mouths is virulently cariogenic when introduced into the mouths of previously germ-free animals. These experiments with gnotobiotes have confirmed that the most potent causes of dental caries are a limited number of strains of the *S. mutans* group which are able to form cariogenic plaque (Table 3.2). However, simple clinical observation of the sites (interstitially and in pits and fissures) where dental caries is active shows that the bacteria responsible are not those floating free in the saliva. Dental caries develops only at the interface between tooth and dental plaque in stagnation areas. Stagnation areas allow plaque activity to develop undisturbed and hence are the sites of carious attack (Fig. 3.3).

Table 3.2	Essential properties of cariogenic bacteria

- Acidogenic
- Able to produce a pH low enough (usually pH <5) to demineralise tooth substance
- Able to survive and continue to produce acid at low pH
- Possess attachment mechanisms for firm adhesion to smooth tooth surfaces
- Able to produce adhesive, insoluble plaque polysaccharides (glucans)

Bacterial polysaccharides

The ability of *S. mutans* to initiate smooth surface caries and

Fig. 3.3 The stagnation area in an occlusal pit. A ground section of a molar showing the size of the stagnation area in comparison with a toothbrush bristle placed above it. The complete inaccessibility of the stagnation area to cleaning is obvious.

form large amounts of adherent plaque depends on its ability to polymerise sucrose into sticky, high molecular weight, dextran-like, extracellular polysaccharides (*glucans*).

Glucans enable streptococci to adhere to one another and to the tooth surface via specific receptors. They enable *S. mutans* to become attached to the teeth and plaque to persist there. Production of sticky, insoluble, extracellular glucan by strains of *S. mutans* from sucrose is strongly related to their cariogenicity. Their cariogenicity depends as much on their ability to form large amounts of insoluble extracellular glucans as on their ability to produce acid.

Bacterial plaque polysaccharides play an essential role in the pathogenesis of dental caries. The proportions of the different types of polysaccharide, and the overall amounts formed, depend both on the kinds of bacteria present and the different sugars in the diet.

On a sucrose-rich diet the main extracellular polysaccharides are glucans. Fructans formed from fructose are produced in smaller amounts. They are more soluble and less important in forming cariogenic plaque. Acid-producing microorganisms that do not produce insoluble polysaccharides do not appear to be able to initiate caries of smooth surfaces. Even mutant strains of *S. mutans* which produce more soluble polysaccharides seem not to be cariogenic. Polysaccharides thus contribute to the adhesiveness, bulk and resistance to solution of plaque.

In the past, lactobacilli were thought to be the main cause of dental caries because they are numerous in the saliva and can be isolated from carious cavities. They are also acidogenic. However, they are present only in relatively small numbers in dental plaque until after caries has developed.

Fig. 3.2 Extensive caries of decidous incisors and canines. This pattern of caries is particularly associated with the use of sweetened dummies and sweetened infant drinks.

In gnotobiotes, lactobacilli are weakly cariogenic but some can produce fissure caries where adherent plaque formation is less important. Overall there is little evidence that lactobacilli are clinically important in initiating dental caries but they may contribute to tooth destruction after the process has started.

Many other microorganisms can also be found in plaque. The role of many of them is not known. Strains of actinomyces are also found, particularly when caries is rampant, but appear capable only of producing root surface lesions.

Though bacteria are responsible for acid production, *bacterial plaque* enables large concentrations of them to adhere to the teeth and prevents effective buffering of bacterial acids by saliva.

Important points about microbiological aspects of dental caries are summarised in Table 3.3.

Fig. 3.4 Bacterial plaque. A decalcified section showing darkly staining plaque lying on enamel and within a carious cavity. The plaque has remained intact and adherent to the enamel throughout the processes to which the specimen was subjected in preparation for sectioning.

Table 3.3 Microbiological aspects of dental caries

- Dental caries is a bacterial disease
- The organisms mainly responsible for its initiation are specific strains of *Streptococcus mutans*
- The cariogenicity of *S. mutans* has been established by inoculating it into the mouths of otherwise germ-free animals (gnotobiotes)
- The presence of *S. mutans* in human mouths is associated with caries activity
- Other bacteria, including lactobacilli and other strains of streptococci, are only weakly cariogenic or are non-cariogenic despite being able to produce acid

The cariogenicity of *S. mutans* depends on properties summarised in Table 3.4.

Table 3.4 Cariogenic properties of *Streptococcus mutans*

- It produces lactic acid from sucrose
- It can live at a pH as low as 4.2
- It forms large amounts of extracellular, sticky and insoluble glucan plaque matrix
- It adheres to pellicle and contributes to plaque formation

BACTERIAL PLAQUE

Plaque is a tenaciously adherent deposit that forms on tooth surfaces. It consists of an organic matrix containing a dense concentration of bacteria (Figs 3.4–3.6).

In microbiological terms, plaque is a *biofilm*. Biofilms consist of a hydrated viscous phase formed from bacteria and their extracellular polysaccharide matrices. In such a film, molecules and ions exist in concentrations that can be widely different from those of the surrounding fluid phase (saliva). Bacteria in biofilms can also exhibit cooperative activity and behave differently from the same species in isolation in a culture medium. As a consequence, a biofilm may be resistant to antimicrobials or

Fig. 3.5 This scanning electronmicrograph of plaque shows the large number of filamentous organisms and, in addition, many cocci clustered amongst them. (By kind permission of Dr Sheila J Jones.)

to immunological defences to which the individual bacteria are normally sensitive. Bacterial plaque is therefore a distinct entity and not a mere collection of bacteria. In particular, the ability of dental plaque to concentrate and retain acid was recognised long before the special properties of biofilms were discovered.

Clinically, plaque becomes visible, particularly on the labial surfaces of the incisors, when toothbrushing stops for 12–24 hours. It appears as a translucent film with a matt surface

Fig. 3.6 This scanning electronmicrograph at higher power shows cocci attached to filamentous organisms to produce the corn-cob type of arrangement sometimes seen in plaque. (By kind permission of Dr Sheila J Jones.)

Fig. 3.7 Stephan curves. This is the usual form of curves obtained when changes in reaction to bacterial plaque are measured directly. When the pH falls below the critical level, enamel may become demineralised. Patients with active caries tend to show a lower fall in pH, as in the lower curve. Noteworthy features are the very rapid fall in pH and the slow recovery to the normal level in spite of the very short time the sugar is in the mouth. Carbohydrates which are retained on the teeth will have a more prolonged effect still.

that dulls the otherwise smooth and shiny enamel. It can be made obvious when stained with disclosing agents. Little plaque forms under conditions of starvation but it forms rapidly and abundantly on a high-sucrose diet.

Plaque resists the friction of food during mastication, and can only be readily removed by toothbrushing. However, neither toothbrushing nor fibrous foods will remove plaque from inaccessible surfaces or pits.

Adhesion of bacteria to the teeth, from which they would otherwise be washed away, is an essential requirement for the colonisation of, and attack on, the enamel. Attachment depends on complex mechanisms and on such molecules as glucans and/or glucosyltransferase. Components of plaque which act as adhesion receptors include a group of *proline-rich proteins* (*PRPs*) from the saliva.

The process of plaque formation starts with deposition of structureless, cell-free pellicle of salivary glycoprotein which becomes colonised by bacteria, particularly *S. sanguis* and *S. mutans* strains, within 24 hours. It is built up by formation of bacterial polysaccharides and progressively colonised by other bacteria.

Acid production in plaque

Sucrose diffuses rapidly into plaque, and acid production quickly follows. These changes have been measured directly in the human mouth using microelectrodes in direct contact with plaque and show that, after rinsing the mouth with a 10% glu-

cose solution, the pH falls within 2–5 minutes, often to a level sufficiently low to decalcify enamel. Even though no more sucrose may be taken and the surplus is washed away by the saliva, the pH level remains at a low level for about 15–20 minutes. It returns only gradually to the resting level after about an hour (Fig. 3.7). The rapidity with which the pH falls reflects the speed with which sucrose can diffuse into plaque and the activity of the concentration of enzymes produced by the vast numbers of bacteria in the plaque. The slow rate of recovery to the resting pH (shown in the so-called Stephan curves) is a critical factor in caries production, and depends mainly on factors summarised in Table 3.5.

Table 3.5 Factors contributing to maintenance of low plaque pH

- Rapid production of a high concentration of acid within the plaque, temporarily overcomes local buffering
- Escape of acid into the saliva, delayed by the diffusion-limiting properties of plaque
- Diffusion of salivary buffers into plaque hampered by the diffusion-limiting properties of plaque
- Continued acid production from bacterial intracellular polysaccharides

Acid production is alone responsible for initiation of the carious attack. Lactic acid is mainly responsible. It is quantitatively the predominant acid during plaque activity, has a lower pK constant and causes a greater fall in pH than equimolar solutions of acetic or propionic acids which may also be detected in plaque.

Plaque minerals

In addition to bacteria and their polysaccharides, salivary components also contribute to the plaque matrix. Calcium, phosphorus and, often, fluorides are present in significant amounts. There is some evidence of an inverse relationship between calcium and phosphate levels in plaque and caries activity or sucrose intake. The ability of plaque to concentrate calcium and phosphorus is used in mineralising mouthwashes. The level of fluoride in plaque may be high, ranging from 15 to 75 p.p.m. or more, and is largely dependent on fluorides from dentifrices or from drinking water. Plaque fluoride is mostly bound to organic material in the plaque but, at low pH levels, may become available and active in ionic form.

SUCROSE AS A PLAQUE SUBSTRATE

Direct measurement of pH changes on the tooth surface shows that ingestion of sucrose leads to a burst of plaque activity that may cause the pH to fall low enough to attack enamel. However, if sucrose is taken as a sweet drink, any surplus that cannot be metabolised at the time is washed away. By contrast, if sucrose is taken repeatedly at short intervals, it maintains a supply of substrate that enables bacterial acid production to remain persistently at a destructive level. A greater effect may be caused by carbohydrate in sticky form, such as a caramel, which clings to the teeth, dissolves slowly and releases substrate over a long period. The frequency with which substrate is made available is therefore important.

The effects of maintaining plaque activity by repeated administration of small quantities of sucrose have been demonstrated by use of animal feeding devices to dispense metered quantities of sucrose in diets at fixed intervals. These show that a given amount of sucrose is more cariogenic when fed in small increments at intervals, thus maintaining maximal plaque activity, than the same amount fed as a single dose.

Effects of sucrose on oral bacteria

Colonisation by cariogenic bacteria, especially *S. mutans*, is highly dependent on the sucrose content of the diet which enables adherent polysaccharides to be produced. In the absence of sucrose, *S. mutans* cannot usually be made to colonise the teeth of experimental animals. In humans, the plaque counts of *S. mutans* also appear to depend on the sucrose content of the diet. Severe reduction in dietary sucrose causes *S. mutans* to decline in numbers or disappear from plaque. Sucrose is particularly important for the production of insoluble plaque polysaccharides. Its importance in this activity may depend on the high energy of its glucose–fructose bond which allows synthesis of polysaccharides by glucosyltransferase without any other source of energy. Sucrose is thus the main substrate for such polysaccharides and is also the main sugar present in the diet. Other sugars are less readily formed into

cariogenic glucans but if plaque is already present they can be metabolised to acid.

Experimental evidence for the essential contribution of sucrose to caries activity is summarised in Table 3.6.

Table 3.6 Experimental evidence for the critical contribution of sucrose to caries activity

- In caries-susceptible animals a sucrose-rich diet promotes caries production
- Caries is not induced in susceptible animals if sucrose is fed only by stomach-tube — its effect is entirely local
- Sucrose promotes colonisation of the teeth by *S. mutans*
- Sucrose diffuses rapidly into plaque and is converted into acid
- Sucrose in sticky form clings to the teeth and remains available to bacteria for a longer period and is more cariogenic
- Sucrose contributes greatly to production of adhesive and insoluble plaque polysaccharides
- Frequent feeds of small quantities of sucrose are more cariogenic than the same total amount fed on a single occasion
- Desalivation, by delaying clearance of sugars, enhances caries activity

The importance of sucrose in human caries is shown by epidemiological studies and a few interventional studies (Table 3.7).

Table 3.7 Epidemiological evidence of sucrose as the cause of dental caries

- Low caries prevalence in populations with low sucrose intakes
- The decline in caries prevalence during wartime sugar shortages
- The rise of caries prevalence with increasing availability of sucrose
- Archaeological evidence of low caries prevalence in eras before sucrose became freely available
- Low caries prevalence in disorders of sucrose metabolism (hereditary fructose intolerance)

Dental caries has been most prevalent in well-nourished, Westernised communities, such as Britain, the USA and others with similar life styles where large quantities of sucrose (particularly as sweets or snack-bars) are eaten. There have been many studies of poor communities living on traditional diets with little or no sucrose content and a low caries prevalence has been shown (for example) in parts of China and Africa, the Seychelles, Tristan da Cunha, Alaska and Greenland. Many studies were carried out on Eskimo races who were caries-free when consuming their traditional diet of seal or whale meat, and fish. Similarly in South African races, despite a high-starch carbohydrate diet, caries was found in fewer than 9% of those examined, but greatly increased when there was access to a modern diet.

In such studies no association has been found between malnutrition and caries. Generally the reverse is true, and, when nutrition is poor, caries is infrequent. These diets also vary widely in content, from rice as the staple in China or coarsely ground cereals in Africa to a mainly meat and fish diet among Eskimos. The common feature of these diets, sharply differentiating them from Westernised diets, is low or negligible consumption of sucrose.

Britain is an example of a country where consumption of sucrose is exceptionally high, and where the rest of the diet is more than adequate. A survey in England and Wales in 1973 showed, for example, that (despite the benefits of a National Health Service) 78% of 8-year-old children had active decay and many teeth which had been filled or lost from this cause. A survey in 1978 showed that dentate adults had on average only 13 sound and unfilled teeth.

In Britain and other countries the incidence of caries has risen roughly parallel with rising consumption of sucrose. The incidence of caries has risen in spite of the much greater consumption of so-called 'protective' foods (dairy products, meat and fruit) in recent years. As a consequence of this more varied diet, carbohydrates overall have formed a smaller proportion of the diet. Nevertheless, sucrose forms a higher proportion of the carbohydrate component.

Where there has been a change from simple natural diets to a Westernised diet, as in Alaska, caries has increased sharply, and Eskimo children now have a caries incidence at least as high as other American children. A similar state of affairs is developing in Africa as sweet eating and between-meals sweet snack-bars have become popular. In Nigeria many of the older adults are still totally caries-free but the prevalence of dental caries among children and young people who have picked up sweet-eating habits is rising rapidly. This effect has also been impressively documented in the population of Tristan da Cunha who, up to the late 1930s, lived on a simple meat, fish and vegetable diet with a minimal sucrose content and had a very low caries prevalence. With the adoption of Westernised diet, the caries prevalence had risen eightfold in some age groups by the mid-1960s. Even in Europe, in the 1930s and 1940s there were isolated communities, such as the Outer Hebrides or the Lötschental in Switzerland, where dental caries prevalence rose twentyfold or more when sucrose and sweets became freely available.

The effect of limiting sucrose consumption has been shown on a vast scale in wartime. Those countries which suffered food shortages during the 1939–1945 war had severe restrictions, mainly of meat, fats and sucrose, but much greater overall consumption of starchy carbohydrates. In occupied Norway, where shortages were particularly severe, dental caries declined dramatically during and after the war, but when sucrose became more plentiful later, caries prevalence progressively rose (Fig.3.8).

In Japan also, rising caries prevalence has been associated with increased sucrose consumption. Towards the end of the second world war sucrose consumption and caries levels were very low. More recently, Japan was one of the few countries where sucrose consumption, from 16.5 kg per head in 1961, nearly doubled by 1970. Caries prevalence rose in parallel.

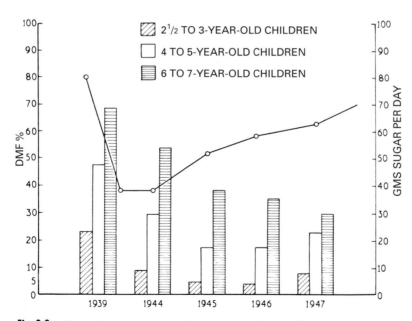

Fig. 3.8 The wartime restrictions on diet, and caries in Norway. The continuous line (above) shows an estimate of the individual daily sugar consumption during and after the war. The heights of the columns show the incidence of caries in children of various ages. Rationing of sugar started in 1938 but it is apparent that the incidence of caries declined slowly and continued for a short time after sugar became freely available. The greatest reduction in caries was in the youngest group of children whose teeth were exposed to the wartime diet for the shortest periods; the mothers of these children, on the other hand, had been exposed to the wartime diet throughout pregnancy and for a long period before this. (Mainly after Toverud G 1949 Journal of the American Dental Association 39:127.)

Unlike most other countries, this picture has not been significantly masked by use of fluoride toothpastes where the market share of fluoride toothpastes was only 15%.

Caries has become epidemic only in relatively recent years as sucrose became cheaper and widely available. In Britain, there was a sudden, widespread rise in sucrose consumption in the middle of the nineteenth century. This resulted both from the falling cost of production and the abolition of a tax on sugar in 1861. Evidence from exhumed skulls confirms the low prevalence of caries before sucrose became widely available and the steady rise in prevalence thereafter.

Patients unable to metabolise fructose as a result of an enzyme deficiency cannot tolerate fructose-containing foods, including disaccharides such as sucrose where fructose forms part of the molecule. These children therefore learn to avoid all sucrose-containing foods and have an unusually low incidence of caries.

Experimental studies on humans

In the Vipeholm study over 400 adults were studied in a closed institution. They received a basic low-carbohydrate diet to establish a baseline of caries activity for each group. They were then divided into seven groups which were each allocated different diets. A control group received the basic diet. Two groups received supplements of sucrose at mealtimes, either in solution or as sweetened bread. The four remaining groups received sweets (toffees, caramels or chocolate) which were eaten between meals.

The effects of sucrose in different quantities and of different degrees of adhesiveness, and of eating sucrose at different times, were thus tested over a period of 5 years. Caries activity was greatly enhanced by the eating, between meals, of sticky sweets (toffees and caramels) that were retained on the teeth (Fig. 3.9). Sucrose at mealtimes only had little effect. The incidence of caries fell to its original low level when toffees or caramels were no longer given, and caries activity was very slight in the control group having the low-carbohydrate diet.

In another large-scale clinical experiment in Turku (Finland) an experimental group was allowed a wide range of foods sweetened with xylitol (a sugar alcohol) but no sucrose. The control group was allowed as much sugary (sucrose-containing) foods as desired. After 2 years the experimental group showed 90% less caries than those who had been allowed sucrose.

Essential factors incriminating sucrose as the most cariogenic substrate are summarised in Table 3.8.

Use of sugar substitutes (artificial sweeteners) in place of sucrose greatly lowers caries activity. The cariogenicity of sugars and artificial sweeteners is summarised in Table 3.9.

SUSCEPTIBILITY OF TEETH TO CARIES

Teeth may be resistant to decay because of factors affecting the

THE EFFECTS ON DENTAL CARIES FREQUENCY OF SUPPLEMENTS OF SWEET FOODS DURING OR BETWEEN MEALS

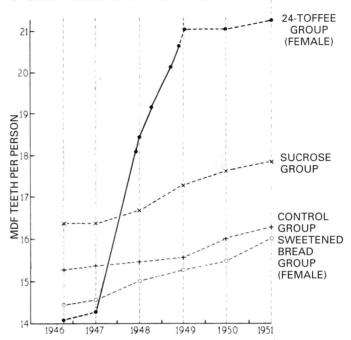

Fig. 3.9 The Vipeholm dental caries study. A simplified diagram showing the results in some of the groups of patients and in particular the striking effect on caries activity of sticky sweets eaten between meals when compared with the eating of sweetstuffs at mealtimes. The broken lines indicate those who consumed sugar only at meals, the continuous line shows those who consumed sugar both at and between meals. (After Gustafsson et al 1954 Acta Odontologica Scandinavica 11:232.)

Table 3.8 Factors determining the cariogenicity of sucrose

- Sucrose forms up to a third of the carbohydrate content of many persons' diets
- It promotes colonisation of teeth by S. mutans
- Its disaccharide bond provides enough energy to react with bacterial enzymes to form extracellular glucan matrix
- Its small molecule allows it to diffuse readily into plaque
- Bacterial metabolism of sucrose to acid is rapid

structure of the tooth during formation. Serious efforts were made in the past to confirm the misguided belief that dental caries was due to hypocalcification of the teeth and was essentially a vitamin deficiency disease. This simplistic view, of course, ignored the extensive epidemiological findings that the best-nourished populations had the worst record for dental disease, while poverty-stricken communities on deficient diets had a low caries prevalence.

Developmentally hypoplastic or hypocalcified teeth are also not particularly susceptible to caries. However, newly erupted teeth are generally caries-susceptible, apparently because of a hypomineralised enamel structure which becomes progressively less vulnerable by deposition of materials from saliva (maturation).

Table 3.9 Sugars and non-sugar sweeteners

Compound	Nature and uses	Cariogenicity
Sucrose	A disaccharide sugar (β1–4-linked glucose–fructose)	Highest of all sugars
Glucose, fructose	Monosaccharide sugars	Slightly less cariogenic than sucrose
Lactose and galactose	Monosaccharide (lactose) and disaccharide (galactose) sugars	Less cariogenic than sucrose
Glucose syrups and maltodextrins	Hydrolysis products of starch used as bulk sweeteners	Less cariogenic than sugars
Hydrogenated glucose syrup and lycasins	Hydrolysis products of starch which are then hydrogenated; used as bulk sweeteners	Less cariogenic than sugars
Isomalt	Mixture of two unusual 12-carbon sugars	Low cariogenicity
Xylitol, sorbitol, mannitol, lactitol, etc.	Sugar alcohols (polyols) sometimes used as bulk sweeteners	Non-cariogenic
Saccharin, aspartame, thaumatin, acesulfame K and cyclamate	Non-sugar intense sweeteners	Non-cariogenic

Effects of fluorides

Fluorides from drinking water and other sources are taken up by calcifying tissues during development. When the fluoride content of the water is 1 p.p.m. or more the incidence of caries declines substantially. Fluoride may affect caries activity by a variety of mechanisms (Table 3.10). Exposure to fluoride during dental development affects the structure of the developing teeth. This is shown by mottling of the enamel produced by excessive levels of fluoride. However, it is believed that the lower incidence of dental caries where water is fluoridated is due to its continued environmental effect on the teeth in reducing solubility of the enamel and promoting remineralisation. These effects may be more important than the effect of fluoride on structure.

Fluoride is the only nutrient which has been proved to have this protective action. Despite the difficulties in distinguishing the degree of resistance of the teeth from the virulence of their cariogenic environment, it has become clear that fluorides have had a major impact on caries prevalence. There has undoubtedly been a significant decline in the prevalence of dental caries in countries where drinking water has been fluoridated. In Britain, as a result of widespread use of fluoridised dentifrices, there has also been so great a decrease in the disease as significantly to affect the nature of dental practice. These changes cannot be related to any comparable decline in sucrose consumption.

Table 3.10 Actions of fluoride on dental caries

- Fluoride is incorporated into the teeth during development
- Fluoride acts mainly after eruption in early lesions by reducing enamel solubility and favouring remineralisation
- A constant supply of small amounts of fluoride is most effective in reducing dental caries
- Fluoride *may* reduce acid generation in plaque

SALIVA AND DENTAL CARIES

The immediate environment of the teeth is bacterial plaque, but saliva is the medium in which plaque develops and works. Though saliva inevitably plays some part in the process of caries, it is a complex secretion whose rates of flow, composition and properties are not easy to correlate with caries activity.

Salivary flow is highly important in clearing cariogenic foods from the mouth. In animals, removal or inactivation of major salivary glands leads to increased caries activity roughly in proportion to the reduction in saliva production. The same effect is seen in humans with xerostomia due to salivary gland disease.

Rate of flow and buffering power

The buffering power of saliva depends mainly on its bicarbonate content and is increased at high rates of flow. It affects the buffering power of dental plaque to some degree and helps to prevent the pH from falling to very low levels. A rapid flow rate, with greater salivary buffering power, may be associated with low caries activity. In Down's syndrome, caries activity is low in spite of gross accumulation of plaque and immunodeficiencies, probably because of the high rate of salivation with greater buffering power. Whilst a rapid flow of saliva of low viscosity assists clearance of foodstuffs from the mouth, other physical properties of different salivas have not been shown to have a significant relationship to caries activity.

Antibacterial activities

Saliva contains thiocyanates, a lysozyme-like substance and other theoretically antibacterial substances. Nevertheless, the mouth teems with bacteria, and there is no evidence that non-specific antibacterial substances in saliva have any significant effect on caries activity.

Immunological defences

IgA is secreted in saliva and small amounts of IgG enter the mouth from the gingival crevice. Persons who suffer from defects in non-specific host defences (complement and neutrophils) or specific immunological defences (IgA deficiency, Down's syndrome or AIDS) do not appear to suffer an excess of dental caries. Nevertheless, an immunological host resistance to dental caries is detectable experimentally in humans and appears to act by reducing the number of *S. mutans* in plaque. The effect does not appear to be very potent and is easily overwhelmed if the diet is high in sucrose or if levels of the relevant antibody are low.

Immunological defences against *S. mutans* could be mediated by salivary IgA or serum IgG from the crevicular fluid. Although salivary IgA is capable of preventing caries in experimental animals, it appears to play no significant role in humans. Immunisation of monkeys against *S. mutans* generates protective serum IgG. Serum IgG also appears to protect against *S. mutans* in humans but the response varies widely between individuals.

It has been shown that dripping a solution of monoclonal antibody against *S. mutans* on to the teeth prevents recolonisation by *S. mutans* in humans. However, plaque must be removed before treatment by using chlorhexidine and oral hygiene. This effect of antibody lasts for several months after applications and this 'passive immunisation' may reduce caries significantly.

Key facts about the effects of saliva on plaque activity are summarised in Table 3.11.

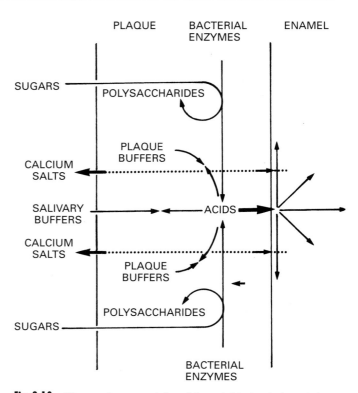

Fig. 3.10 Diagramatic representation of the main biochemical events in dental plaque, initiating caries. (From McCracken A W, Cawson R A 1983 Clinical and oral microbiology. McGraw-Hill.)

Table 3.11 **Key facts about the effects of saliva on plaque activity**

- Salivary components contribute to plaque formation
- Sucrose in saliva is taken up by plaque
- The buffering power of saliva may limit the fall in pH caused by acid formed in plaque
- The buffering power of saliva is related to the rate of secretion High flow rates *may* be associated with lower caries activity
- Gross reduction in salivary secretion leads to increased caries activity when a cariogenic diet is eaten
- IgA is present in saliva but has little effect on caries activity

The main biochemical events in dental plaque in the development of dental caries are summarised diagrammatically in Figure 3.10.

PATHOLOGY OF ENAMEL CARIES

Enamel is the usual site of the initial lesion unless dentine or cementum becomes exposed by gingival recession. Enamel, the hardest and densest tissue in the body, consists almost entirely of calcium apatite with only a minute organic content. It therefore forms a formidable barrier to bacterial attack. However, once enamel has been breached, infection of dentine can spread with relatively little obstruction. Preventive measures must therefore be aimed primarily at stopping the attack or at making enamel more resistant.

The essential nature of the carious attack on enamel is permeation of acid into its substance. The crystalline lattice of cal-

cium apatite crystals is relatively impermeable but part of the organic matrix of enamel, which envelops the apatite crystals, has a relatively high water content and is permeable to hydrogen ions. Permeation of enamel by acid causes a series of submicroscopic changes. This process of enamel caries is dynamic and, initially at least, consists of alternating phases of demineralisation and remineralisation, rather than a continuous process of dissolution.

Enamel caries develops in four main phases (Table 3.12). These stages of enamel caries are distinguishable microscopically and are also clinically significant. In particular, the early (white spot) lesion is potentially reversible, but cavity formation is irreversible and demands restorative procedures to replace the lost tissue.

Table 3.12 **Stages of enamel caries**

- The early (submicroscopic) lesion
- Phase of non-bacterial enamel crystal destruction
- Cavity formation
- Bacterial invasion of enamel

The early lesion

The earliest visible change appears as a white opaque spot that

Fig. 3.11 Early enamel caries, a white spot lesion, in a deciduous molar. The lesion forms below the contact point and in consequence is much larger than an interproximal lesion in a permanent tooth (see Fig. 3.20).

Fig. 3.12 Early interproximal caries. Ground section in water viewed by polarised light. The body of the lesion and the intact surface layer are visible. The translucent and dark zones are not seen until the section is viewed immersed in quinoline.

Fig. 3.13 Early interproximal caries. Ground section viewed by polarised light after immersion in quinoline. Quinoline has filled the larger pores, causing most of the fine detail in the body of the lesion to disappear (Fig. 3.12), but the dark zone with its smaller pores is accentuated.

Fig. 3.14 The same lesion (Figs 3.12 and 3.13) viewed dry under polarised light to show the full extent of demineralisation. (Figs 3.12–3.14 by kind permission of Professor Leon Silverstone and the Editor of Dental Update 1989;10:262.)

forms just adjacent to a contact point. Despite the chalky appearance the enamel is hard and smooth to the probe (Fig. 3.11). The microscopic changes under this early white spot lesion are seen in undecalcified sections but more readily when polarised light is used. Microradiography confirms the degree of demineralisation seen in the different zones.

The initial lesion is conical in shape with its apex towards the dentine, and a series of four zones of differing translucency can be discerned. Working back from the deepest, advancing edge of the lesion, these zones consist first of a *translucent zone* most deeply; immediately within this is a second *dark zone*; the third consists of the *body of the lesion* and the fourth consists of the *surface zone* (Fig. 3.12–3.14).

These initial changes are not due to bacterial invasion but to bacterial lactic or other acids causing varying degrees of demineralisation and remineralisation in the enamel. The features of these zones are summarised in Table 3.13.

The *translucent zone* is the first observable change. Its appearance results from formation of submicroscopic spaces or pores apparently located at prism boundaries and other junctional sites such as the striae of Retzius. When the section is mounted in quinoline, it fills the pores, and since it has the same refractive index as enamel the normal structural features disap-

Table 3.13 Key features of the enamel zones preceding cavity formation

Zone	Key features	Comments
Translucent zone	Earliest and deepest demineralisation. 1% mineral loss	Broader in progressing caries; narrow or absent in arrested or remineralised lesions
Dark zone	2–4% mineral loss but overall a zone of remineralisation just behind the advancing front	Broader in arrested or remineralised lesions; narrow in advancing lesions
Body	5–25% mineral loss	Broader in progressing caries; replaced by a broad dark zone in arrested or remineralised lesions
Surface zone	1% mineral loss. A zone of remineralisation resulting from the diffusion barrier and mineral content of plaque. Cavitation is loss of this layer, allowing bacteria to enter the lesion	Relatively constant width; a little thicker in arrested or remineralising lesions

Fig. 3.15 Early interproximal caries. A microradiograph of the same section as in figures 3.12–14, showing radiolucency following the same pattern, the intact surface zone and accentuation of the striae of Retzius. (Kindly lent by the late Professor A I Darling.)

pear and the enamel appears translucent. Microradiography confirms that the changes in the translucent zone are due to demineralisation.

The *dark zone* is fractionally superficial to the translucent zone. Polarised light microscopy shows that the volume of the pores in this zone has risen to 2–4% of the enamel volume. This change is due mainly to formation of more small pores. Two different-sized pores thus coexist in the dark zone: but the small ones are so minute that molecules of quinoline are unable to enter, and the tissue has become transformed into a molecular sieve. The small pores therefore remain filled with air, and this appears to produce the zone's dark appearance. Microradiography confirms that the dark zone has suffered a greater degree of demineralisation. However, when the lesion is exposed to saliva or synthetic calcifying solutions in vitro, the dark zone actually extends further. This may indicate that formation of the dark zone may be due not merely to creation of new porosities but possibly also to remineralisation of the large pores of the translucent zone so that they become micropores impermeable to quinoline. It is widely believed therefore that these changes in the dark zone are evidence of remineralisation, as discussed later.

The *body of the lesion* extends from just beneath the surface zone to the dark zone. By transmitted light the body of the lesion is comparatively translucent compared with normal enamel and sharply demarcated from the dark zone. In the body of the lesion, the striae of Retzius appear enhanced, particularly when mounted in quinoline and viewed under polarised light.

Polarised light examination also shows that the pore volume is 5% at the periphery but increases to at least 25% in the centre. Microradiography, which detects demineralisation in excess of 5%, shows that the area of radiolucency corresponds closely with the size and shape of the body of the lesion. By contrast, the surface zone appears relatively radiopaque (Fig. 3.15). Alternating radiopaque and radiolucent lines, about 30 μm apart, can also be seen passing obliquely through the subsurface region. These lines show apparently preferential demineralisation and probably represent the striae of Retzius.

The *surface zone* represents one of the most important changes in enamel caries in terms of prevention and management of the disease. It shows the paradoxical feature that it has not merely remained intact during this stage of the attack but remains more heavily mineralised and radiopaque than the deeper zones. It has a pore volume of only 1%.

When the surface zone is removed and the enamel is exposed to an acid buffer, the more highly mineralised surface zone reappears over the deeper changes described earlier. The surface zone therefore appears to form partly by remineralisation. Remineralising salts may come either from those concentrated in the plaque or from precipitation of calcium and phosphate ions diffusing outwards as the deeper zones are demineralised.

In pit and fissure caries the same changes take place but as acid diffuses out into the enamel the lesion forms a ring round the pit. However, in a two-dimensional view, the same zones as

Fig. 3.16 Undecalcified section showing early enamel lesions in the enamel surrounding and deep to an occlusal pit.

Fig. 3.17 Chalky enamel. An electronphotomicrograph of chalky enamel produced by the action of very dilute acid. The crystalites of calcium salts remain intact in the prism sheaths, while the prism cores and some of the interprismatic substance have been destroyed. The same appearance is seen in chalky enamel caused by early caries. (From a picture kindly lent by Dr K Little.)

Fig. 3.18 The organic matrix of developing enamel. An electronphotomicrograph of a section across the lines of the prisms before calcification showing the matrix to be more dense in the region of the prism sheaths than in the prism cores or interprismatic substance. (From a photograph kindly lent by Dr K Little.)

in smooth surface caries are seen on either side of the fissure (Fig. 3.16).

As noted earlier, the initial attack on enamel appears to be by highly mobile hydrogen ions permeating the organic matrix, enabling them to attack the surface of the apatite crystals. The apatite crystals become progressively smaller. Microdissection of the translucent zone, has shown that the apatite crystals have declined in diameter from the normal of 35–40 nm to 25–30 nm, and in the body of the lesion to 10–30 nm. In the dark zone, by contrast, enamel crystals appeared to have grown to 50–100 nm, and in the surface zone to 35–40 nm. Demineralisation and remineralisation may thus be alternating processes. However, as the lesion progresses and cavitation develops, demineralisation predominates.

In broad general terms, therefore, enamel crystallites are progressively dissolved until disintegration becomes visible microscopically. There is also evidence of preferential destruction of the prism cores, and experimentally a similar effect is seen when enamel is exposed to dilute acid (Fig. 3.17 and 3.18). Irrespective of the precise nature of these changes, bacteria do not physically penetrate enamel until acid destruction of it has provided pathways large enough for them to enter (Figs 3.19 and 3.20).

Cavity formation

Once bacteria have penetrated the enamel, they reach the amelodentinal junction and spread laterally to undermine the enamel. This has three major effects. First, the enamel loses the support of the dentine and is therefore greatly weakened. Second, it is

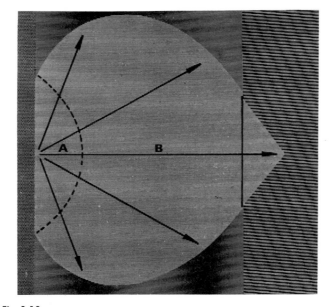

Fig. 3.19 Diagram summarising the main features of the precavitation phase of enamel caries as indicated here in this final stage of acid attack on enamel before bacterial invasion, decalcification of dentine has begun. The area (A) would be radiolucent in a bite-wing film but the area (B) could be visualised only in a section by polarised light microscopy or microradiography. Clinically the enamel would appear solid and intact but the surface would be marked by an opaque white spot over the area (A) as seen in Figure 3.11 (From McCracken A W, Cawson R A 1983 Clinical and oral microbiology. McGraw-Hill.)

Fig. 3.20 Early cavitation in enamel caries. The surface layer of the white spot lesion has broken down, allowing plaque bacteria into the enamel.

destroyed from beneath. Third, spread of bacteria along the amelodentinal junction allows them to attack the dentine over a wide area (Fig. 3.21). Thus the primary lesion provides the bridgehead for the attack on enamel, but undermining of the enamel determines the area of a cavity. Clinically, this may be evident when there is no more than a pinhole lesion in an occlusal pit, but cutting away the surrounding enamel shows it to be widely undermined (Fig. 3.22).

As undermining of the enamel continues, it starts to collapse under the stress of mastication and to fragment around the edge of the (clinically obvious) cavity. By this stage, bacterial attack on the dentine is well established.

Fig. 3.21 Enamel caries. Infection has spread along the amelodentinal junction undermining and invading the deep surface of the enamel. The terminations of the dentinal tubules are also infected but destruction, at this stage, is mainly at the expense of the enamel.

Fig. 3.22 Caries of an occlusal fissure. The chalky appearance of the enamel indicates that there is well-advanced secondary enamel caries and widepread involvement of the dentine beneath the apparently intact surface.

Bite-wing radiographs also show early demineralisation of the enamel (Fig. 3.23).

The process of enamel caries is summarised in Table 3.14.

Table 3.14 Stages of enamel caries
• Permeation of the organic matrix by hydrogen ions causes submicroscopic changes
• Early (precavitation) damage appears as a series of zones of differing translucency
• Microradiography confirms that these changes represent areas of increasing demineralisation
• The surface zone is largely formed by remineralisation
• There is alternating demineralisation and remineralisation but demineralisation predominates as cavity formation progresses
• Bacteria cannot invade enamel until demineralisation provides pathways large enough for them to enter

PATHOLOGY OF DENTINE CARIES

The *initial (non-bacterial) lesion* forms deep to carious enamel before any cavity has formed (Fig. 3.24). Diffusion of acid into the dentine leaves its collagenous matrix intact at this stage.

Fig. 3.23 Bite-wing radiograph showing interproximal caries below many of the contact points.

However, once bacteria have penetrated the enamel, they spread along the amelodentinal junction to attack the dentine over a wide area. The lesion is therefore conical with its apex towards the pulp.

Spread of infection is facilitated by the dentinal tubules which form a pathway open to bacteria. After demineralisation, the dentine matrix is progressively destroyed by proteolysis.

Streptococci play the major role in the attack on enamel, but lactobacilli may be important in dentine caries. As the lesion progresses, the bacterial population becomes increasingly mixed and their relative contributions to dentine destruction become more difficult to disentangle.

At first, the decalcified dentine retains its normal morphology, and no bacteria can be seen. Once the amelodentinal junc-

tion has been reached, pioneer bacteria extend down the tubules, soon fill them and spread along any lateral branches (Fig. 3.25). The tubules become distended into spindle shapes by the expanding masses of bacteria and their products, which the softened matrix cannot confine (Fig. 3.26). As a result, adjacent, less heavily infected tubules become bent. Later still, the intervening tubule walls are destroyed and collections of bacteria in adjacent tubules coalesce to form irregular *liquefaction foci*. These in turn coalesce to form progressively more widespread tissue destruction.

In some areas bacteria also spread laterally and, occasionally, large bacteria-filled clefts form at right angles to the tubules (Fig. 3.27). Clinically, these clefts may allow carious dentine sometimes to be excavated in flakes in a plane parallel to the surface.

The main events in dentine caries are summarised in Table 3.15.

Table 3.15 Key events in the development of dentine caries

- Non-bacterial, precavitation demineralisation of matrix
- Migration of pioneer bacteria along tubules
- Distortion of tubules by expanding masses of bacteria
- Proteolysis of intervening matrix forming liquefaction foci
- Progressive disintegration of remaining matrix tissue

Protective reactions of dentine and pulp under caries

The reactions in dentine are mainly due to odontoblast activity,

Fig. 3.24 This diagram summarises the sequential changes in enamel from the stage of the initial lesion to early cavity formation and relates the different stages in the development of the lesion with the radiographic appearances and clinical findings. (Diagram kindly lent by the late Professor I A Darling and reproduced by courtesy of the Editor of the British Dental Journal 1959; 107:27–30.)

Fig. 3.26 Caries of dentine. A specimen showing infected tubules and fusiform masses of bacteria which have expanded into the softened tissue. Adjacent tubules in the demineralised dentine have been bent and pushed aside by these masses.

Fig. 3.25 Infection of the dentinal tubules. This electronphotomicrograph shows bacteria in the lumen of the tubules. Between the tubules is the collagenous matrix of the dentine. (From a picture kindly lent by Dr K Little.)

so that dentine and pulp should be considered as one tissue. These reactions are not specific and may be provoked by other irritants such as attrition, erosion, abrasion and restorative procedures. Reactionary changes in dentine start even before cavity formation in enamel but are more likely to develop significantly under slowly progressing caries.

Reactionary changes in dentine are summarised in Table 3.16. These changes start to develop early but at best can only slow the advance of dental caries. Even sclerotic dentine is vulnerable to

bacterial acid and proteolysis and, once bacteria have penetrated the normal dentine, they can invade any reactionary dentine to reach the pulp.

Clinically, these reactive changes make the dentine immediately under a carious cavity less permeable but it is still vulnerable to demineralisation. Reactionary dentine may allow deep restorations to be made without exposing the pulp.

Root surface caries

When the neck of the tooth becomes exposed by recession of the gingival margin in later life a stagnation area may be

Fig. 3.27 Clefts in carious dentine. The main body of the lesion is to the left. Infection is tracking along the tubules but in this case has also spread across the tubules, forming heavily infected clefts. Within the clefts, strips of dentine split from the rest of the tissue are lying in the mass of organisms. Further clefts are starting to form from the left-hand edge of the lesion and the appearances suggest that there are lines of weakness in the dentine, along which infection spreads easily.

Table 3.16 Reactionary changes in dentine

Response	Key facts
Tubular sclerosis (translucent zone) (Fig. 3.28)	Peritubular dentine reduces the size of the dentinal tubules, preventing bacterial penetration and generating a more heavily mineralised dentine. Tubular sclerosis usually forms in a band about halfway between the pulp and amelodentinal junction. It forms a translucent zone which may be visible radiographically and is detectable with hand instruments when excavating caries
Regular reactionary dentine (Fig. 3.29)	Forms at the pulp dentine interface and retains the tubular structure of dentine. Forms in response to mild stimuli and may obliterate pulp horns, increasing the dentine thickness between caries and pulp. Unfortunately it often forms most on the floor and sides of the pulp chamber where it is of little value in defence against caries
Irregular reactionary dentine (Figs 3.30 and 3.31)	Forms in response to moderate or severe insult by caries and correspondingly ranges from dentine with irregular tubules to a disorganised bone-like mineralised tissue ('eburnoid')
Dead tracts (Fig. 3.32)	Formed when odontoblasts die and their tubules become sealed off. If peritubular dentine formation was extensive before odontoblast death, the dead tract may be sclerotic and inhibit advance of caries. If not, it may allow more rapid progress

Fig. 3.29 Chronic caries and reactionary dentine formation. Infection has penetrated the full thickness of the crown but the slowness of this process has allowed time for the formation of a substantial thickness of secondary dentine. The pulp has therefore remained vital and uninflamed and deep cavity preparation is feasible.

Fig. 3.30 Secondary (reactionary) dentine and caries. Regular, tubular, secondary dentine has formed under a carious cavity. A line marks the junction of the primary and secondary dentine where the tubules change direction. Bacteria spreading down the tubules of the primary tissue have extended along the junction and into the tubules of the reactionary dentine.

Fig. 3.28 A translucent zone. The dentinal tubules are seen in cross-section. Those in the centre of the picture have become obliterated by calcification of their contents; only the original outline of the tubules remains visible and the zone appears translucent to transmitted light. On either side are patent tubules filled with stain. (Kindly lent by Dr G C Blake, and reproduced by courtesy of the Honorary Editors, Proceedings of the Royal Society of Medicine 1958; 51:678.)

formed and the cementum attacked. Cementum is readily decalcified and presents little barrier to infection. The cementum therefore softens beneath the plaque over a wide area, producing a saucer-shaped cavity, and the underlying dentine is soon involved. Cementum is invaded along the direction of Sharpey's fibres. Infection spreads between the lamellae along

Fig. 3.31 Regular reactionary dentine below occlusal caries. Bacteria extend more than half the distance from the ameiodentinal junction to the pulp and the underlying pulp horn has been obliterated by reactionary dentine. The reactionary dentine bulges into the pulp. Note the lack of inflammation in the pulp.

the incremental lines, with the result that the dentine becomes split up and progressively destroyed by a combination of demineralisation and proteolysis. Further progress of caries in the underlying dentine is essentially similar to that in other parts of the tooth.

Arrested caries and remineralisation

Precavity (white spot) interstitial caries may become arrested when the adjacent tooth is removed so that the stagnation area is removed. The lesion may become remineralised by minerals from the saliva.

Dentine caries may occasionally be arrested as a result of destruction of so much enamel that a wide area of dentine becomes exposed. If this surface is then subjected to attrition, plaque deposition may be prevented. More frequently, but still uncommonly, dentine is exposed by attrition and remains caries-free for the same reason. It becomes smooth, polished and stained.

Under favourable conditions caries can be reversed and early lesions can remineralise. Use of fluorides and consumption of a less cariogenic diet may cause a surface lesion in enamel to heal entirely. Even under natural conditions, approximately 50% of interproximal enamel lesions may show no radiographic evidence of progression for 3 years. Similarly, in some patients, secondary caries may not necessarily develop at the margins of restorations overhanging the enamel.

Fig. 3.32 A dead tract. The empty tubules below the worn incisal edge have been filled with a stain to which they are permeable from the surface, so that the whole zone appears black. At the proximal end of the tubules the dead tract has been sealed off by impermeable reactionary dentine through which the stain cannot penetrate. The pulp is thus protected from irritants penetrating along the dentinal tubules.

Adult and childhood caries

In adults, caries usually progresses slowly and a small cavity may take several years to develop. By contrast, childhood caries, particularly of deciduous teeth, may be so rapid that the pulp becomes exposed long before the tooth is due to be shed.

Pulpitis

Pulpitis follows penetration of dentine by bacteria or their metabolites and represents the breakdown of the protective hard dental tissues and opening of the soft tissues to infection.

SUGGESTED FURTHER READING

Brathall D 1992 Caries, views and perspectives. Scand J Dent Res 100:47–51
Van Houte J 1994 Role of micro-organisms in caries etiology. J Dent Res 73:672–681
Woodward M, Walker A R P 1994 Sugar consumption and dental caries: evidence from 90 countries. Br Dent J 176:297–302

Pulpitis, apical periodontitis, resorption, hypercementosis

PULPITIS

Pulpitis is the most common cause of dental pain and loss of teeth in younger persons. The usual cause is caries penetrating the dentine but there are other possibilities (Table 4.1). Pulpitis, if untreated, is followed by death of the pulp and spread of infection through the apical foramina into the periapical tissues. This in turn causes periapical periodontitis. Dental caries is by far the most common cause and is usually obvious unless it has extended under the edge of a restoration.

Table 4.1 Causes of pulpitis

- Dental caries
- Traumatic exposure of the pulp
- Fracture of a crown or cusp
- Cracked tooth syndrome
- Thermal or chemical irritation

Exposure during cavity preparation allows bacteria to enter the pulp and usually also damages it mechanically (Fig. 4.1).

Fracture may either open the pulp chamber or leave so thin a covering of dentine that bacteria can enter.

A tooth, particularly a restored premolar, may split, usually under masticatory stress (Fig. 4.2). These minute cracks are often invisible, but allow bacteria into the pulp chamber. The affected tooth may sometimes be identified by applying pressure to the occlusal fissure with a ball-ended burnisher to open up the crack. Pulp pain usually then results. Alternatively the crack may be made visible with oblique transillumination or, possibly more easily, by wetting the crown of the tooth with a dye such as fluorescein and visualising it with ultraviolet light.

Over-rapid cavity cutting, especially of deep cavities, can cause immediate damage to the pulp. Large unlined metal restorations may also allow continuous low-grade thermal stimuli to damage the pulp over a longer period. Some restorations without a protective lining, particularly, in the past were sufficiently irritant to kill the pulp.

Fig. 4.1 Traumatic exposure. The pulp has been exposed during cavity preparation and dentine chippings and larger fragments have been driven into the pulp. The tooth was extracted before a strong inflammatory reaction has had time to develop but it is clear that some inflammatory cells have already localised around the debris which will have introduced many bacteria to the pulp.

Clinical features

Acute pulpitis

In the early stages the tooth is hypersensitive. Very cold or hot food causes a stab of pain which stops as soon as the irritant is removed. As inflammation progresses, pain becomes more persistent and there may be prolonged attacks of toothache. The pain may start spontaneously, often when the patient is trying to get to sleep.

The pain is partly due to the pressure on the irritated nerve endings by inflammatory infiltrate within the rigid pulp chamber and partly due to release of pain-producing substances from the damaged tissue. The pain at its worst is excruciatingly severe, sharp and stabbing in character. It is little affected by simple analgesics.

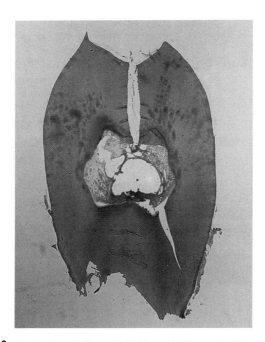

Fig. 4.2 Cracked tooth. The pulp died beneath this crack which was undetected clinically but which has opened up after decalcification of the tooth.

Fig. 4.3 Pulpal hyperaemia. While bacteria are still some distance from the pulp, acid permeating along the dentinal tubules gives rise to hyperaemia, oedema and a light cellular inflammatory infiltrate in the pulp.

The pulps of individual teeth are not precisely represented on the sensory cortex. Pulp pain is therefore poorly localised and may be felt in any of the teeth of the upper or lower jaw of the affected side. Rarely, pain may be referred to a more distant site such as the ear. Pulp pain is not provoked by pressure on the tooth. The patient can chew in comfort unless there is a large open cavity allowing fragments of food to press on the pulp through the softened dentine. Many pulps under large carious cavities die painlessly. The first indication is then development of periapical periodontitis, either with pain or seen by chance in a radiograph. In other cases there are bouts of dull pain, brought on by hot or cold stimuli or coming on spontaneously. There are often prolonged remissions.

Pathology

Pulpitis is caused by a mixed infection which usually enters from the mouth via a carious cavity.

Acute closed pulpitis

Histologically, there is initial hyperaemia limited to the area immediately beneath the irritant (Fig. 4.3). Infiltration by inflammatory cells and destruction of odontoblasts and adjacent mesenchyme follow. A limited area of necrosis may result in formation of a minute abscess, localised by granulation tissue (Figs 4.4–4.8). Later, inflammation spreads until the pulp is obliterated by dilated blood vessels and acute inflammatory cells (Fig. 4.9). Necrosis follows.

Fig. 4.4 Acute pulpitis. The dark streaks in the dentine show where bacteria have penetrated from an interproximal cavity into the pulp. Acute pulpitis has led to suppuration and a bead of darkly stained pus fills the affected cornu.

Chronic closed pulpitis

The main features are a predominantly mononuclear cell infiltrate and a more vigorous connective tissue reaction. A small area of pulpal necrosis and pus formation may be localised by a well-defined wall of granulation tissue, and a minute abscess may thus form. The remainder of the pulp may then appear normal.

Rarely, inflammation may be well localised beneath an exposure so that a partial calcific barrier forms beneath the lesion, or considerable amounts of reactionary dentine continue to form round the opening. Such changes are particularly likely to follow pulp capping. Calcific barriers (seen radiographically as 'dentine bridges') are frequently poorly formed, and inflamma-

Fig. 4.5 Acute pulpitis. In this more advanced lesion, there is an exposure of the left cornu and destruction of the main body of the pulp, which has been replaced by an abscess filling the pulp chamber.

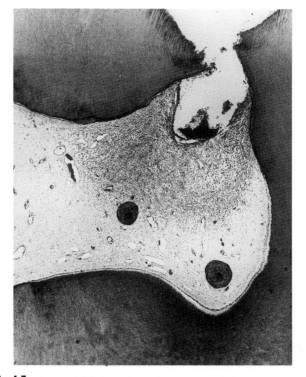

Fig. 4.7 Acute pulpitis. There is a carious exposure, destruction of a cornu of the pulp with formation of an abscess cavity and an extending inflammatory reaction. Nevertheless, immediately beyond (bottom of the picture), virtually normal pulpal tissue remains. Two small pulp stones are present in the pulp.

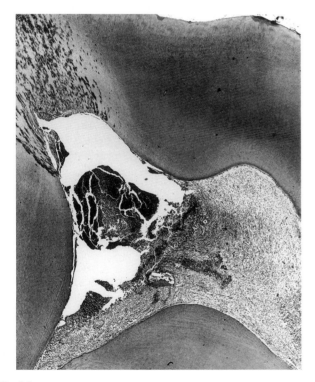

Fig. 4.6 Acute caries and pulpitis. Infection has penetrated to the pulp before any reactionary dentine has formed. Part of the pulp has been destroyed, and an abscess has formed, containing a bead of pus. This is a relatively early stage and destruction is not yet widespread.

Fig. 4.8 Acute spreading pulpitis. At the coronal tip of the pulp is a bead of pus, while the rest of the pulp chamber is filled with polymorphonuclear leukocytes and oedema. In the lower part of the picture are greatly dilated vessels stuffed with blood cells.

tion progresses beneath them (Figs 4.10 and 4.11). However, in successful cases, formation of a complete barrier of tubular reactionary dentine may allow preservation of the remainder of the pulp.

The chief factor hampering pulpal survival is its enclosure within the rigid walls of the pulp chamber and, in fully formed teeth, the limited aperture for the apical vessels. In acute inflammation, these vessels can readily be compressed by inflammatory oedema and thrombose. The blood supply of the pulp is thus cut off and dies. This may be rapid in the case of

Fig. 4.9 Advanced acute pulpitis. The outline of an abscess wall is still visible beneath the collection of pus, but infection and inflammation have spread beyond: no trace of pulp structure can be seen and the pulp chamber is filled with inflammatory cells and exudate.

Fig. 4.11 Chronic pulpitis. This higher power view shows the calcific barrier in more detail, in particular its irregular structure and failure to hold back the infection.

acute pulpitis, or delayed in chronic lesions. The relatively prolonged survival of chronically inflamed pulps is shown by the persistence of symptoms over a long period. However, pulp death is the end-result.

Open pulpitis

Occasionally the pulp survives, but is chronically inflamed,

Fig. 4.10 Chronic pulpitis. Successive layers of secondary dentine have been formed and destroyed in turn; their remains are seen at the right-hand edge of the cavity. A barrier of irregular calcified tissue covers the pulp, and beneath this a localised chronic pulpitis has developed. In spite of the prolonged and massive infection there is only local inflammation, and a fibrous reaction can be seen.

beneath a wide exposure, despite the heavy infection (Fig. 4.12). This is traditionally believed to be associated with open apices which allow an adequate blood supply.

Chronic hyperplastic pulpitis (pulp polyp). Rarely, despite wide exposure and heavy infection, the pulp not merely survives but proliferates through the opening. This may even happen in fully formed teeth.

Clinically, a pulp polyp appears as a dusky red or pinkish soft nodule protruding into the cavity. It is painless but may be tender and bleed on probing. It should be distinguished from proliferating gingival tissue extending over the edge of the cavity by tracing its attachment (Fig. 4.13).

Histologically, few odontoblasts survive and the pulp becomes replaced by granulation tissue (Fig. 4.14). As this mass grows out into the cavity in the tooth it can become epithelialised and covered by a layer of well-formed stratified squamous epithelium. This protects the mass and allows inflammation under it to subside and fibrous tissue to replace

Fig. 4.14 Chronic open pulpitis. A hyperplastic nodule of granulation tissue is growing out through a wide exposure of the pulp. The masses of inflammatory cells and the many new vessels are characteristic of granulation tissue.

Fig. 4.15 Pulp polyp. In this broken down molar, granulation tissue is proliferating from the pulp cavity and has acquired an epithelial covering over much of its surface. Note also the internal resorption as a result of pulpal inflammation.

Fig. 4.12 Pulp polyp. In this tooth with chronic open pulpitis granulation tissue has proliferated to fill the pulp chamber and its superficial layers contain a dense inflammatory infiltrate.

the granulation tissue. This degree of pulpal proliferation can be seen in teeth with fully formed roots (Fig. 4.15).

Treatment. Open pulpitis is usually associated with gross cavity formation and it is rarely possible to save the tooth, despite the vitality of the pulp.

Management

The chances of survival of the pulp are poor and treatment options are limited (Table 4.2).

Table 4.2 Pulpitis — treatment options
● Extraction
● Endodontic treatment
● Pulp capping (Fig. 4.16)

Fig. 4.13 Pulp polyp. An inflamed nodule of granulation tissue can be seen growing from the pulp chamber of this broken down first permanent molar.

Fig. 4.16 Pulp capping. A wide exposure has been capped. Reactionary dentine production has continued, forming rounded masses extending across from either side and narrowing the exposure. A localised chronic inflammatory reaction has developed on the surface of the pulp, but the amount of secondary dentine formation indicates that vitality has been retained for a long period. The exposure appears to have been too wide for successful capping and the material used is unknown.

Key features of pulpitis are summarised in Table 4.3.

Table 4.3   Pulpitis — key features
● Pulpitis is caused by infection or irritation of the pulp, usually by caries
● Severe stabbing pain in a tooth, triggered by hot or cold food or starting spontaneously, indicates acute irreversible pulpitis
● Pulp pain is poorly localised
● Chronic pulpitis is often symptomless
● Untreated pulpitis usually leads to death of the pulp and spread of infection to the periapical tissues

PULP CALCIFICATIONS

Pulp stones

Rounded masses of dentine may form within the pulp and can be seen in radiographs as small opacities. In the past they were thought to cause symptoms but are developmental anomalies. For unknown reasons, they are common in the teeth of patients with Ehlers–Danlos (floppy joint) syndrome, a genetic defect of collagen formation.

Fig. 4.17 Pulp stones. A rounded nodule of calcified tissue in which some irregular tubules may be seen is present in the pulp. Smaller stones and amorphous calcifications surround the main mass (trichrome stain).

Histologically, pulp stones consist of dentine which may show complete or incomplete tubule formation (Fig. 4.17). A distinction used to be drawn between free and attached pulp stones. However, this is frequently an illusion caused by a plane of section which fails to pass through the connection between the pulp stone and the pulp wall.

Diffuse calcification

Amorphous dystrophic calcifications may sometimes be seen histologically in the pulp and are thought to be an age-related degenerative change.

Pulp stones and diffuse calcification are of no clinical significance except insofar as they may obstruct endodontic treatment. Otherwise they can be ignored.

PERIAPICAL PERIODONTITIS

Periapical inflammation is usually due to spread of infection following death of the pulp (Table 4.4). It characteristically causes tenderness of the tooth in its socket. Local (periapical) periodontitis must be distinguished from chronic (marginal) periodontitis,

Table 4.4   Causes of apical periodontitis
● Infection
● Trauma
● Chemical irritation

in which infection and destruction of the supporting tissues spread from chronic infection of the gingival margins (Ch. 5). Infection is far the most common cause. The usual sequence of events is caries, pulpitis, death of the pulp and periodontitis.

The pulp sometimes dies from a blow which damages the apical vessels. The necrotic pulp probably becomes infected by bacteria from the gingival margins, leading to apical periodontitis. A high filling, or biting suddenly on a hard object, sometimes causes an acute but usually transient periodontitis.

During endodontic treatment, instruments may be pushed through the apex or side of the root, damaging the periodontal membrane and carrying infected debris from the pulp chamber into the wound.

Irritant antiseptics used to sterilise a root canal can escape through the apex and damage the surrounding tissues. A root-canal filling may also extend beyond the apex with similar effect.

Fig. 4.18 Oedema due to acute apical periodontitis. An acute periapical infection of a canine has perforated the buccal plate of bone causing oedema of the face; this quickly subsides when the infection is treated.

ACUTE APICAL PERIODONTITIS

Clinical features

The patient may give a history of pain due to previous pulpitis. When periodontitis develops, escape of exudate into the periodontal membrane causes the tooth to be extruded by a minute amount and the bite to fall more heavily on it. The tooth is at first uncomfortable, then increasingly tender, even to mere touch. Hot or cold substances do not cause pain in the tooth. As inflammation becomes more severe and pus starts to form, pain becomes intense and throbbing in character. There is often a large carious cavity or filling in the affected tooth, or it may be discoloured due to death of the pulp earlier. At this stage the gingiva over the root is red and tender, but there is no swelling while inflammation is confined within the bone.

Radiographs give little information because bony changes have had too short a time to develop. Immediately round the apex the lamina dura may appear slightly hazy and the periodontal space may be slightly widened. When acute periodontitis is due to exacerbation of a chronic infection, the original lesion can be seen as an area of radiolucency at the apex.

Exudate may penetrate overlying bone and periosteum a day or so after the onset of pain, allowing relief of the pressure. Pain quickly abates but exudate, if it cannot escape, distends the soft tissues to form a swelling. When an upper canine is affected, the swelling quickly spreads to the face and eyelid and may close the eye on that side (Fig. 4.18). In spite of the alarming appearance, the swelling is due only to oedema. It subsides when the tooth is extracted or the infection is drained.

The regional lymph nodes may be enlarged and tender, but general symptoms are usually slight or absent.

Inflammation typically remains localised. Further spread of infection can cause inflammation of the surrounding bone (osteomyelitis) or cellulitis (Ch. 6), but only exceedingly rarely.

Fig. 4.19 Acute apical periodontitis. In this early acute lesion inflammatory cells, mainly neutrophil polymorphonuclear leukocytes, are seen clustered around the apex of a non-vital tooth. The inflammatory cells are spreading around and into bone and there has not yet been time for significant bone resorption to develop.

Pathology

Acute apical periodontitis is a typical acute inflammatory reaction with engorged blood vessels and packing of the tissue with neutrophils (Fig. 4.19). These changes are initially localised to the immediate vicinity of the apex as a consequence of the rich blood supply to this area. The immediately adjacent lamina dura becomes resorbed and an abscess cavity may form if not aborted by treatment (Table 4.5).

Table 4.5 Possible complications of acute apical periodontitis

- Suppuration
- Regional lymphadenopathy
- Spreading infection

Treatment

Extraction of the diseased tooth removes the source of infection and drains the exudate. This is the simplest and most effective treatment. Antibiotics should not be given for simple acute periodontitis if immediate dental treatment is available. Alternative treatment is to retain the tooth by endodontic treatment, which also serves to drain the infection.

CHRONIC APICAL PERIODONTITIS

Clinical features

Chronic periodontitis is a low-grade infection. It may follow an acute infection that has been inadequately drained and incompletely resolved. The tooth is non-vital and may be slightly tender to percussion but otherwise symptoms may be minimal. Frequently, chronic periodontitis is first recognised as a rounded area of radiolucency at the apex of a tooth (an 'apical granuloma') in a routine radiograph (Fig. 4.20). The area is usually about 5 mm in diameter and has well-defined margins. A distinct cortex is sometimes interpreted as early cyst formation, but this cannot be distinguished without a biopsy.

Fig. 4.20 Chronic apical abscess. Periapical bone resorption has developed as a result of inflammation. The area of radiolucency corresponds with the histological changes seen in the next figure.

PATHOLOGY

Chronic periodontitis is a typical chronic inflammatory reaction characterised by lymphocytes, macrophages and plasma cells. Infection is confined by inflammatory cells, and granulation tissue surrounds the area (Table 4.6). The granulation tissue grows into a rounded mass (a 'granuloma'), and osteoclasts resorb the bone to accommodate it (Figs 4.21 and 4.22).

Despite absence of symptoms, there is no spontaneous healing because of the persistent reservoir of infection in the root canal. Instead, granulation tissue proliferates round the focus of irritation at the tooth apex, and surrounding bone is resorbed to

Fig. 4.21 Chronic periapical abscess. At the apex of the non-vital tooth is an abscess cavity surrounded by a thick fibrous wall densely infiltrated by inflammatory cells, predominantly neutrophils. Periapical bone has been resorbed and the trabeculae reorientated around the mass.

Fig. 4.22 High power of an apical granuloma showing neutrophils, lymphocytes and plasma cells in loose oedematous fibrous tissue.

Table 4.6 Possible complications of chronic apical periodontitis

- Periapical granuloma formation
- Radicular cyst formation
- Suppuration and sinus formation

Fig. 4.24 Epithelial proliferation in an apical granuloma. Inflammation induces proliferation of odontogenic epithelium in rests of Malassez. This change may lead to cyst formation (Ch. 7).

Fig. 4.23 Apicectomy. The tip of the apex has been excised, allowing the root canal to be sealed effectively; the periapical tissues have entirely healed; inflammatory changes have disappeared; new bone trabeculae have replaced the tissue lost and a scar has formed over the end of the root canal filling.

Fig. 4.25 Chronic periapical infection with an abscess pointing buccally on the alveolar mucosa. A pus-filled nodule is present over the apex of the central incisor which has died as a result of trauma, as indicated by the coronal fracture.

leave a round area of radiolucency. Healing only follows extraction, effective endodontic treatment or apicectomy (Fig. 4.23).

Variable degrees of proliferation of the epithelial rests of Malassez in a periapical granuloma at the apex of a dead tooth are common (Fig. 4.24). Epithelial proliferation may be sufficient to lead ultimately to cyst formation and is the most common cause of jaw cysts.

This epithelium forms irregular strands or loops. Sometimes a microscopic cyst cavity, with a lining of hyperplastic epithelium, forms and represents the earliest stage of radicular cyst. In other cases the epithelium is scanty or destroyed by the inflammation.

Periapical granulomas usually remain localised within the bone. Occasionally, there is abscess formation and pus may reach the surface by resorption of the bone (usually on the buccal surface of the gingiva) immediately over the apex of the tooth. A nodule of granulation tissue forms in response to the irritation by pus and marks the opening of the sinus (Fig. 4.25).

An uncommon complication, but sometimes the first sign of periapical periodontitis, is the tracking of a sinus on to the skin surface. This most frequently happens on or near the chin as a result of a long-forgotten blow and death of a lower incisor (Fig. 4.26). In such cases the crown of the damaged tooth is usually discoloured (Fig. 4.27) and may be chipped. A radiograph shows the periapical area of bone destruction. Many patients fail to

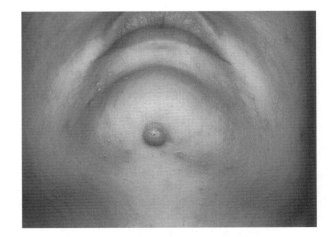

Fig. 4.26 A persistent skin sinus from a lower incisor rendered non-vital by a blow some time previously. This young woman was seen and treated unsuccessfully for 2 years by her doctor, surgeons and dermatologists before anyone looked at her teeth.

Fig. 4.27   Non-vital incisor teeth, in this case as a result of trauma. Haemorrhage and products of autolysis of the pulp discolour the dentine and darken the teeth.

associate the sinus with dental infection but competent endodontic treatment causes the sinus to heal remarkably quickly.

Treatment

According to the state of the rest of the dentition, extraction or endodontic treatment are the main options. Competent endodontic treatment leads to healing even if cystic change has started. Persistence of chronic periodontitis after root canal treatment is usually due to technical faults, and apicectomy may be required (see Fig. 4.23).

RESORPTION OF TEETH

The deciduous teeth are progressively loosened and ultimately shed as a result of progressive resorption of the roots as a physiological process arising from the pressure of the underlying successors. Resorption of permanent teeth is always pathological.

Whenever resorption takes place, there is usually some attempt at repair by apposition of cementum or bone. During resorption of deciduous teeth a period of resorption is followed by one of repair, so that clinically the looseness of these teeth varies before they are shed.

Resorption is rarely important but very occasionally it results from some destructive disease such as a tumour. Hypercementosis is also rarely important but may occasionally be a cause of difficult extractions.

Pathology

Pressure is probably the main factor. However, in some cases no cause is apparent. Resorption is mainly carried out by osteoclasts which, during active phases, may be seen in lacunas in the hard tissue with which their cytoplasm appears to merge (Fig. 4.28). When resorption is very slow, osteoclasts may not be seen and, being intermittent in their action, disappear during

Fig. 4.28   Resorption during periapical periodontitis. Active osteoclastic resorption of dentine is continuing in the presence of inflammatory exudate. This is a common change but usually minor in extent.

inactive periods. Inflammatory mediators such as prostaglandins and cytokines may also contribute to bone resorption.

Resorption of deciduous teeth

Resorption of deciduous teeth occasionally leads to a few minor complications.

Ankylosis.   In the resting stages of resorption excessive repair tissue may be deposited until the root becomes fused to the adjacent bone. This may prevent the tooth from being shed and the permanent successor from erupting. If not removed, the ankylosed tooth becomes partially submerged by the continued growth of the surrounding alveolar ridge. The tooth should be removed, surgically if necessary, to allow the successor to erupt.

Separation of an apex.   Resorption may be irregular, so that part of the tooth is cut off. The fragment remains buried or eventually appears on the surface.

Failure of resorption.   Absence or misplacement of a permanent successor is the usual cause. The deciduous tooth may then remain in the arch for many years.

Resorption of permanent teeth

Resorption of permanent teeth is usually limited in extent but may rarely destroy a large part of them. There are various causes (Table 4.7).

Cementum is most readily resorbed, while enamel is the most resistant. When an impacted tooth presses on the roots of

Table 4.7   Important causes of resorption of permanent teeth

- Periapical periodontitis. The most common cause but is usually slight
- Impacted teeth pressing on the root of an adjacent tooth
- Unerupted teeth. Over the course of years these may undergo resorption or hypercementosis, or both
- Replanted teeth. These are sometimes rapidly and grossly resorbed
- Neoplasms. Resorption of related teeth is a typical sign of an intraosseous neoplasm such as an ameloblastoma
- Idiopathic resorption, peripheral and internal

Fig. 4.29   Resorption of a buried tooth. In this specimen from an elderly patient, a buried canine has undergone complete resorption of the crown during the course of many years. Fragments of enamel remaining can be seen as spaces in the connective tissue against the root of the lateral incisor. Inflammatory changes are absent.

Fig. 4.30   Idiopathic internal resorption. A central incisor showing gross resorption that has widely enlarged the pulp chamber and perforated the labial aspect of the crown. Infection has entered, and the pulp has been replaced by granulation tissue. Extensive bony repair tissue has been laid down apical to the exposure.

another, these are resorbed, but sometimes the crown of the impacted tooth may be destroyed (Fig. 4.29).

Idiopathic resorption

Internal resorption (pink spot) is a curious and uncommon condition in which dentine is resorbed from within the pulp. Resorption tends to be localised, producing the characteristic sign of a well-defined rounded area of radiolucency in the crown (Fig. 4.30). This may affect an incisor tooth, and a rounded pink area appears where the vascular pulp has become visible through the attenuated hard tissue. The cause is unknown but it may possibly be a late result of damage to the blood supply of the pulp by a blow.

Idiopathic internal resorption can also affect any part of other teeth but causes no signs until the pulp is opened and allows access to infection. Alternatively, resorption may be detected by chance in a routine radiograph.

Peripheral resorption may be localised or generalised. Very rarely resorption may start, for unknown reasons, on the surface of the root near the apex, and affect many teeth. Over the course of years, more than half the root may be destroyed. The lost tissue is partially repaired by bone-like tissue.

Localised root resorption is also uncommon and of unknown cause. A limited area of the root is attacked from its external surface and resorption goes on until the pulp is reached (Fig. 4.31). Treatment is ineffective.

Pathology

Vascular granulation tissue replaces part of the periodontal ligament or pulp. Osteoclasts border the affected dentine or enamel. Inflammatory changes may be superimposed if the pulp chamber has been opened by destruction of its walls. Irregular repair with bone or cementum may take place.

Treatment

Idiopathic resorption is usually untreatable. However, if a pink spot in an incisor tooth is noticed at an early stage endodontic treatment should be carried out before the pulp chamber becomes exposed.

Fig. 4.31   Idiopathic external resorption. A localised area of destruction of dentine produced by osteoclastic activity. The cavity is filled with proliferating connective tissue. The pulp shows no reaction and the sparing of the circumpulpal dentine until a late stage is a characteristic feature of external resorption.

Fig. 4.32   Hypercementosis in Paget's disease. An irregular craggy mass of bone-like cementum has been formed over thickened regular and acellular cementum.

HYPERCEMENTOSIS

Apposition of excessive amounts of cementum is not uncommon and is due to several possible causes (Table 4.8).

Table 4.8   Causes of hypercementosis
● Ageing
● Periapical periodontitis. A common cause but minor in amount. Close to the apex there is usually a little resorption, but coronally, cementum is laid down, forming a shoulder
● Functionless and unerupted teeth. Hypercementosis and resorption may alternate
● Paget's disease. Alternating, irregular apposition and resorption, with apposition predominating, produce an irregular mass of cementum on the root with a histological 'mosaic' pattern
● Cementoblastoma (Ch.8) and cementofosseus dysplasia

Increased thickness of cementum is not itself a disease, and no treatment is necessary. If hypercementosis is gross, as in Paget's disease, extractions become difficult (Fig. 4.32).

Concresence

Rarely hypercementosis causes fusion of the roots of adjacent teeth (Figs 4.33 and 4.34). It is rarely noticed until an attempt is made to extract one of the teeth. The two teeth are then found to move in unison, and surgical intervention becomes necessary.

Fig. 4.33   Concrescence. Two upper molars fused together by cementum.

CHRONIC (NON-CARIOUS) INJURIES TO TEETH

Attrition

Attrition results more rapidly from a gritty diet and is seen in those from developing countries or in ancient skulls. Attrition may also be seen in the elderly and can result from a subconscious tooth-grinding habit which may be nocturnal and may be associated with pain dysfunction syndrome (Ch. 11).

Fig. 4.36 Abrasion. This elderly patient has worn grooves into the teeth by vigorous toothbrushing for many years. The pulps have retreated behind successive layers of reactionary dentine. The incisal edges also show attrition.

Fig. 4.34 Concrescence. Histological section of teeth shown in the previous figure reveals that the teeth are joined by cementum and not dentine.

Fig. 4.37 Severe abrasion. Vigorous toothbrushing over the course of many years has cut so deeply into several teeth that they have fractured off. Note how the gingival margins resist the abrasion well and remain firm, pale and healthy as a result of effective plaque removal.

Fig. 4.35 Attrition. Increased wear on the occlusal surfaces of the teeth, in this case as a result of an abrasive diet. The site of the pulp of several teeth is marked by reactionary dentine which is porous and easily stained. Teeth remain vital.

Attrition can flatten the masticatory surfaces and expose the dentine. Reactionary dentine formation in response to this slow process protects the pulp (Fig. 4.35).

Abrasion

Abrasion of the necks of the teeth is seen mainly in the elderly as a consequence of overvigorous toothbrushing or use of an abrasive dentifrice. The exposed dentine is shiny and smooth. Eventually, grooves worn into the necks of the teeth can be so deep as to extend into the pulp chamber but reactionary dentine protects the pulp (Figs 4.36 and 4.37). The crown of the tooth may even break off without exposing the pulp.

Fig. 4.38 Erosion. Saucer-shaped defects on the labial enamel resulting from acid drinks being trapped between the upper lip and teeth.

Fig. 4.39 Mixed pattern tooth loss. In this case, as in most cases of severe abrasion, an element of erosion is present. Note the shiny polished surface produced by abrasion.

Erosion

Erosion is progressive dissolution of tooth substance by exposure to acids. It appears to be a growing problem as a result of overconsumption of soft drinks or fruit juices, or both (Fig. 4.38).

Chronic regurgitation of gastric secretions, typically as a consequence of chronic pyloric stenosis, can cause a characteristic erosion, particularly of the palatal surfaces of the upper teeth (Fig. 29.1). Similar damage can result from self-induced vomiting. The latter is characteristic of bulimia, a psychological disorder in which there are episodes of binge gorging followed by self-induced vomiting to maintain a thin figure.

In the past, industrial exposure to corrosive chemicals was a significant cause of dental erosion.

SUGGESTED FURTHER READING

Bergenholtz G 1981 Inflammatory response of the dental pulp to bacterial irritation. J Endod 7:100–104

Brook I, Frazier E H, Gher M E 1996 Microbiology of periapical abscesses and associated maxillary sinusitis. J Periodontol 67:608–610

Currie W J R, Ho V 1993 An unexpected death associated with an acute dentoalveolar abscess. Br J Oral Maxillofac Surg 31:296–298

Lewis M A O, MacFarlane T W, McGowan D A 1986 Quantitative bacteriology of acute dentoalveolar abscesses. J Med Microbiol 21:101–104.

Morse D R, Furst M L, Belot R M et al 1987 Infectious flare-ups and serious sequelae following endodontic treatment: a prospective randomized trial on antibiotic prophylaxis in cases of asymptomatic pulpal – periapical lesions. Oral Surg Oral Med Oral Pathol 64:96–109

Trowbridge H O 1981 Pathogenesis of pulpitis resulting from dental caries. J Endod 7:52–60

Wright E F, Gullickson D C 1996 Identifying acute pulpalgia as a factor in TMD pain. J Am Dert Assoc 127:773–780

Gingivitis and periodontitis

THE NORMAL PERIODONTAL TISSUES

The gingival tissues comprise a series of anatomical regions (Table 5.1).

Table 5.1 Anatomical regions of normal healthy gingival tissue

- *Junctional epithelium.* Extends from the amelocemental junction to the floor of the gingival sulcus and forms the epithelial attachment to the tooth surface
- *Sulcular epithelium.* Lines the gingival sulcus and joins the epithelial attachment to the free gingiva
- *Free gingiva.* Coronal to the amelocemental junction and attached gingiva, and includes the tips of the interdental papillae
- *Attached gingiva.* Extends apically from the free gingiva to the mucogingival junction and is bound down to the superficial periodontal fibres and periosteum

---

Histologically, gingival epithelium is stratified squamous: the free and attached gingiva are parakeratinised. The epithelial attachment consists of flattened stratified squamous epithelium adhering to enamel (Fig. 5.1). The attachment apparatus consists of a basal lamina and hemidesmosomes. The attachment to the enamel appears histologically as a clear cuticle. It forms an effective seal, protecting the underlying connective tissues. The epithelial attachment is so firmly adherent to the tooth surface that mechanical damage, which would otherwise pull the epithelium from the tooth, tears the epithelial cells apart (Fig. 5.2). This epithelium has a relatively high turnover rate and the epithelial attachment is probably actively maintained and reformed. This enables the attachment to migrate apically until it becomes attached to cementum when periodontitis becomes established.

The attached gingiva is firmly bound down to the underlying bone to form a tough mucoperiosteum. Its stippled appearance is due to the intersections of its underlying epithelial ridges at the junction with the connective tissue.

The alveolar mucosa is continuous with the attached gingiva but is sharply demarcated by its smooth surface, darker colour and increasing separation from the bone.

Fig. 5.1 Gingival sulcus and epithelial attachment. This sagittal section of a specimen from a woman of 27 shows the normal appearances. Enamel removed by decalcification of the specimen has left the triangular space. The epithelial attachment forms a line from the top of the papilla to the amelocemental junction; its enamel surface, the actual line of attachment, is sharply defined. The gingival sulcus, minute in extent, is formed where the papilla curves away from the line of the enamel surface. Here there is a very scanty inflammatory infiltrate and slight hyperplasia of the sulcular epithelium.

Gingival and periodontal fibres

The principal fibres of the periodontal ligament form fibrous bundles interspersed by loose connective tissue containing blood vessels and nerves. These components provide a viscoelastic supportive mechanism resisting both compressive and tensile forces on the teeth. The normal thickness of the periodontal ligament is about 0.1–0.3 mm.

The principal fibres are arranged in a series of fairly well-defined groups (Table 5.2).

The periodontal ligament fibres are embedded in cementum at their inner ends and in the lamina dura at their outer ends. New fibres replacing those which have aged, or forming in response to new functional stresses, are attached by apposition

Fig. 5.2 The strength of the epithelial attachment. On this tooth the epithelial attachment has migrated on to the surface of the cementum as a result of periodontal disease. The epithelium has been torn away from the tooth but the tear is within the junctional epithelium, leaving some of its cells still adherent to the cementum and attached by a clear cuticle. A similar strength is seen when the junctional epithelium is attached to enamel.

Table 5.2 Principal fibres of the periodontal ligament

- *Oblique fibres* form a suspensory ligament from socket to root in coronal to apical directions
- *Horizontal fibres* form a dense group attaching neck of tooth to rim of socket
- *Transeptal fibres* of the horizontal group are not attached to alveolar bone but pass superficially to it and join adjacent teeth together. They protect the interdental gingiva by resisting forces that would otherwise separate the teeth and open the contact points
- *Gingival fibres* form a cuff round the neck of the tooth, supporting the soft tissues. They resist separation of the gingivae from the tooth and help to prevent formation of pockets

---

of further layers of cementum which becomes thicker with age. The lamina dura is a layer of compact bone, continuous, at the mouths of the sockets, with the cortical bone of the jaw. The radiographic appearance of the lamina dura has limited diagnostic value in periodontics as its presence largely depends on the alignment of the beam.

Gingival fluid (exudate)

In health, a minute amount of fluid can be collected from the gingival margins. It differs in composition from saliva, which contains IgA, while gingival fluid has a variable but significant content of IgG, IgM and leukocytes. Unlike saliva, gingival fluid is not a secretion (there are no glands in this region) but is

inflammatory exudate. It therefore increases greatly with the degree of inflammation.

Nomenclature and classification of periodontal disease

The term *periodontal disease* usually refers only to plaque-related inflammatory disease of the dental supporting tissues. A wide variety of diseases of the oral mucosa can also affect the gingivae occasionally, so that conditions as diverse as tuberculosis or lichen planus can produce lesions in this area. Such conditions do not play any significant part in the development of periodontal disease in its commonly accepted sense.

Chronic gingivitis is, with few exceptions, the preliminary stage of the development of chronic periodontitis, but clinically no sharp dividing line can be drawn between chronic gingivitis and the onset of periodontitis (Fig. 5.11) . Nevertheless, the distinction is important in that chronic gingivitis can generally be cured by plaque control. By contrast, bone loss and tooth support due to chronic periodontitis are largely irreversible.

The main *clinical* types of periodontal disease are grouped together on the basis of what seems to be the predominant pathological process (Table 5.3).

Table 5.3 Types of periodontal disease

I. Gingivitis and periodontitis
- Chronic gingivitis (common plaque-related type)
- Chronic periodontitis (common, plaque-related adult type)

II. Less common types of gingivitis
- Acute ulcerative gingivitis
- HIV-associated gingivitis

III. Uncommon types of periodontitis
- Prepubertal periodontitis
- Juvenile periodontitis
- Rapidly progressive periodontitis
- HIV-associated periodontitis

IV. Miscellaneous periodontal disorders
- Gingival hyperplasia
  Familial
  Drug-related
- Periodontal atrophy
- Periodontal (lateral) abscess
- Pericoronitis

V. Other diseases which may affect the periodontal tissues
- Acute leukaemic periodontal destruction
- Herpetic gingivostomatitis (Ch. 12)
- Wegener's granulomatosis (Ch. 28)

CHRONIC GINGIVITIS

Clinical features

Chronic gingivitis is asymptomatic, low-grade inflammation of the gingivae, which become red and slightly swollen with oedema (Fig. 5.3). Plaque, deposited along the gingival margins, is readily detectable. In most patients, chronic gingivitis is due to

Fig. 5.3 Gingivitis. A florid, bright-red band of gingival inflammation as a result of very poor oral hygiene. Thick accumulations of plaque are visible on all tooth surfaces.

local factors and, in particular, ineffective toothbrushing. It should be curable by effective oral hygiene.

Chronic hyperplastic gingivitis is a term sometimes given to chronic gingivitis in which inflammatory oedema is prominent. However, there is no soft tissue hyperplasia. Maintenance of strict oral hygiene brings resolution.

Systemic disorders can exacerbate chronic gingivitis but rarely play a significant role (Table 5.4).

Table 5.4 Factors contributing to or exacerbating chronic gingivitis

Local
Poor tooth cleaning technique
Dental irregularities providing stagnation areas
Restorations or appliances causing stagnation areas

Systemic
Pregnancy
Down's syndrome
Poorly-controlled diabetes mellitus

Pathology

Gingivitis is an inflammatory response to plaque bacteria. By definition, inflammation is restricted to the gingival margins and does not affect the periodontal ligament or bone (Fig. 5.4).

The development of chronic adult periodontitis has been arbitrarily divided into three histological stages (Tables 5.5 and 5.6), the third of which refers to chronic periodontitis. It must be appreciated that these stages are largely based on animal studies and cannot be so clearly identified in humans.

Variations in plaque bacteria with stage of disease

Healthy (uninflamed) gingivae. The plaque is supragingival and thin (10–20 cells thick). Gram-positive bacteria predominate and include *Actinomyces* species, *Rothia*, viridans

Fig. 5.4 Chronic gingivitis. The epithelial attachment remains at the level of the amelocemental junction and inflammatory cells are concentrated in the gingiva.

Table 5.5 'Initial stage' chronic gingivitis

- Develops within 24–48 hours of exposure to plaque
- Plaque related to gingival sulcus
- Vasodilatation
- Infiltration predominantly of neutrophils
- Leakage of exudate into gingival sulcus

Table 5.6 Established chronic gingivitis

- Dense, predominantly plasmacytic infiltrate
- Infiltrate fills but limited to interdental papillae
- Destruction of superficial connective tissue fibres
- Deepened gingival crevice
- Epithelial attachment remains at or near amelocemental junction
- Alveolar bone and periodontal ligament remain intact

streptococci and *Staphylococcus epidermidis*. In elderly patients in periodontal health, Gram-positive bacteria, particularly streptococci, form the largest single group (50% of the predominant cultivable flora), while Gram-negative bacteria only account for 30%. The latter include *Porphyromonas* and *Fusobacterium* species.

Early (and experimental) gingivitis. If toothbrushing is neglected for several days, plaque grows in thickness and is typically 100–300 cells thick. In the earliest stages bacteria proliferate but the plaque remains Gram-positive in character and *Actinomyces* species become predominant.

Chronic gingivitis. With the passage of time, persistence of plaque leads to chronic inflammation, and Gram-negative organisms become increasingly prominent. *Veillonella*, *Fusobacterium* and *Campylobacter* species become conspicuous.

Calculus

Calculus is calcified plaque. The calcification is less significant than the bacterial content, which induces inflammation and, later, tissue destruction. However, calculus distorts the gingival crevice and by increasing the stagnation area probably promotes even greater bacterial proliferation (Fig. 5.5). Supragingival calculus mainly forms opposite the orifices of the major salivary glands in the lower incisor and upper first molar areas. It cannot be removed by the patient and provides a rough plaque-retentive surface.

Management

Chronic gingivitis is readily recognisable from the clinical features already described. Gentle probing shows absence of pocketing and radiographs show intact crestal alveolar bone. The diagnosis is confirmed by resolution of gingivitis when effective oral hygiene measures (including calculus removal and effective toothbrushing habits) become established (Figs 5.6 and 5.7). Any exacerbating factors must also be dealt with if possible.

Pregnancy gingivitis

Pre-existing gingivitis may become more severe in the first 2

Fig. 5.6 Accumulation of plaque stained after 24 hours by disclosing solution.

Fig. 5.7 The effects of toothbrushing in the same patient. Plaque remains interdentally in most areas, explaining why gingivitis is often localised here.

Fig. 5.5 Subgingival calculus showing the layered structure resulting from incremental deposition. The calculus has a brown colour as a result of blood and bacterial pigment within it. A thick layer of plaque adheres to the deep surface.

months of pregnancy (see Fig. 31.9). Inflammatory erythema and oedema typically become more severe and a localised vascular lesion (a *pregnancy tumour*) may develop. The latter has the same structure as a pyogenic granuloma (Ch. 19).

Pregnancy gingivitis can be much ameliorated or abolished by a strict oral hygiene regimen, and improves after parturition. However, if a pregnancy tumour persists, it should be excised.

Down's syndrome

In Down's syndrome (Ch. 33), gingivitis is exacerbated by

excessive plaque formation. Difficulties in establishing effective toothbrushing habits in these handicapped children worsens the problem. The multiple immunodeficiencies typical of this disorder contribute. Progress to periodontitis and early tooth loss are frequent consequences.

Diabetes mellitus

In poorly controlled diabetes, periodontal health may deteriorate sharply. In well-controlled diabetes, acceleration of gingivitis may not be noticeable. However, it appears that, overall, diabetics suffer somewhat more severe periodontal disease and slightly earlier tooth loss than healthy, control populations. The neutrophil defect typical of this disease is probably the main factor involved.

CHRONIC PERIODONTITIS

Clinical features

Chronic periodontitis (the 'advanced lesion') is the chief cause of tooth loss in later adult life, but symptoms are typically minimal. Many patients remain unaware of the disease until teeth become loose.

Gingivitis persists and patients may complain of gingival bleeding or an unpleasant taste. Later, gingival recession or loosening of the teeth may become conspicuous. Periodontitis is a potent cause of foul-smelling breath. The congested gingival margins become purplish-red, flabby and swollen. The interdental papillae 'split' and can be separated from the teeth. Later, the papillae are destroyed and the gingival margin tends to become straight with a swollen, rounded edge.

Pressure on the gingival margins causes bleeding, and sometimes pus can be expressed from round the necks of the teeth. Bacterial plaque and calculus are widespread (Fig. 5.8).

Loss of attachment leads to pocketing, which allows a probe to be passed down between teeth and gingiva. In pockets the rough surface of subgingival calculus can be felt. Eventually, teeth become increasingly loose and dull to percussion.

Radiography

The earliest change is loss of definition and blunting of the tips of the alveolar crests. Bone resorption usually progresses in a regular manner and its level remains the same along a row of teeth. A straight line can be drawn along the crest of the alveolar bone (horizontal bone loss, Fig. 5.9). Complex patterns of bone loss may also be seen, probably due to the effects of variable degrees of loss of attachment superimposed upon the underlying anatomical features. Thus, in areas where bone is thin, destruction results in horizontal bone loss, but where alveolar bone is thicker, partial destruction gives rise to vertical or angular bone defects.

Aetiology and pathology

Conditions promoting stagnation and maintenance of infection

Fig. 5.9 Severe horizontal bone loss in advanced chronic adult periodontitis.

Fig. 5.8 Advanced chronic periodontitis. There is severe destruction of alveolar bone and the teeth are drifting apart; thick plaque covers the necks of the teeth and the gingival margins are swollen. A periodontal abscess is pointing between the lower right central and lateral incisor.

Fig. 5.10 Site variation in disease severity as a result of local plaque retention. The mesial and distal aspects of the same tooth are shown. On the right the adjacent tooth is present; plaque is present beneath the contact point and is associated with pocketing and a dense inflammatory infiltrate. On the left, the distal tooth has been removed; the area is accessible to cleaning, plaque is absent, inflammatory changes have virtually disappeared and there is no appreciable pocketing.

at the gingival margins have been discussed earlier. Persistence of infection at the gingival margins leads to progressive inflammation and destruction of the supporting tissues. Usually, local factors are most important in the progress of chronic periodontitis (Fig. 5.10), but, for reasons which are unclear, there is wide individual response.

The main features of the pathology of chronic periodontitis are summarised in Table 5.7.

Table 5.7 Pathological processes in chronic periodontitis

- Chronic inflammation
- Destruction of periodontal ligament fibres
- Resorption of alveolar bone
- Migration of the epithelial attachment towards the apex
- Formation of pockets around the teeth
- Formation of subgingival plaque and calculus

Plaque

Bacterial plaque, a dense mat of bacteria (Table 5.8), extends from the gingival margins into pockets.

Subgingival calculus

Extension and calcification of plaque leads to formation of sub-

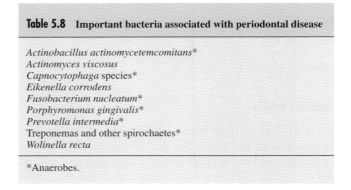

Table 5.8 Important bacteria associated with periodontal disease

*Actinobacillus actinomycetemcomitans**
Actinomyces viscosus
Capnocytophaga species*
Eikenella corrodens
*Fusobacterium nucleatum**
*Porphyromonas gingivalis**
*Prevotella intermedia**
Treponemas and other spirochaetes*
Wolinella recta

*Anaerobes.

gingival calculus within periodontal pockets. The deposits are thin, more widely distributed, harder, darker and more firmly attached than supragingival calculus. Calculus appears laminated histologically, with altered staining, probably due to breakdown products from blood cells oozing into the pockets (Fig. 5.12). Subgingival calculus helps to perpetuate chronic periodontitis. It forms a reservoir of bacteria, helping to sustain inflammation, and acts as a barrier to healing.

Chronic inflammation

Plasma cells typically predominate but are accompanied by lymphocytes and neutrophils which migrate into pockets. Inflammatory cells infiltrate the connective tissue and spread between the principal fibres (Fig. 5.12). Dense masses of these cells accumulate, especially under the epithelium in the connective tissue apposed to plaque and calculus.

Pocketing

Pocketing, a characteristic feature of chronic periodontitis, is due to the slower destruction of gingival soft tissues than of periodontal ligament and bone. Less frequently, where gingival tissue is thin, it may be lost at the same rate as the supporting tissues, and gingival recession results. Pockets round the teeth provide a protected environment in which bacteria grow more freely. There is no effective drainage and the wall of the pocket presents a large area where bacteria or their products can irritate the tissues. Pockets also favour the growth of anaerobes, which probably contribute greatly to tissue destruction.

Pockets surround the teeth (Fig. 5.13). One wall is formed by cementum, the other by soft tissue replacing the destroyed bone and periodontal fibres. The outer wall consists of connective tissue infiltrated by chronic inflammatory cells and lined by epithelium continuous with the gingival epithelium at the pocket mouth. The epithelial attachment forms the deep boundary (Fig. 5.14). The epithelium is often hyperplastic but blood vessels may extend through it almost to its surface.

Fig. 5.11 Transition from chronic gingivitis to periodontitis. No pocket has yet formed but the epithelial attachment has extended on to the cementum and inflammation has spread deeper still.

'Ulceration' of the lining is often described but rarely seen histologically.

Epithelial migration

The epithelial attachment migrates from enamel on to cementum, forming the floor of the pocket (Fig. 5.15). The attachment to cementum is strong, and a clear refractile cuticle can sometimes be seen joining the epithelium to the root surface. The

Fig. 5.12 Established chronic periodontitis. In this woman of 33, there were heavy deposits of plaque, shallow pockets have developed and the epithelial attachment has extended considerably more deeply along the cementum. The pockets have a thick, intact epithelial lining and inflammatory cells do not extend significantly beyond the deeper limits of the epithelial attachment. Much subgingival calculus is present and there has been considerable bone loss.

length of the epithelial attachment is variable but may extend several millimetres apically.

Destruction of periodontal fibres

Periodontal fibres are destroyed progressively from the gingival

Normal supporting tissues

False pocket

Infrabony pocket (vertical or angular bone loss)

Suprabony pocketing (horizontal bone loss)

Gingival recession

Fig. 5.13 Pocket formation in periodontal disease. A simplified diagram to show the relationship between periodontal soft tissues and alveolar bone in the different types of periodontal disease.

Fig. 5.14 An infrabony pocket. The pocket, with a thick epithelial lining, has extended deeply between the root and alveolar bone on the left, and to a slight extent on the right.

Fig. 5.15 Early transition between gingivitis and periodontitis. The junctional epithelium has migrated on to the surface of the cementum.

margin down to the level of the floor of the pocket. More deeply, the fibres retain their normal appearance.

Destruction of alveolar bone

Bone destruction starts at the alveolar crest. The usual level of the remaining bone is just deep to the floor of the pocket where the superficial fibres of the periodontal ligament are attached. The zone of inflammation is separated from the underlying bone by a zone of fibrous tissue. This so-called fibrous walling-off is typical of chronic periodontitis and invariably present (Figs 5.16 and 5.17). It has been suggested that the inflammatory lesion may extend beyond this to affect the alveolar bone and remaining periodontal ligament during periods of active disease, but histological evidence of this is lacking. Osteoclasts are rarely seen, probably because their action is intermittent and the rate of bone destruction extremely slow.

Role of specific bacteria in destructive periodontitis

With formation of pockets and subgingival plaque there is enormous proliferation of bacteria of all kinds. Subgingival plaque

Fig. 5.16 Advanced periodontitis. The epithelial attachment has migrated a considerable distance apically from the amelocemental junction but inflammatory cells remain localised around the pocket wall and do not extend to involve the crest of the alveolar bone interdentally.

Fig. 5.17 Advanced periodontitis. The pocket has extended well below the amelocemental junction, and heavy deposits of subgingival plaque (P) can be seen on either side of the gingival tissue. It will be obvious that the inflammatory infiltrate is concentrated in the vicinity of the plaque (above dotted line) and the connective tissue immediately above the alveolar bone is virtually free of inflammatory cells.

appears to have a dense zone attached to the tooth surface where the bacteria are mainly Gram-positive. By contrast, plaque related to the pocket wall is less densely packed but involves many Gram-negative bacteria, including anaerobes and spirochaetes. Bacteria particularly associated with destructive disease include *Porphyromonas gingivalis, Actinobacillus actinomycetemcomitans, Bacteroides intermedius, Wolinella recta*, spirochaetes with axial filaments, or in other cases *Eikenella corrodens*, and other corroding bacteria whose colonies cause pitting ('corrosion') of the surface of culture media. Also present are *Fusobacterium nucleatum* and as yet unidentified anaerobic vibrios and spirochaetes. Where there is severe and relatively acute bone loss associated with severe inflammation, in young adults, for example, *Actinobacillus actinomycetemcomitans* and *Porphyromonas gingivalis* appear to be particularly important. Where inflammation is minimal in spite of extensive bone loss there may be greater numbers of *Prevotella melaninogenica* and *Eikenella corrodens*. Many of the bacteria implicated in destructive periodontitis are dangerous pathogens and in other circumstances can cause severe or lethal systemic infections. For example, *Capnocytophaga ochraceus, Selenomonas sputigena* and *Eikenella corrodens* have been implicated in life-threatening infections, particularly in patients with granulocytopenia.

In human periodontal disease, it remains unclear which particular types of bacteria are responsible for tissue destruction. However, inoculation of specific bacteria into the mouths of germ-free animals has yielded somewhat unexpected results. Thus, various Gram-positive bacteria typically produced large amounts of plaque but Gram-negative bacteria did not. Certain

bacteria of either group could induce or accelerate periodontal tissue damage but there was typically little inflammation or lymphocytic infiltration of the tissues. In Gram-positive infections also, few osteoclasts were seen. However, *Actinomyces viscosus*, in particular, produces a bone-resorbing factor. Gram-negative bacteria also stimulated osteoclastic activity, and numerous osteoclasts were seen at the sites of tissue destruction.

That individual species of bacteria may be responsible for periodontal tissue destruction is also suggested by the finding in monkeys, that the severity of periodontal damage correlates well with the numbers of *Porphyromonas gingivalis* which can be isolated. Further, antimicrobial treatment that suppressed *P. gingivalis* led to healing and bone regeneration. Greater numbers of *P. gingivalis* also appear to be associated with enhanced periodontal disease activity in humans.

Bacterial mediators of tissue damage

Periodontal destruction may result from the actions of bacterial products or indirectly from immunologically mediated processes or both in varying degree. Bacterial products (virulence factors) that may contribute to tissue damage include enzymes, toxins and bone-resorbing factors.

Enzymes. Destruction of periodontal fibres may be due to collagenases. *Prevotella* species, for example, produce collagenase, trypsin, fibrinolysin, hyaluronidase, chondroitin sulphatase, heparinase, aribonuclease and deoxyribonuclease. Cytotoxic metabolic products such as indole, ammonia and hydrogen sulphide may also contribute. *Porphyromonas* species, especially *P. gingivalis*, are regularly associated with human destructive periodontitis.

Toxins. Certain strains of *Actinobacillus actinomycetemcomitans* produce a powerful leukotoxin, while *P. gingivalis* and *Prevotella intermedia* produce an epitheliotoxin.

Endotoxin, a lipopolysaccharide (LPS) component of Gram-negative bacteria cell walls, is released after cell lysis. It can liberate lysosomal enzymes from phagocytes and activate complement via the alternative pathway. Endotoxins can therefore mediate an inflammatory response. Endotoxins from some bacteria can enhance osteoclastic resorption to variable degrees and in this respect, endotoxin from *P. gingivalis* is ten times more potent than that from *A. actinomycetemcomitans*. The Gram-positive cell wall component, lipoteichoic acid (LTA), is also a potent mediator of inflammation and enhances bone resorption.

Bone resorbing factors. *Actinomyces viscosus* produces factors which induce decalcification of bone in vitro. Lipopolysaccharide can also induce bone resorption under experimental conditions, as can crude soluble extracts of human supragingival plaque and some other bacterial products. Bacterial factors can also cause bone resorption by stimulating release of, or acting synergistically with, lymphokines, osteoclast-activating factors and prostaglandin E_2.

Interference with host defence mechanisms

Other virulence factors act by interfering with host defences. Substances (leukotoxins) cytotoxic for human leukocytes are produced by *A. actinomycetemcomitans* in particular. This bacterium is involved in juvenile periodontitis and can also cause osteomyelitis and infective endocarditis in humans. Other bacterial factors potentially capable of damaging host defences are immunoglobulin proteases. *Neisseria gonorrhoeae* can produce IgA proteases which helps it overcome mucosal defences and contributes to the inability of infected persons to develop protective immunity. Several of the oral viridans streptococci have also been shown to produce IgA proteases. Lipopolysaccharides, dextran and levan may also be immunosuppressive, but under different circumstances may be immunopotentiating.

Immunological processes in periodontal disease

Immunological mechanisms are involved in periodontal disease, as they are in every microbial disease. Antibodies are produced against plaque bacterial antigens. These may, for example, mediate opsonisation and killing of bacteria by neutrophils and macrophages. Complement is also activated by antigen–antibody complexes and contributes to the inflammatory reaction. In the process of inflammation, microbes are killed but there may also be some damage to host tissues in so-called innocent bystander damage.

Many T lymphocytes are also present and may be involved in cell-mediated reactions to plaque pathogens. Other hypersensitivity reactions may also participate.

However, it must be appreciated that the immunological reactions in chronic periodontitis are essentially protective. With loss of normal immune competence, as in conditions of neutropenia for example, periodontal destruction may be greatly accelerated. Severely destructive periodontitis may also be seen in AIDS.

The remarkable feature of periodontal disease is that, despite the presence of innumerable major pathogens in periodontal pockets, tissue destruction is so slow. In an otherwise healthy person it is not uncommon for half a century to pass before 1 cm of alveolar bone is lost. This represents a loss of an average of 0.2 mm of bone loss a year.

Progress of chronic periodontitis

Chronic periodontitis, once established, is self-perpetuating. Pockets cannot drain effectively and favour proliferation of bacteria. The epithelial lining, plaque and subgingival calculus effectively obstruct healing. Further destruction of periodontal fibres and alveolar bone causes the pockets to deepen. The natural termination of the process is loosening and exfoliation of the teeth.

General principles of management of chronic periodontitis

The main components of the management of periodontal disease are summarised in Table 5.9.

Table 5.9 General principles of management of periodontal disease

- Control of bacterial plaque
- Establishment of healthy gingiva accessible to plaque control
- Minimisation of periodontal tissue loss
- Use of antibiotics in selected cases
- Mucogingival surgery in selected cases

It may be depressing for readers who have steeped themselves in the complexities of the immunology of periodontal disease to find that its management largely depends on time-honoured manual methods of plaque control.

Effective daily plaque removal by the patient is imperative for success. Conscientious toothbrushing and interdental cleaning with aids such as floss, wooden sticks or small brushes, as necessary, are required. These simple measures will bring about complete resolution of simple gingivitis, as mentioned earlier.

Anything hampering plaque control, particularly calculus and faulty restorations, should be dealt with. Other conditions promoting stagnation (Table 5.10) may be more difficult to eliminate.

Table 5.10   **Factors promoting stagnation and persistence of plaque**

- Calculus
- Overhanging restorations
- Food packing due to faulty contact points
- Irregularities of the teeth
- Mouthbreathing
- Pocketing

Treatment of periodontal pockets

Successful treatment depends upon thorough supragingival and subgingival plaque removal. The latter may be achieved by *subgingival scaling* or *root planing*, which also removes some cementum, to ensure plaque elimination from surface irregularities. The aim is to produce a root surface to which the detached gingival tissue may adhere. Such methods should result in resolution of inflammation in the pocket wall. The junctional epithelial attachment to the root surface may extend in length coronally, and there is usually shrinkage of the gingival margin, thus exposing more root surface. The clinical result is greater recession, shallower probing depth and less bleeding on probing. Failure to achieve clinical improvement is due to either a lapse in plaque control by the patient or failure to remove subgingival plaque (Table 5.11).

Table 5.11   **Factors compromising subgingival plaque removal**

- Excessive pocket depth
- Distorted root morphology and furcations
- Inaccessible root surfaces (e.g. distal surfaces of posterior teeth)
- Operator skill

Failure of benefit from root planing is shown by:

- Bleeding or exudation of pus on probing the depth of pocket
- Increasing probing depths
- Radiographic deterioration of bone levels

Subgingival scaling or root planing will not remove subgingival plaque entirely and may force pocket bacteria into the tissues. However, competent performance of these procedures reduces bacterial bulk, changes the composition of the flora and frequently produces clinical improvement.

When root planing fails, mucogingival surgery may be used to excise pockets to enable the patient to keep the root surfaces clean. The earliest form of resective surgery was gingivectomy.* This is still a useful procedure, particularly in patients with false pockets due to fibrous gingival hyperplasia and unresponsive to non-surgical treatment. However gingivectomy is unsuitable (1) for pockets extending beyond the mucogingival junction such that excision would remove all the keratinised gingiva, and (2) if the base of the pocket is apical to the bone crest (infrabony pockets, see Fig. 5.13). Gingivectomy for deep pocketing also exposes the necks of the teeth and produces a 'horse-tooth' appearance unacceptable to most patients.

Flap operations

Surgical approaches usually depend on elevation of flaps and are designed to remove the inner lining of the pocket whilst preserving the outer keratinised gingiva. Remaining inflamed tissue is curetted away and the root surfaces are cleaned. The flaps are then sutured back around the necks of the teeth. The flap can be replaced at or near the preoperative level or it can be repositioned apically so that it just covers the alveolar crest. The former approach requires that the flap must reattach to the denuded root surface, whereas the latter aims to eliminate the pocket. Apical placement of the flap may produce an aesthetically undesirable result, and exposure of complex root forms may not facilitate plaque control by the patient.

Reattachment surgery

The ultimate goal of this technique is the promotion of new cementum apposition to anchor periodontal fibres to a healthier root surface. This ideal result ('new attachment') would obviously be the most satisfactory method of treatment. Unfortunately it has been largely unsuccessful, mainly as a consequence of rapid re-epithelialisation of the root surface and production of a long junctional epithelium. Until recently, methods designed to retard or redirect epithelial migration at the healing dentogingival junction have not been successful. A new connective tissue attachment will probably only form if cells from the remaining healthy periodontal ligament repopulate the root surface. Insertion of a barrier membrane between the flap and root surface may prevent epithelial and gingival connective tissue ingrowth ('guided tissue regeneration'). Histological evidence suggests that new attachment that forms after this procedure is only in relatively small amounts.

Limitations of periodontal surgery

Periodontal surgery may be of little benefit when multirooted teeth have furcation involvement. When one root is more

---

*Gingivectomy dates back at least 800 years when Crusaders whose gums were so swollen by scurvy, that they had to be cut away to enable them to eat.

severely affected than another, resection of the affected root or half the tooth (hemisection) may be successful.

Overall, however, clinical trials comparing gingivectomy and various flap procedures have shown minimal differences in results under conditions where the standard of plaque control is high. If plaque control is poor they are equally ineffective and may lead to greater loss of periodontal support. Most patients with periodontal disease can be successfully treated with a non-surgical approach, and similar results have been obtained when surgical and non-surgical treatment have been compared. Surgery may have advantages when treating deep pockets, while the non-surgical approach is better for shallower pockets.

Antibiotics for control of plaque bacteria

Antibiotics reaching periodontal plaque cause considerable disturbance of the bacterial flora and have the potential for destroying important pathogens. It might seem that this effect would be transient, but it must be borne in mind that the complex interdependent ecosystem of plaque bacteria associated with periodontal disease is built up over a period of years. A possible limitation is the development of resistance by plaque bacteria. Though this undoubtedly happens, anaerobes generally do not lose antibiotic sensitivity as readily as many aerobes. In the USA especially, antibiotics have been used experimentally, particularly for the management of periodontal disease responding poorly to conventional treatment. Overall, tetracyclines seem to be the most effective. They have the widest spectrum of activity of all antibiotics, and the side-effects, particularly of topical applications, are minimal. Even when given systemically, tetracyclines may reach concentrations in the gingival sulcus several times greater than serum levels. They also bind to calcified tissues such as cementum. In various studies, tetracyclines appear to have produced significant changes in the composition of plaque. They have brought clinical improvement, particularly when combined with conventional treatment such as root planing.

Tetracycline-containing plastic fibres have also been placed in the gingival sulcus for direct delivery of a high local concentration of the drug. Putative plaque pathogens such as *Porphyromonas* species and other anaerobes were not found to have repopulated the plaque within the period of follow-up. Though the use of antibiotics in the management of periodontal disease is not universally accepted, it seems likely that they can produce long-term reduction in plaque pathogenicity. By interfering with complex bacterial ecosystems, less harmful species may proliferate. With the small doses used in topical applications, significant adverse effects seem unlikely to be troublesome.

However, some long-term studies have shown little or no benefit from the use of tetracyclines over scaling and root planing alone.

Treatment of advanced periodontal disease

Once pocketing has extended beyond the point where treatment

can be beneficial, the teeth should be extracted. Deep pockets are a source of sepsis which may have remote effects such as infective endocarditis. Deep pockets are most frequent in elderly patients, who have the highest susceptibility to and mortality from infective endocarditis. At the local level, if infection is allowed to persist, excessive resorption of the alveolar bone may cause difficulties in retaining dentures.

Prognosis in periodontal disease

Reliable predictions about the results of treatment cannot be made but some factors obviously affect the outcome (Table 5.12). Much depends on the level of oral hygiene maintained by the patients and whether they are sufficiently strongly motivated to cooperate in a long regimen of treatment. The degree of attachment loss, as shown by pocket depth and radiographic assessment, clearly determines whether teeth can be saved. However, in patients with the same amount of destruction of supporting tissues, the older the patient the better the prognosis, as the disease is of slower progress. Dental factors such as tooth type, root length, root anatomy and degree of furcation involvement can significantly affect the response to periodontal surgery. If, in addition, the teeth are heavily restored or have had faulty endodontic treatment or have already been lost, extensive periodontal treatment may be inappropriate.

Table 5.12 **Factors affecting prognosis of periodontal disease**

- Oral hygiene status and motivation
- Degree of bone loss
- Age
- Tooth factors
- Host resistance

Despite intensive investigation, there remains, for no clear reasons, a 'high-risk' group for periodontitis who suffer more extensive bone loss than others of similar age.

PERIODONTAL (LATERAL) ABSCESS

Periodontal abscess is a complication of chronic periodontitis and results from acute infection of a pocket. It sometimes follows treatment such as root planing when trauma to the pocket lining implants bacteria into the tissues. Otherwise the causes are uncertain but an abscess may result from some change in the pocket flora or damage by a foreign body, such as a fish bone driven through the floor of a pocket. Food packing down between the teeth with poor contact points may also contribute. Drainage through the pocket mouth is poor, and made worse by inflammatory oedema and soft-tissue swelling.

Fig. 5.18 Periodontal abscess. The abscess is pointing on the alveolar mucosa well above the attached gingiva. The probe is inserted deeply in the pocket communicating with the abscess.

Clinical features

The onset is rapid. Gingival tenderness progresses to throbbing pain. The tooth affected is vital and tender to percussion. The overlying gingiva is red and swollen. Pus may exude from the pocket, but a deep periodontal abscess may point on the alveolar mucosa, forming a sinus (Fig. 5.18). Generalised chronic periodontitis is usually associated. The vitality of the tooth and its less severe tenderness usually distinguish a lateral abscess from acute apical periodontitis. The great depth of the pocket, from which pus may exude, helps to make the diagnosis clear.

Radiographic changes are not visible until after about a week. A radiolucent area may then be seen beside the tooth.

Pathology

The bony wall of the pocket is actively resorbed by many osteoclasts. There is dense infiltration by neutrophils and pus formation (Fig. 5.19). The pocket deepens rapidly by destruction of periodontal fibres, sometimes to the apex of the tooth. Alveolar bone in the floor of the original pocket is destroyed, and the pocket extends between the tooth and alveolar bone. An intrabony pocket may thus form.

Treatment

A periodontal abscess should be drained. Infected tissue can be removed by subgingival curettage, and the root surfaces thoroughly debrided. Occasionally incision through the overlying gingiva is needed. However, if periodontal disease is severe and widespread, it may be appropriate to extract the affected tooth.

LOCALISED JUVENILE PERIODONTITIS ('PERIODONTOSIS')

Juvenile periodontitis is uncommon, having a prevalence of

Fig. 5.19 Acute periodontal abscess. There is well-advanced chronic periodontitis, but acute inflammatory changes have developed in this pocket with disruption of periodontal ligament and alveolar bone extending to the apex with formation of an abscess and a deep intrabony pocket from a man of 55.

about 1:1000, with males and females equally affected. Its onset may be around puberty or earlier.

The main features are rapid breakdown of the periodontal tissues of permanent first molars and incisors. There is also a rare, more generalised form, which appears to be a less clearly definable disease entity. Several systemic diseases can cause premature periodontal destruction but the term 'juvenile periodontitis' is reserved for cases in which clinically significant organic disease is absent.

Aetiology

There is a familial predisposition but the immediate cause may be a specific bacterial infection and an associated neutrophil defect. The bacterium commonly found in the diseased sites is *A. actinomycetemcomitans*, strains of which produce a potent leukotoxin. Antibodies to this bacterium and the leukotoxin are found in the serum and gingival fluid. Neutrophils from many patients have a defect in chemotaxis and reduced surface receptor-binding capacity. The defect may be genetically determined, while acquisition of the organism is probably from other family members.

Clinical features

The incisor and first molar teeth are usually the most severely affected. Gingivitis is minimal or absent and the main feature

Fig. 5.20 Localised juvenile periodontitis. Drifting of upper central incisors due to gross loss of attachment. There is some marginal inflammation but oral hygiene is good and the clinical appearance belies the periodontal destruction.

Fig. 5.21 Juvenile periodontitis. Patient aged 17 years showing severe bone destruction around first permanent molars. Probing depths exceeded 10 mm. One first permanent molar was affected on the contralateral side but in this case the central incisors were spared.

is drifting and loosening of teeth, most noticeably in the front of the mouth. The teeth may also tilt or become extruded (Fig. 5.20).

Radiography

Deep, angular bone loss and displacement of the anterior teeth are typical findings (Fig. 5.21). The remarkable symmetry seen in this condition is often such as to make each side of the mouth appear almost as mirror images.

Pathology

Little material has become available for histological examination but there is degeneration of principal periodontal fibres, which become replaced by a loose oedematous network of connective tissue, without significant inflammatory infiltration (Figs 5.22 and 5.23). Alveolar bone is resorbed.

Fig. 5.22 Juvenile periodontitis. Severe loss of alveolar bone and apical migration of the epithelial attachment but with only a small amount of plaque.

Treatment

Severely affected teeth may require extraction. Currently, early surgical treatment and tetracycline administration are advised. Surgical excision of the pocket lining may help to eradicate bacteria colonising the epithelial lining and, possibly, bacteria within the diseased tissue. Tetracycline is effective against *A. actinomycetemcomitans* and is given for 2–3 weeks. This treatment may be dramatically successful in the early stages of the disease.

There is a tendency for the condition to slow down or burn out in some individuals in their twenties. This is referred to as *post-juvenile periodontitis*.

Other causes of early-onset periodontal destruction

Very rarely, severe periodontal destruction may affect the

Fig. 5.23 Juvenile periodontitis. A higher power view of the periodontal ligament showing loss of the principal fibre bundles. In their place is loose, cellular connective tissue without any functional orientation of the fibres. The epithelial rests of Malassez have drifted laterally away from the surface of the root. At the bottom of the picture (about two-thirds of the way down the root) there is some bone, but even here the normal structure of the periodontal ligament has disappeared and the fibres between bone and root run vertically.

deciduous and permanent dentition in a condition termed *prepubertal periodontitis*. These children have profound neutrophil or monocyte dysfunction or both and suffer from other infections such as otitis media. Another form of generalised severe periodontitis which affects young individuals in their twenties and early thirties may also be associated with a phagocyte defect and is referred to as 'rapidly progressive periodontitis'. Recognised causes of premature periodontal destruction are summarised in Table 5.13. All (except Down's syndrome) are uncommon or rare but are important to distinguish from 'idiopathic' juvenile periodontitis, in that the underlying disorder may threaten the patient's health or life.

Immunodeficiencies

Some types of immunodeficiency disease are associated with premature destructive periodontitis. Down's syndrome, in which there are multiple immunodeficiencies, is the most common example. Agranulocytosis and acute leukaemia may also be associated with necrotising gingivitis and periodontal tissue destruction. Agranulocytosis is mainly a disease of adults, while the common childhood type of acute leukaemia (acute lymphocytic leukaemia) typically does not show periodontal

Table 5.13 Systemic causes of premature periodontal tissue destruction

- Immunodeficiencies
  Down's syndrome (Ch. 34)
  Leukopenia (Ch. 22)
  Severe, uncontrolled diabetes mellitus
  HIV infection
- Genetic syndromes
  Hypophosphatasia
  Papillon–Lefèvre syndrome
  Ehlers–Danlos syndrome (type VIII)
  Eosinophilic granuloma (Langerhans' cell histiocytosis, Ch. 9)

destruction. The importance of cyclic neutropenia has been somewhat exaggerated and early-onset periodontitis is by no means always associated. It should be emphasised that early-onset periodontitis in patients with immunodeficiency disorders (unlike 'idiopathic' juvenile periodontitis) is typically associated with abnormal susceptibility to non-oral infections.

Hypophosphatasia

Hypophosphatasia is a rare genetic disorder which can have severe skeletal effects as a result of failure of development of mature bone. There may also be failure of cementum formation causing loosening or exfoliation of the teeth without signs of gingivitis or periodontitis. Premature loss of the deciduous teeth, especially the incisors, is characteristic and occasionally the only overt manifestation of the disease.

Papillon–Lefèvre syndrome

The main features are hyperkeratosis of the palms and soles but the mechanisms of early onset periodontal destruction remain controversial. *A. actinomycetemcomitans* has frequently been implicated. An associated neutrophil defect has also sometimes been detected.

Ehlers–Danlos syndrome (type VIII)

Ehlers–Danlos syndrome is an important cause of floppy joint syndromes and its main effects are on the temporomandibular joint. However, in the type VIII variant, which is inherited as an autosomal dominant, there is bruising, soft and hyperextensible skin, and hypermobile joints. Early-onset periodontal disease is related to a defect in collagen formation but the molecular defect is unknown. Teeth are commonly lost by the age of 30 years.

Langerhans' cell histiocytosis (eosinophilic granuloma)

Eosinophilic granuloma may cause a distinctive type of periodontal destruction which involves the gingival soft tissues and exposes the roots of the teeth. There is also widespread destruction of the bone of the jaw with formation of a tumour-like mass (Ch. 9).

ACUTE PERICORONITIS

Incomplete eruption of a wisdom tooth produces a large stagnation area under the gum flap. It can easily become infected, causing pericoronitis. Several factors (Table 5.14) may contribute. Pericoronitis is caused by a mixed infection and various pathogens of dental plaque, particularly anaerobes, can be causative.

Table 5.14 Factors contributing to pericoronitis

- Impaction of food and plaque accumulation under the gum flap
- An upper tooth biting on the gum flap
- Acute ulcerative gingivitis (rarely)

Clinical features

Young adults are affected. The main symptoms are soreness and tenderness around the partially erupted tooth (Figs 5.24 and 5.25). There is pain, swelling, difficulty in opening the mouth, lymphadenopathy, sometimes slight fever and, in severe cases, suppuration and abscess formation. Swelling and difficulty in opening the mouth may be severe enough to prevent examination of the area.

Management

Food debris should be removed from under the gum flap by irrigation. The position of the affected tooth, its relationship to the

Fig. 5.24 Pericoronitis. A form of gingivitis in which a pocket has formed between the gingiva or operculum and the crown of an unerupted tooth.

Fig. 5.25 Pericoronitis. A section through the operculum over an unerupted molar reveals the very large blue-staining deposits of microbial plaque which lie below.

second molar and any complicating factors should be determined by radiography.

In mild cases it may be enough for patients to keep the mouth clean and to use hot mouth rinses whenever symptoms develop, until the inflammation subsides. This may happen naturally by further eruption or by extraction of the tooth after the infection has been overcome.

If radiographs show that the third molar is badly misplaced, impacted or carious, it should be extracted after inflammation has subsided.

When an upper tooth is biting on the flap it is often preferable to extract it, especially if the lower tooth is ultimately to be removed. If there are strong reasons for retaining the upper tooth, the cusps should be ground away sufficiently to prevent it from traumatising the flap. Trichloracetic acid used very sparingly on a cotton-wool pledget, followed by glycerine, is often useful to reduce the operculum.

In severe cases, particularly when there is fever and lymphadenopathy, metronidazole or penicillin or both should be given.

Spread of infection (cellulitis or osteomyelitis) may follow extraction of the tooth while infection is still acute, but is rare.

ACUTE ULCERATIVE GINGIVITIS (ACUTE NECROTISING ULCERATIVE GINGIVITIS)

Acute ulcerative gingivitis is a distinct and specific disease which can cause significant periodontal tissue damage but does not often contribute to chronic periodontal disease. The following account describes the disease in HIV-negative persons.

Clinical features

The incidence of ulcerative gingivitis has declined sharply in the Western world since the second world war. It typically affects apparently healthy young adults, usually those with neglected mouths.

Typical features are summarised in Table 5.15.

Table 5.15 Typical features of acute ulcerative gingivitis
• Young adult males mainly affected • Often cigarette smokers and/or with minor respiratory infection • Cratered ulcers starting at the tips of the interdental papillae • Ulcers spread along gingival margins • Gingival soreness and bleeding • Foul breath • No significant lymphadenopathy • No fever or systemic upset • Smears from ulcers dominated by spirochaetes and Gram-negative fusiform bacteria • Responds to oral hygiene and metronidazole in immunocompetent patients

Crater-shaped or punched-out ulcers form initially at the tips of the interdental papillae (Fig. 5.26). Ulcers are sharply defined with surrounding erythema and oedema; their surface is covered by a greyish or yellowish tenacious slough (Fig. 5.27). Removal of the slough causes free bleeding.

Lesions remain restricted to the gingivae and supporting tissues. They mainly spread along the gingival margins and deeply, destroying interdental soft and hard tissues, but rarely extend across the attached gingiva. Deep spread can cause rapid destruction of both soft tissues and bone, producing triangular spaces between the teeth (Fig. 5.28).

If treatment is delayed, the end-result can be considerable distortion of the normal gingival contours, promoting stagnation and possibly recurrences or chronic periodontal disease.

In the past particularly, localised spread to immediately adjacent oral mucosa was occasionally seen, but acute ulcerative gingivitis is *not* an oral mucosal infection.

Fig. 5.26 Early acute ulcerative gingivitis. The interdental papillae are swollen due partly to pre-existing chronic gingivitis and partly to the acute inflammatory oedema. Blood and slough exude from the gingival margins, and an early ulcer at the tip of the papilla between the upper canine and lateral can be seen.

Fig. 5.27 Acute ulcerative gingivitis. The characteristic features of the ulcers are shown in this enlarged photograph. The ulcers start at the tips of the interdental papillae, are crater-shaped, have a pale margin and are covered by a slough. Removal of the slough leaves a raw bleeding surface.

Fig. 5.28 Advanced ulcerative gingivitis. The gingival and periodontal tissues, especially of the lower central incisors, have been destroyed, leaving triangular spaces between the teeth. The condition can be said to have reached the stage of acute periodontitis.

Aetiology

The bacteria responsible are a complex of spirochaetes and fusiforms (Fig. 5.29). These organisms may be present in small numbers in the healthy gingival flora. With the onset of ulcerative gingivitis, both bacteria proliferate until they dominate the bacterial picture in smears from the lesions. This overwhelming proliferation of the spirochaete and fusobacterium at the site of tissue destruction, invasion of the tissues by spirochaetes seen by electron microscopy and the sharp fall in their numbers with effective treatment indicate that they are the responsible agents. Nevertheless, it is still uncertain whether this spirochaetal complex is the sole cause of ulcerative gingivitis and other bacteria have been implicated (Table 5.16).

Despite doubts about the precise bacterial cause of acute ulcerative gingivitis, it is clearly an anaerobic infection and responds rapidly to metronidazole.

Host factors

Ulcerative gingivitis is a disease of otherwise healthy young

Fig. 5.29 *Treponema vincentii* and *Fusobacterium nucleatum.* A smear from a patient with acute ulcerative gingivitis. The loose irregular shape of the spirochaetes and the plumper curved fusiform bacilli can be seen among other bacilli and cocci.

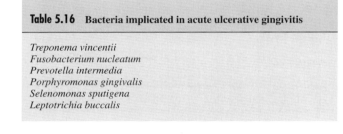

Table 5.16 Bacteria implicated in acute ulcerative gingivitis

Treponema vincentii
Fusobacterium nucleatum
Prevotella intermedia
Porphyromonas gingivalis
Selenomonas sputigena
Leptotrichia buccalis

adults, usually with neglected, dirty mouths. However, ulcerative gingivitis may also develop in children having immunosuppressive treatment and in patients with HIV infection (see below).

Local factors appear to be important and ulcerative gingivitis does not appear to be transmissible. Ulcerative gingivitis ('trench mouth') was almost epidemic among the troops in the 1914–1918 war and civilians subjected to bombing in the 1939–1945 war. Malnutrition has been excluded as a factor during these periods but being shelled or bombed can (reasonably enough) be regarded as stressful. Other evidence also suggests that chronic anxiety may be a predisposing factor in this infection. Smoking and upper respiratory infections have also been implicated. However, ulcerative gingivitis is relatively rarely seen in Britain now (Table 5.17) and the aetiology remains uncertain.

Table 5.17 Differential diagnosis of acute ulcerative gingivitis

- Primary herpetic gingivostomatitis
- HIV-associated acute ulcerative gingivitis (see below)
- Gingival ulceration in acute leukaemia or aplastic anaemia

Treatment

Oral hygiene (debridement) is essential. *Metronidazole* (200 mg

by mouth, taken after food three times a day for 3 days) greatly accelerates resolution. Side-effects are few, apart from interaction with alcohol, and rarely significant.

Follow-up treatment — rehabilitation of the mouth. Once the acute phase has subsided, the state of oral hygiene should be brought to as high a standard as possible to lessen the risk of recurrence.

HIV-ASSOCIATED GINGIVITIS

HIV-positive persons can suffer severe necrotising ulcerative gingivitis as their immune function declines. Clinically, it resembles ulcerative gingititis in HIV-negative persons but rapidly progresses to HIV-associated periodontitis.

A distinctive HIV-associated gingivitis is a relatively uncommon manifestation but can be an early sign and precede other opportunistic infections. It appears as a distinct erythematous band extending along the free and attached gingiva. Clinically, it resembles so-called desquamative gingivitis (Ch. 13) rather than common chronic gingivitis, but profuse bleeding is charactistic (Table 5.18).

The aetiology of HIV-associated gingivitis is unclear, especially as the bacteria isolated from it are similar to those from advanced chronic periodontitis.

Table 5.18 Typical features of HIV-associated gingivitis

- Well demarcated band of erythema along free and attached gingiva
- Resembles 'desquamative gingivitis' clinically
- Profuse bleeding
- Bacteria similar to those from periodontal pockets

HIV-ASSOCIATED PERIODONTITIS

HIV-associated ulcerative gingivitis, as described earlier, is associated with soft-tissue necrosis and rapid destruction of the periodontal tissues. It is typically intensely painful. There is little deep pocketing because soft tissue and bone are lost virtually simultaneously. More than 90% of the attachment can be lost within 3–6 months, and the soft-tissue necrosis can lead to exposure of bone and sequestration.

The pain of HIV-associated periodontitis is usually aching in character and felt within the jaw rather than in the gingivae. It may be felt before tissue destruction becomes obvious. HIV-associated gingivitis and periodontitis are usually generalised but are sometimes localised to one or more discrete areas.

Bacteriologically HIV-associated periodontitis resembles that of classical periodontitis in HIV-negative persons. It is typically associated with a low CD4 count and a poor prognosis for the patient.

Fig. 5.30 Acute herpetic gingivostomatitis. There is diffuse reddening of the attached gingiva with ulceration in the lower incisor region extending beyond the attached gingiva. Two vesicles lie on the upper left alveolar mucosa. Herpetic infection affects all oral mucosae but has a predilection for the gingiva. It is discussed further in Chapter 12.

Management

Debridement and removal of any sequestra under local anaesthesia, chlorhexidine mouth rinses, systemic metronidazole and analgesics may be effective. Additional broad-spectrum antibiotics have been recommended by some but increase the risk of thrush, to which these patients are particularly susceptible. If thrush is present or develops, antifungal drugs are required.

HERPETIC GINGIVOSTOMATITIS

In children particularly, primary herpetic stomatitis is associated with acute gingivitis. The gingivae are conspicuously erythematous and oedematous (Fig. 5.30). Herpetic ulcers may form on the tips of the interdental papillae or on any other anatomical regions of the gingivae, but are not an essential feature. Unlike ulcerative gingivitis, herpetic vesicles and ulcers extend widely over the oral mucosa. Lymphadenopathy is associated; systemic upset may be severe.

Smears from the lesions show typical viral-damaged cells and the gingivitis resolves with control of the virus. This may be hastened by use of acyclovir (Ch. 12).

MISCELLANEOUS PERIODONTAL DISORDERS

Gingival swelling

Gingival swelling may be due to fibrous hyperplasia or to non-fibrous inflammatory or other infiltrations (Table 5.19).

Hereditary gingival fibromatosis

Gingival fibromatosis is a feature of several heritable disorders. All are rare but the most common type is an autosomal dominant syndrome in which gingival fibromatosis may be associated with hypertrichosis and mental retardation.

Table 5.19 Causes of gingival enlargement

- Fibrous gingival hyperplasia
  Genetic
  Drug-associated
    Phenytoin
    Calcium channel blockers
    Cyclosporin
- Non-fibrous gingival enlargement
  Chronic 'hyperplastic' gingivitis
  Pregnancy gingivitis
  Leukaemic infiltration
  Wegener's granulomatosis
  Sarcoidosis
  Orofacial granulomatosis
  Scurvy

Fig. 5.31 Hereditary gingival fibromatosis. Fibrous overgrowth of the gingiva covers the clinical crowns of the teeth in an affected adolescent.

Gingival enlargement may precede eruption of the teeth or may not develop until later in childhood. The gingivae may be so grossly enlarged as completely to bury the teeth and are pale, firm and smooth or stippled in texture (Fig. 5.31). The facial features may also be coarse and thickened, simulating acromegaly, and there may be excessive hairiness (hypertrichosis). Epilepsy or mental retardation are rare features.

Histologically, the gingival tissue consists of thick bundles of collagenous connective tissue with little or no inflammatory exudate.

The excess gingival tissue can only be removed surgically but is likely to reform. Gingivectomy should be delayed as long as possible, preferably until after puberty when the rate of growth of the tissues is slower. Maintenance of oral hygiene is important to prevent infection becoming established in the deep false pockets. However, inflammation is frequently insignificant.

Drug-induced hyperplasia

Long-term use of the antiepileptic drug phenytoin (Epanutin*) can cause gingival hyperplasia. The overgrowth principally

---

*Phenytoin is sometimes referred to as Dilantin by a generation that has not caught up with current drug names. Dilantin is an American proprietary name for phenytoin and does not exist in Britain.

Fig. 5.32 Gingival hyperplasia due to phenytoin. Characteristic features are fibrous swelling of the interdental papillae, which become bulbous but remain firm and pale. The stippling of the attached gingiva becomes exaggerated. Localised gross enlargement such as that around the upper central incisor may result where the enlarged tissue forms a plaque trap.

Fig. 5.33 Acute myelomonocytic leukaemia. The gingival margins are swollen, soft and have a deep red or red-purple colour.

involves the interdental papillae, which become bulbous and overlap the teeth (Fig. 5.32). Typically the gingivae are firm and pale, and the stippled texture is exaggerated, producing an orange-peel appearance.

Infection appears to contribute and overgrowth of the gingivae can sometimes be kept under control by rigorous oral hygiene. Frequently, however, gingivectomy becomes necessary or is demanded by patients who are embarrassed by what they regard as a stigma of their disease.

Clinically similar changes are seen with use of calcium channel blockers such as nifedipine and diltiazem (for hypertension or angina), and with the immunosuppressive drug cyclosporin. Histologically they all resemble the genetic type of gingival hyperplasia.

NON-FIBROUS GINGIVAL SWELLINGS

Chronic 'hyperplastic' and pregnancy gingivitis have been discussed earlier.

Wegener's granulomatosis

Wegener's granulomatosis (Ch. 28) is an uncommon, frequently lethal disease of which the typical features are granulomatous ulceration of the nasopharynx, pulmonary cavitation and renal damage. Occasionally, the first sign is a characteristic form of proliferative gingivitis, bright or dusky red in colour and with a granular surface, to which the term 'strawberry gums' has been applied. Recognition of this type of gingivitis and confirmation of the diagnosis by biopsy, which shows the characteristic giant cells, may be life-saving by enabling treatment to start exceptionally early.

Sarcoidosis and orofacial granulomatosis

As discussed in Chapters 28 and 29, these diseases can give rise to gingival swelling in which granuloma formation is seen histologically. They cannot be distinguished by gingival biopsy alone.

Fig. 5.34 Acute myelomonocytic leukaemia. The gingival swelling is seen to be due to packing of the gingivae with leukaemic cells. The leukaemic cells are defective and tissues break down as a result of poor resistance to infection.

Acute leukaemia

Gingival swelling is most frequently seen in acute myelomonocytic leukaemia. The abnormal white cells are unable to perform their normal defensive function and cannot control infection at the gingival margins. The abnormal leucocytes pack the area until the gingivae become swollen with leukaemic cells (Fig. 5.34). These cells are so defective that infection progresses, causing ulceration and breakdown of the tissues.

Clinically the gingivae are swollen, shiny, pale or purplish in colour and frequently ulcerated (Fig. 5.33). Other signs of leukaemia (pallor, purpura or lassitude) may also be seen.

Topical antibiotics or chlorhexidine and improved oral hygiene may lead to regression of the swelling (Fig. 5.35), but the patient's general prognosis is poor.

Fig. 5.36 Advanced periodontitis with recession. Recession has exposed approximately half of the root length, predisposing to root surface caries. Considerable deposits of plaque and supragingival calculus adhere to the exposed roots.

Fig. 5.35 Acute leukaemia. Gross swelling causing the gingival margins to reach the incisal edges of the teeth as seen in the upper picture. The lower picture shows the effects of an antibiotic mouth rinse (tetracycline with amphotericin) and oral hygiene. The swelling has entirely subsided and the gingivae have regained their normal firm texture and pale colour, indicating that plaque is responsible for much of the gingival swelling in acute leukaemia. The underlying malignant disease is, of course, unaffected.

Fig. 5.37 Periodontitis with recession. In this case of advanced periodontitis gingival recession has kept pace with bone resorption, producing an excessively long clinical crown. There are large deposits of supragingival calculus and a dense inflammatory infiltrate in the gingiva.

Scurvy

Grossly swollen and congested gingivae are a classical sign of scurvy, but only of advanced disease and are rarely seen, even among the very few scorbutic patients who are not edentulous.

The gingival swelling is the result of a combination of chronic inflammation and an exaggeration of the inflammatory congestion due to scorbutic purpura. The diagnosis should only be made on clear evidence of dietary deficiency and of purpura. In these cases treatment with vitamin C and adequate oral hygiene relieves the gingival condition.

GINGIVAL RECESSION

Recession of the gingivae and eventual exposure of the roots is common (Figs 5.36 and 5.37). It is usually but not invariably associated with ageing, as susceptibility to it varies. The major predisposing factor is thinness of the gingival tissue. This is readily damaged by trauma from forceful toothbrushing and plaque-induced inflammation. One hypothesis suggests that epithelial proliferation of the junctional epithelium in inflammation results in an epithelial 'bridge' extending to the external gingival epithelium across the narrow band of inflamed connective tissue. This is followed by remodelling of the gingival margin. It seems likely that plaque-induced loss of attachment in areas of thick tissue can lead to pocket formation, whereas thin tissue is destroyed entirely. The resulting receded gingival margins often appear relatively uninflamed.

Gingival abrasion

Abrasion causes recession of the gingivae and damage to the teeth. Early changes may be seen in some young adults, and severe examples in later life. Forceful toothbrushing with a stiff brush used with a sawing motion across the teeth and use of an abrasive dentifrice is the usual cause. Grooves are worn into the

Fig. 5.38 Abrasion. Severe damage caused by vigorous toothbrushing over the course of many years. The teeth have been cut so deeply that many have snapped off but the gingival margins have resisted the heavy wear and remain firm, pale and healthy.

necks of the teeth, and reactionary dentine forms beneath. Eventually the necks of teeth may be cut so deeply that the crowns break off, but the pulp remains covered by reactionary dentine (Fig. 5.38). The gingival margins recede but they remain conspicuously firm, pale and healthy where they are worn away. Nearby, there may be chronic gingivitis interstitially where the toothbrush fails to reach.

Treatment of gingival recession

Recession of the gingivae sometimes causes patients to fear that they will soon lose their teeth. In older patients, where enough alveolar bone remains, the teeth can remain in useful

Fig. 5.39 Adaptive changes in the periodontal ligament. The second molar has erupted at an angle and oblique stresses are imposed on the supporting tissues. The periodontal membrane is compressed at the sites of the arrows where there is resorption of bone and widening of the periodontal ligament.

Fig. 5.40 Higher power view of the periodontal ligament from the previous figure near the gingival margin. There is resorption of the normally smooth lamina dura by osteoclasts and superficial resorption of the tooth. Such minor degrees of surface resorption of the teeth are relatively common and usually repair without causing problems.

function for many years and patients can be reassured. The main requirement is to keep the gingival margins plaque-free, especially in the enlarged interstitial spaces. In the case of abrasive gingival recession, the patient must also be shown how to keep the teeth clean without causing further damage. Various surgical procedures have been devised to correct localised areas of gingival recession or to produce thicker zones of gingiva which, it is hoped, are more resistant to recession.

An early result of abrasion is exposure of the dentine, which may be hypersensitive. Many treatments for it have been introduced, but their number betrays their limitations. Traditional remedies are topical applications of strong astringents such as zinc chloride or silver nitrate. Proprietary preparations such as Tresiolan and Durophat may be more effective.

Adaptive changes by the periodontal tissues

Malpositioned teeth, such as those which erupt at an angle, may have oblique stresses imposed on them by mastication. As a result the periodontal ligament may be stretched laterally on one side of the tooth and compressed on the other. On the compression side there may be some resorption of the lamina dura and sometimes of the root (Figs 5.39 and 5.40). Repair usually takes place without significant complications and the tooth can remain reasonably functional.

SUGGESTED FURTHER READING

Bozzo L, Almeida O P E, Scully C, Aldred M J 1994 Hereditary gingival fibromatosis. Report of an extensive four-generation pedigree. Oral Surg Oral Med Oral Pathol 78:452–454

Corbet E F, Davies W I R 1993 The role of supragingival plaque in the control of progressive periodontal disease. J Clin Periodontol 20:307–313

Fine D H 1994 Microbial identification and antibiotic sensitivity testing, an aid for patients refractory to periodontal therapy. J Clin Periodontal 21:98–106

Grossi S G, Zambon J J, Ho A W et al 1994 Assessment of risk for periodontal disease. I. Risk indicators for attachment loss. J Periodontol 65:260–267

Grossi S G, Genco R J, Machtei E E et al 1995 Assessment of risk for periodontal disease. II. Risk factors for alveolar bone loss. J Periodontol 66:23–29

Holmstrup P, Westergaard J 1994 Periodontal disease in HIV-infected patients. J Clin Periodontol 21:270–280

Hornung G M, Cohen M E 1995 Necrotizing ulcerative gingivitis, periodontitis, and stomatitis: clinical staging and predisposing factors. J Periodontol 66:990–998

Ishikawa I, Umeda M, Laosrisin N 1994 Clinical, bacteriological and immunological examinations and the treatment process of two Papillon–Lefèvre patients. J Clin Periodontol 65:364–371

Jeffcoat M K, Chesnut C H 1993 Systemic osteoporosis and oral bone loss. Evidence shows increased risk. J Am Dent Assoc 124:49–56

Johnson B D, Engel D 1986 Acute necrotising ulcerative gingivitis: a review of diagnosis, etiology and treatment. J Periodontol 57:141–150

Liljenberg B, Lindhe J, Berglundh T et al 1994 Some microbiological, histopathological and immunohistochemical characteristics of progressive periodontal disease. J Clin Periodontol 21:720–727

Linden G J, Mullaly B H 1994 Cigarette smoking and periodontal destruction in young adults. J Periodontol 65:718–723

Löe H, Brown J 1991 Early onset periodontitis in the United States of America. J Periodontol 62:608–616

Luke D A 1992 The structure and function of the dentogingival junction and periodontal ligament. Br Dent J 172:187–190

Margiotta V, Pizza I, Pizza G, Barbaro A 1996 Cyclosporin- and nifedipine-induced gingival overgrowth in renal transplant patients: correlations with periodontal and pharmacological parameters, and HLA-antigens. Oral Pathol Med 25:128–134

Nery E B, Eson R G, Lee K K et al 1995 Prevalence of nifedipine-induced gingival hyperplasia. J Periodontol 66:572–578

Plagmann H-C, Kocher T, Kuhrau N, Caliebe A 1994 Periodontal manifestation of hypophosphatasia. A family case report. J Clin Periodontol 21:710–716

Praytino S W, Addy M, Wade W G 1993 Does gingivitis lead to periodontitis in young adults? Lancet 342:471–472

Renvert S, Dahlén G, Wikström M 1996 Treatment of periodontal disease based on microbiological diagnosis. Relation between microbiological and clinical parameters during 5 years. J Periodontol 67:562–571

Robinson P G, Winkler J R, Palmer G et al 1994 The diagnosis of periodontal conditions associated with HIV infection. J Periodontol 65:236–243

Smith G L F. Diagnosis of periodontal disease activity by detection of key microbial antigens. J Clin Periodontol 21:615–620

Socransky S S, Haffajee A D 1991 Microbial mechanisms in the pathogenesis of destructive periodontal disease: a critical assessment. J Periodontol 26:322–331

Socransky S S, Haffajee A D 1992 The bacteriology of destructive periodontal disease: current concepts. J Periodontol 63:322–331

Timmerman M F, van der Weijden G A, van Steenbergen T J M et al 1996 Evaluation of the long-term efficacy and safety of locally applied minocycline in adult periodontitis patients. J Clin Periodontol 23:707–716

Williams D M, Hughes F J, Odell E W, Farthing P M 1992 Pathology of periodontal disease. Oxford University Press, Oxford

Major Infections of the mouth, jaws and perioral tissues

Severe oral and perioral infections are uncommon. Oral bacteria can also cause systemic infections, of which the main example is infective endocarditis. This can occasionally follow extractions or some other procedures.

ACUTE OSTEOMYELITIS OF THE JAWS

Osteomyelitis of the jaws is mainly a disease of adults, with several potential sources of infection (Table 6.1). Important predisposing causes are summarised in Table 6.2.

Table 6.1 Acute osteomyelitis of the jaws — potential sources of infection

- Periapical infection
- A periodontal pocket involved in a fracture
- Acute gingivitis or pericoronitis (even more rarely)
- Penetrating, contaminated injuries (open fractures or gunshot wounds)

Table 6.2 Important predisposing conditions for osteomyelitis

Local damage to or disease of the jaws
- Fractures, including gunshot wounds
- Radiation damage
- Paget's disease or osteopetrosis (Ch. 5)

Impaired immune defences
- Acute leukaemia
- Poorly-controlled diabetes mellitus
- Sickle cell anaemia
- Chronic alcoholism or malnutrition

The effect of immunodeficiency is variable and acute osteomyelitis of the jaw is uncommon in HIV infection.

Clinical features

Most patients are adult males with infection of the mandible.

Osteomyelitis of the maxilla is a rare disease of neonates or infants after either birth injuries or uncontrolled middle ear infection.

Early complaints are severe, throbbing, deep-seated pain, and swelling, with external swelling due to inflammatory oedema. Later, distension of the periosteum with pus, and finally subperiosteal bone formation, cause the swelling to become firm. The overlying gingiva is red, swollen and tender.

Associated teeth are tender. They may become loose and pus may exude from an open socket or gingival margins. Muscle oedema causes difficulty in opening the mouth and swallowing. Regional lymph nodes are enlarged and tender, and anaesthesia or paraesthesia of the lower lip is characteristic.

Frequently the patient remains well but in the acute phase there may be fever and leucocytosis. A severely ill or very pale patient suggests underlying disease which requires investigation.

Radiographic changes do not appear until after at least 10 days. Loss of trabecular pattern and areas of radiolucency indicate bone destruction. These areas have ill-defined margins and have a fluffy or moth-eaten appearance (Fig. 6.1). Areas of dead

Fig. 6.1 Osteomyelitis of the mandible following dental extractions. The outlines of the extraction sockets can be seen, together with dense sequestra of bone lying in a poorly circumscribed radiolucency.

bone appear as relatively dense areas which become more sharply defined as they are progressively separated as sequestra. Later, in young persons particularly, subperiosteal new bone formation causes a buccal swelling and appears as a thin, curved strip of new bone below the lower border of the jaw in lateral radiographs.

Pathology

Oral bacteria, particularly anaerobes such as *Bacteroides*, *Porphyromonas* or *Prevotella* species, are important causes but the infection is often mixed. Staphylococci may be responsible when they enter from the skin via an open fracture.

The mandible has a relatively limited blood supply and dense bone with thick cortical plates. Infection causes acute inflammation in the medullary soft tissues and inflammatory exudate spreads infection through the marrow spaces. It also compresses blood vessels confined in the rigid boundaries of the vascular canals. Thrombosis and obstruction then lead to further bone necrosis. Dead bone is recognisable microscopically by lacunae empty of osteocytes but filled with neutrophils and colonies of bacteria which proliferate in the dead tissue (Fig. 6.2).

Pus, formed by liquefaction of necrotic soft tissue and inflammatory cells, is forced along the medulla and eventually reaches the subperiosteal region by resorption of bone. Distension of the periosteum by pus stimulates subperiosteal bone formation but perforation of the periosteum by pus and formation of sinuses on the skin or oral mucosa are rarely seen now.

At the boundaries between infected and healthy tissue, osteoclasts resorb the periphery of the dead bone, which eventually becomes separated as a sequestrum. Once infection starts to localise, new bone forms around it, particularly subperiosteally.

Where bone has died and been removed, healing is by granulation with formation of coarse fibrous bone in the proliferating connective tissue. After resolution, fibrous bone is gradually

replaced by compact bone and remodelled to restore normal morphology.

Management

The main requirements are summarised in Table 6.3.

Table 6.3   **Summary of treatment of osteomyelitis**

Essential measures
Bacterial sampling and culture
Vigorous (empirical) antibiotic treatment
Drainage
Give specific antibiotics based on culture and sensitivities
Give analgesics
Debridement
Remove source of infection, if possible

Adjunctive treatment
Sequestrectomy
Decortication if necessary
Hyperbaric oxygen*
Resection and reconstruction for extensive bone destruction

*Mainly of value for osteoradionecrosis and possibly, anaerobic infections.

Bacteriological diagnosis. A specimen of pus or a swab from the depths of the lesion must first be taken for culture and sensitivity testing.

Antimicrobial treatment. Immediately a specimen has been obtained, vigorous antibiotic treatment should be started. Initially, penicillin, 600–1200 mg daily can be given by injection (if the patient is not allergic), with metronidazole 200–400 mg 8-hourly. Clindamycin penetrates avascular tissue better and is frequently effective. The regimen is adjusted later in the light of the bacteriological findings.

Debridement. Removal of foreign or necrotic material and immobilisation of any fracture are necessary if there has been a gunshot wound or other contaminating injury.

Drainage. Pressure should be relieved by tooth extraction, bur holes or decortication, as necessary, and exudate drained into the mouth or externally.

Removal of sequestra. Dead bone should not be forcibly separated and vigorous curetting is inadvisable, but in the late stages a loosened sequestrum may have to be removed (Fig. 6.3). Teeth should be extracted only if loosened by tissue destruction.

Adjunctive treatment. Decortication or hyperbaric oxygen therapy or both may be required, particularly in radiation-associated osteomyelitis.

Complications

Anaesthesia of the lower lip usually recovers with elimination of the infection. Rare complications include pathological fracture caused by extensive bone destruction, chronic

Fig. 6.2   High power view of a sequestrum showing non-vital bone (the osteocyte lacunae are empty), and eroded outline with the shape of Howship's lacunae produced by osteoclastic resorption and a dense surface growth of bacteria.

Fig. 6.3 Late-stage chronic osteomyelitis. A sequestrum trapped in a cavity within the bone. It is surrounded by fibrous tissue containing an infiltrate of inflammatory cells. Surgical intervention is needed to remove an infected sequestrum such as this.

Fig. 6.4 Chronic osteomyelitis secondary to radiotherapy. Part of the necrotic portion of the mandible is visible, having ulcerated through the skin.

osteomyelitis after inadequate treatment, cellulitis due to spread of exceptionally virulent bacteria or septicaemia in an immunodeficient patient.

Key features of osteomyelitis of the jaws are summarised in Table 6.4.

Table 6.4 Acute osteomyelitis of the jaws — key features

- Mandible mainly affected, usually in adult males
- Infection of dental origin — anaerobes are important
- Pain and swelling of jaw
- Teeth in the area are tender; gingivae are red and swollen
- Sometimes paraesthesia of the lip
- Minimal systemic upset
- After about 10 days, radiographs show moth-eaten pattern of bone destruction
- Good response to prompt antibiotic treatment and debridement

---

CHRONIC OSTEOMYELITIS

Rarely, inadequately treated acute osteomyelitis may lead to *chronic suppurative osteomyelitis*, which may also be a complication of irradiation (Fig. 6.4). Persistent low-grade infection is associated with bone destruction and granulation tissue formation, but little suppuration.

Chronic osteomyelitis can also arise de novo as a result of infection by weakly virulent bacteria or in avascular bone. Radiographic appearances are variable but sometimes distinctive.

Chronic focal sclerosing osteomyelitis (condensing osteitis)

This is an uncommon bony reaction to exceptionally low-grade periapical inflammation or, alternatively, to unusually strong local tissue resistance.

Patients are typically under 20 years. Infection is most frequently related to a mandibular first permanent molar which is typically grossly carious and non-vital, but causes little or no symptoms.

Radiographs show a radiopaque area up to 2–3 cm in diameter below the apex of one or both roots, which typically retain an intact lamina dura.

Pathology

The main features are dense compact bone with few lacunae, many of which are empty of osteocytes. Prominent resting and reversal lines give it a pagetoid appearance. Scanty fibrous interstitial tissue is infiltrated by a few lymphocytes.

Removal of the offending tooth is followed by slow resolution. An area of sclerotic bone may remain indefinitely.

Diffuse sclerosing osteomyelitis

Diffuse sclerosing osteomyelitis is usually seen in the elderly and most commonly in black people. The microscopic and radiographic appearances are similar to florid cemento-osseous dysplasia (Ch. 10) and are almost certainly due to superimposition of infection on the latter in the sclerotic stage.

The main symptoms are vague pain or an unpleasant taste, with occasional episodes of mild suppuration and fistula formation.

Radiographs show patchy diffuse or nodular sclerosis, resembling the cotton-wool radiopacities of cemento-osseous dysplasia or Paget's disease, often bilaterally.

Pathology

Dense, irregular bone shows a pagetoid ('mosaic') pattern of reversal lines. Connective tissue in the marrow spaces is patchily infiltrated by variable numbers of chronic inflammatory cells. During acute exacerbations, neutrophils become numerous.

Chronic diffuse sclerosing osteomyelitis needs to be distinguished from Paget's and other sclerotic bone diseases.

Removal of any infected teeth and antibiotic therapy are the initial treatment. Often the sclerotic masses form sequestra and, if so, the affected area should be guttered and the dense masses removed. Healing may then follow but because of the bony sclerosis a chronic relapsing course is common.

Chronic osteomyelitis with productive periostitis (non-suppurative osteomyelitis, Garrés osteomyelitis)

This uncommon response to low-grade chronic periapical or perifollicular infection is characterised by reactive subperiosteal new bone formation.

Typically, the lower first permanent molar region of the mandible in young adults is affected. There may be mild pain before a non-tender, bony, hard swelling forms, usually along the lower border or lateral aspect of the jaw.

Radiographs show a carious tooth and a related periapical area of radiolucency or, less commonly, folliculitis round an unerupted tooth. A smooth, convex overgrowth of cortical bone results. The remainder of the jaw may appear normal or radiolucent or osteosclerotic.

Pathology

Osteoid and woven bone forms in fibrous connective tissue. It shows parallel, concentric (onion skin) laminations. Patchy infiltration by chronic inflammatory cells may be found in a deep biopsy.

Removal of the infection leads to gradual remodelling of the jaw.

Chronic specific osteomyelitis

Syphilitic, actinomycotic and tuberculous osteomyelitis of the jaws are recognised entities but largely of historical interest.

SCLEROTIC BONE ISLANDS (IDIOPATHIC OSTEOSCLEROSIS)

Areas of sclerosis in the jaw are sometimes seen by chance in routine, particularly panoramic, radiographs. They should not be mistaken for a low-grade bone infection (particularly if first noticed after a surgical procedure), as they have sometimes been. Operative interference should be avoided as it is more likely to lead to complications and medicolegal claims than to be beneficial.

ALVEOLAR OSTEITIS

Alveolar osteitis (dry socket) can hardly be termed a major

infection but can be mistaken clinically for osteomyelitis, which can rarely follow. It is by far the most frequent painful complication of extractions. Nevertheless, it is uncommon overall.

Aetiology

Alveolar osteitis is frequently unpredictable and without any obvious predisposing cause but numerous possible aetiological factors exist (Table 6.5).

Table 6.5 **Possible aetiological factors for alveolar osteitis**

- Excessive extraction trauma
- Limited local blood supply
- Local anaesthesia
- Oral contraceptives
- Osteosclerotic disease
- Radiotherapy

Difficult disimpactions of third molars frequently lead to painful alveolar osteitis. However, the blood supply to the area often appears to be critical. In healthy persons alveolar osteitis virtually only affects the lower molar region where the bone is more dense and less vascular than elsewhere. Alveolar osteitis is also an expected complication of extractions in Paget's disease and particularly after radiotherapy where endarteritis causes ischaemia of the bone. Alveolar osteitis is also more frequent in susceptible patients, when local anaesthesia is used.

The oestrogen component of oral contraceptives apparently enhances serum fibrinolytic activity and, reportedly, is also associated with a higher incidence of alveolar osteitis.

Clinical features

Women are more frequently affected. Pain usually starts a few days after the extraction, but sometimes may be delayed for a week or more. It is deep-seated, severe and aching or throbbing. The mucosa around the socket is red and tender. There is no clot in the socket, which instead contains saliva and often decomposing food debris (Fig. 6.5). When debris is washed away, whitish, dead bone may be seen or may be felt as a rough area with a probe. Sometimes the socket becomes concealed by granulations growing in from the gingival margins. Pain often continues for a week or two, or occasionally longer. Sequestration of the socket may sometimes be seen radiographically (Fig. 6.6).

Pathology

The initial event is destruction of the clot which normally fills the socket. This was traditionally ascribed to bacterial proteolytic enzymes but is widely believed to be due to excessive local fibrinolytic activity. The alveolar bone and other oral tis-

Fig. 6.5 Dry socket. Typical appearances of chronic alveolar osteitis; the socket is empty and the bony lamina dura is visible.

Fig. 6.6 Sequestration in a severe dry socket. Almost the whole of the lamina dura and attached trabeculae have become necrotic, forming a sequestrum. Healing is delayed while the sequestrum remains in place. Most dry sockets are not associated with sequestration, or with only small sequestra.

sues have a high content of fibrinolysin activators (plasmin) which are released when the bone is traumatised. Nevertheless, once the clot has been destroyed, infection from the mouth is inevitable and anaerobes are likely to play a major role.

Destruction of the clot leaves an open socket in which infected food and other debris accumulates in direct contact with the bone. Bone damaged during the extraction, particularly the dense bone of the lamina dura, also dies. The necrotic bone lodges bacteria which proliferate freely, protected from leucocytes unable to reach them through this avascular material. In the surrounding tissue, inflammation usually localises infection to the socket walls. Dead bone is gradually separated by osteo-

clasts, and sequestra are usually shed in tiny fragments. Healing is by granulation from the base and walls of the socket.

Prevention

Since damage to bone appears to be an important predisposing factor, clearly extractions should be carried out with minimal trauma. Immediately after the extraction the socket edges should be squeezed firmly together and held for a few minutes until the clot has formed. In the case of disimpactions of third molars, where alveolar osteitis is more common, prophylactic antibiotics are often given. Their value is unproven and there is no indication for using antibiotics for routine dental extractions. However, in patients who have had irradiation for oral cancer or osteosclerotic Paget's disease where there is extensive infection, antibiotic cover should be given and the tooth removed surgically, with as little damage as possible to surrounding bone.

There remain a few patients who otherwise appear to be well but are especially prone to alveolar osteitis which follows every extraction under local anaesthesia, including regional blocks. In such patients, dry socket may be preventable if general anaesthesia is used.

Treatment

Local conditions strongly favour persistence of infection, and it is more surprising that the infection is well localised than that it responds poorly to treatment. It is important to explain this to patients and to warn them that they may have a week or more of discomfort. It is also important to explain that the pain is not due, as patients usually think, to a broken root.

Treatment should aim to keep the open socket clean and to protect exposed bone. The socket should be irrigated with mild warm antiseptic, then filled with an obtundant dressing containing some non-irritant antiseptic to prevent food and debris from accumulating. This should be followed by frequent use of hot mouth rinses. Many socket dressings have been formulated but a convenient proprietary preparation is Alvogel. It is easy to manipulate and patients report that it gives a sensation of warmth in place of the pain. Apart from being obtundant and antiseptic, the socket dressing should preferably be soft, adhere to the socket wall and be absorbable. Non-absorbable dressings must be removed as soon as possible to allow the socket to heal. Most cases become free from pain after one or two dressings.

Key features of alveolar osteitis are summarised in Table 6.6.

FASCIAL SPACE INFECTIONS (CERVICOFACIAL CELLULITIS)

Deep fascial space infections cause gross inflammatory exudate and tissue oedema, associated with fever and toxaemia. Before the advent of antibiotics the mortality was high and the disease

Table 6.6 **Alveolar osteitis — key features**

- The most common painful complication of dental extractions
- Loss of clot normally filling extraction socket
- Loss of clot may be due to excessive local fibrinolytic action or bacterial enzymes, or both
- Bare, whitish lamina dura exposed in socket
- Pain relieved by irrigation and repeated dressing of socket
- Dead bone usually shed as crumb-like fragments
- Eventual healing of socket from its base by granulation

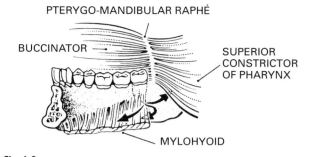

Fig. 6.8 Paths of infection from the third molar. The diagram shows the lingual aspect of the jaw and indicates how infection penetrating from the lingual plate of bone can enter the sublingual space above, or the submandibular space below, the mylohyoid muscle which forms the major structure of the floor of the mouth. Moreover, since this point is at the junction of the oral cavity and pharynx, infection can also spread backwards to reach the lateral surface of superior constrictor, i.e. the lateral pharyngeal space.

Fig. 6.9 Cellulitis. Infection spreading through the tissues is accompanied by a dense infiltrate of neutrophils, here separating muscle bundles in a facial muscle.

Fig. 6.7 Paths of infection spread from lower molars. By penetrating the lingual plate of the jaw below the attachment of mylohyoid (C) infection immediately enters the submandibular space (A). Below the mylohyoid is the main body of the submandibular salivary gland with its deep process curving around the posterior border of the muscle; infection from the third molar can follow the same route to enter the sublingual space (B).

is still life-threatening if treatment is delayed. The main types are sublingual, submandibular (Fig. 6.7) and parapharyngeal. *Ludwig's angina* involves several of these regions.

The characteristic features are diffuse swelling, pain, fever and malaise. The swelling is tense and tender, with a characteristic board-like firmness. The overlying skin is taut and shiny. Pain and oedema limit opening the mouth and often cause dysphagia. Systemic upset is severe, with worsening fever, toxaemia and leucocytosis. The regional lymph nodes are swollen and tender.

In Ludwig's angina particularly, airway obstruction can quickly result in asphyxia.

Pathology

Anaerobic bacteria are primarily responsible and infection mainly spreads from mandibular third molars whose apices are closely related to several fascial spaces (Figs 6.7 and 6.8). Fasciae covering muscles and other structures are normally adherent but can be spread apart by inflammatory exudate. Spaces created in this way are almost avascular and inflammatory exudate carries bacteria widely through them (Fig. 6.9).

Ludwig's angina is a severe form of cellulitis which usually arises from the lower second or third molars. It involves the sublingual and submandibular spaces bilaterally almost simultaneously; it readily spreads into the lateral pharyngeal and pterygoid spaces and can extend into the mediastinum.

The main features are rapidly spreading sublingual and submaxillary cellulitis with painful, brawny swelling of the upper part of the neck and the floor of the mouth on both sides (Fig. 6.10). With involvement of the parapharyngeal space, the swelling tracks down the neck (Figs 6.11 and 6.12), and oedema can quickly spread to the glottis.

Fig. 6.10 Ludwig's angina. Incision and drainage of the front of the neck relieve the pressure of exudate which compromises the airway. The neck is grossly swollen, shiny and dusky in hue; the edges of the wound have pulled apart, indicating the distension of these normally lax tissues.

Fig. 6.12 Ludwig's angina. There is cellulitis and gross oedema of the right submandibular and sublingual spaces extending on to the left side and into the neck and parapharyngeal space. (By kind permission of Professor J D Langdon.)

Fig. 6.11 Facial cellulitis arising from an infected upper tooth. The tissues are red, tense and shiny and the patient is incapacitated by the systemic effects of infection. (By kind permission of Professor J D Langdon.)

Table 6.7 Fascial space infections — key features
• Potentially life-threatening infections due to spread of bacteria into perioral fascial spaces
• Infection usually arises from lower second or third molars
• Ludwig's angina comprises bilateral involvement of sublingual and submandibular spaces and readily spreads into lateral pharyngea and pterygoid spaces
• Affected tissues swollen and of board-like hardness
• Severe systemic upset associated
• Glottic oedema or spread into the mediastinum may be fatal

Swallowing and opening the mouth become difficult, and the tongue may be pushed up against the soft palate. The latter or oedema of the glottis causes worsening respiratory obstruction. The patient soon becomes desperately ill, with fever, respiratory distress, headache and malaise.

Management

The main requirements are immediate admission to hospital, procurement of a sample for culture and sensitivity testing, aggressive antibiotic treatment, securement of the airway by tracheostomy if necessary, and drainage of the swelling to reduce pressure.

Key features of fascial space infections are summarised in Table 6.7.

CAVERNOUS SINUS THROMBOSIS

Cavernous sinus thrombosis is an uncommon life-threatening complication of infection that can sometimes originate from an upper anterior tooth. Blindness or death can result.

Clinically, gross oedema of the eyelid is associated with pulsatile exophthalmos due to venous obstruction. Cyanosis, proptosis, a fixed dilated pupil and limited eye movement rapidly develop. The patient is seriously ill with rigors, a high swinging fever and deteriorating sight.

Early recognition and treatment of cavernous sinus thrombosis is essential. The main measures are antibiotics, drainage of pus and possibly anticoagulant treatment. There is a 50% mortality and 50% of survivors may lose the sight of one or both eyes.

CANCRUM ORIS (NOMA)

Cancrum oris is a gangrenous infection spreading outwards from the mouth to cause extensive facial destruction and, often, a fatal outcome. It has virtually disappeared from developed countries but is still seen in some areas, particularly parts of Africa.

Children under the age of 10 years with poor resistance due to protein-calorie malnutrition, anaemia or infections such as measles, and poor oral hygiene are the main victims.

Cancrum oris starts in the oral cavity as an acute ulcerative gingivitis associated with gross oedema but extends outwards, rapidly destroying soft tissues and bone (Fig. 6.13). Diffuse oedema of the face, foetor and profuse salivation are associated.

Muscle, invaded by spirochaetes and fusiform bacteria, undergoes rapid necrosis associated with a weak inflammatory response (Fig. 6.14). Gangrene causes the skin to turn blue-black and the area becomes increasingly sharply demarcated,

and ultimately sloughs away. As the slough separates, the bone becomes necrotic; sequestration and exfoliation of teeth follow and, in survivors, a gaping facial defect is left (Fig. 6.15).

Management

Essential measures are control of malnutrition or underlying systemic infections, antibiotic treatment (typically with penicillin and metronidazole) and reconstructive surgery once the lesions have fully healed.

ACTINOMYCOSIS

Actinomycosis is a chronic, suppurative infection caused by a filamentous bacterium, usually *Actinomyces israelii*. Though common in the past, it has become rare.

Bacteria causing actinomycosis are common in the normal mouth. Injuries, especially dental extractions or fractures of the jaw, can provide a pathway and sometimes precede infection, but in fact rarely do so. Most patients were previously healthy and it is uncommon even in patients with AIDS. The pathogenesis is therefore unclear.

Clinically, men are predominantly affected, typically between the ages of 30 and 60 years. A chronic soft-tissue swelling near the angle of the jaw in the upper neck is the usual complaint. The swelling is dusky-red or purplish, firm and slightly tender. The skin eventually breaks down as discharging sinuses form. There is often difficulty in opening the mouth but

Fig. 6.13 Cancrum oris. In the maxilla there is extension of necrotising gingivitis into the alveolar process and in the lower arch anteriorly, resulting in destruction of much of the lower lip.

Fig. 6.14 Cancrum oris. Muscle has been invaded by spirochaetes and fusiforms. There is rapid necrosis and only a light inflammatory response of neutrophils.

Fig. 6.15 Cancrum oris. Gross destruction and sloughing of facial tissues as a result of spread of infection from the maxillary gingivae. A molar tooth is visible centrally in the defect. (By kind permission of Professor R D Emslie.)

pain is minimal. Healing leads to scarring and puckering of the skin and, in the absence of treatment, a large fibrotic mass can form, covered by scarred and pigmented skin, on which several sinuses open. However, such a picture is rarely now seen. Currently, the usual clinical features are a persistent subcutaneous collection of pus or a sinus, unresponsive to conventional, short courses of antibiotics.

Pathology

A. israelii spreads by direct extension through the tissues and causes chronic suppurative inflammation. In the tissues, colonies of actinomyces form rounded masses of filaments with peripheral, radially-arranged club-shaped thickenings. Neutrophils mass round the colonies; pus forms centrally, chronic inflammatory cells surround the focus and an abscess wall of connective tissue forms (Fig. 6.16).

The abscess eventually points on the skin, discharging pus in which so-called sulphur granules (colonies of actinomyces) may be visible. The abscess continues to discharge and surrounding tissues become fibrotic. Nevertheless, infection spreads to cause further abscesses. Untreated, the area can become honeycombed with abscesses and sinuses and widespread fibrosis.

Management

Actinomycosis should be suspected if a skin sinus fails to heal

Fig. 6.16 Actinomycosis. This single, complete loculus was from an early case of actinomycosis that followed dental extraction. The colony of actinomyces with its paler staining periphery (a sulphur granule) is in the centre; around it is a dense collection of inflammatory cells, surrounded in turn by proliferating fibrous tissue. It will be apparent that an antibiotic cannot readily penetrate such a fibrous mass and must be given in large doses to be effective.

after a possible focus has been found and eliminated. A fresh specimen of pus is needed. A positive diagnosis can rarely be made without sulphur granules, which may be found by rinsing the pus with sterile saline. The laboratory should be warned that actinomycosis is suspected, to enable appropriate media to be used and the culture maintained long enough for these slow-growing organisms to grow.

Frequently, small amounts of penicillin have been given earlier. These are insufficient to control the infection but make bacteriological diagnosis difficult.

The mainstay of treatment is penicillin, which should be continued from 4 to 6 weeks or occasionally longer, as pockets of surviving organisms may persist in the depths of the lesion and cause relapse. Abscesses should be drained surgically as they form. For patients allergic to penicillin, erythromycin can be given.

THE DEEP MYCOSES

The deep mycoses are rare in Britain but are seen in immunocompromised patients or in those from endemic areas such as South America. Though superficial candidosis is common, there are surprisingly few reports of oral lesions due to deep mycoses in AIDS patients. Cryptococcosis is the most common mycosis in AIDS and is sometimes the presenting symptom.

Clinically, most of the deep mycoses can cause oral lesions at some stage, and often then give rise to a nodular and ulcerated mass, which can be tumour-like in appearance (Table 6.8).

Table 6.8   Some deep mycoses that can affect the mouth
Histoplasmosis Rhinocerebral mucormycosis Rhinocerebral aspergillosis Cryptococcosis Paracoccidioidomycosis (South American blastomycosis)

Microscopically, most deep mycoses give rise to granulomas similar to those of tuberculosis but there may be abscess formation. Characteristic yeast forms or hyphae may sometimes be seen with special stains such as PAS (Figs 6.17–6.19), but microscopy may not be diagnostic and culture of unfixed material may be necessary.

Treatment

Amphotericin remains the most generally effective drug for most deep mycoses but given intravenously can cause renal damage and severe hypersensitivity reactions. Liposomal amphotericin is less toxic and as effective. Ketoconazole and its analogues have mainly been used for maintenance.

Fig. 6.17 Histoplasmosis. Part of an oral biopsy under high power, showing typical round yeast forms with their clear haloes (PAS stain).

Fig. 6.18 Aspergillosis. Tissue densely infiltrated by aspergillus hyphae. In this section stained with PAS stain the septate hyphae appear as unstained tubes with a red PAS-positive wall.

Fig. 6.19 Mucormycosis. Necrotic tissue infiltrated by the broad, knobbly branching hyphae of *Mucor* sp.

SYSTEMIC INFECTIONS BY ORAL BACTERIA

The mouth harbours a great variety of microbes and virulent pathogens, particularly in periodontal pockets, but has high levels of local immunity. Oral bacteria, even some such as *Leptotrichia buccalis*, which were long thought to be harmless, once they reach the bloodstream of immunocompromised patients can cause septicaemias, which can be fatal.

Infective endocarditis

A special example of a systemic infection of dental origin is infective endocarditis, which can occasionally follow dental operations, particularly extractions, and cause irreparable damage to heart valves (Ch. 27).

Lung and brain abscesses

Some of these abscesses are due to oral anaerobic bacteria which are probably aspirated during sleep to cause a lung abscess and a secondary brain abscesses. Isolated brain abscesses caused by oral bacteria are recognised but difficult to explain.

Immunodeficiency states

In severe immunodeficiency states, such as immunosuppression for organ transplants, lymphoreticular diseases or neutropenia due to cytotoxic chemotherapy, bacteraemias of oral origin can sometimes cause septicaemias. Viridans streptococcal bacteraemia is a recognised complication of neutropenia, but is not due to dental manipulations. Mucosal ulceration due to cytotoxic drugs is believed to be the portal of entry.

If antibiotic cover is thought necessary for dental operations, particularly extractions or periodontal treatment, a combination of amoxycillin 3 g plus metronidazole 400 mg by mouth, 1 hour before operations, may possibly offer some protection and can be repeated 6 hours later, if thought desirable. However, there is no definitive prophylactic regimen, as the causes are varied and unpredictable.

Prosthetic joint replacements

There is no evidence of a significant risk of infection of prosthetic joints from dental operations.

SUGGESTED FURTHER READING

Bochud P-Y, Clandra T, Francioli P 1994 Bacteremia due to viridans streptococci in neutropenic patients: a review. Am J Med 97:256
Cawson R A, Binnie W H, Eveson J W 1994 Color atlas of oral disease, 2nd edn. Mosby-Wolfe, London.
Cawson R A, Langdon J D, Eveson J W 1996 Surgical pathology of the mouth and jaws. Wright, Oxford
Chow A W 1992 Life-threatening infections of the head and neck. Clin Infect Dis 14:991–1004
Cohen M E, Simecek J W 1995 Effects of gender-related factors on the incidence of localized alveolar osteitis. Oral Surg Oral Med Oral Pathol Oral. Radiol Endod 79:416–422
Diamond R D 1991 The growing problem of mycoses in patients

SUGGESTED FURTHER READING (*cont'd*)

infected with the human immunodeficiency virus. Rev Infect Dis 13:480–486

Glueck C J, McMahon R E, Bouquot J et al 1996 Thrombophilia, hypofibrinolysis, and alveolar osteonecrosis of the jaws. Oral Surg Oral Med Oral Pathol Oral Radiol Endod 81:557–566

Griffin J M, Bach D E, Nespeca J A, Marshall K J 1983 Noma. Report of two cases. Oral Surg 56:605–607

Har-El G, Aroesty J H, Shaha A, Lucente F E 1994 Changing trends in deep neck abscess. A retrospective study of 110 patients. Oral Surg Oral Med Oral Pathol 77:446–450

Indresano A T, Haug R H, Hoffman M J 1992 The third molar as a cause of deep space infections. J Oral Maxillofac Surg 50:33–35

Jansma J, Vissink A, Spijkervet F K L et al 1992 Protocol for the prevention and treatment of oral sequelae resulting from head and neck radiation therapy. Cancer 70:2171

Koorbusch G F, Fotos P, Goll T K 1992 Retrospective study of osteomyelitis. Etiology, demographics, risk factors and management in 35 cases. Oral Surg Oral Med Oral Pathol 74:149–154

McDonnell D 1993 Dense bone islands. A review of 107 patients. Oral Surg Oral Med Oral Pathol 76:124–128

Maximew W G, Wood R E, Liu F-F 1991 Postradiation dental extractions without hyperbaric oxygen. Oral Surg Oral Med Oral Pathol 72:270–274

Ogundiya D A, Keith D A, Mirowski J 1989 Cavernous sinus thrombosis and blindness as a complication of an odontogenic infection. Report of a case and review of the literature. J Oral Maxillofac Surg 47:1317

Pascale R Del Valle G A, Moreau P et al 1995 Viridans streptococcal bacteraemia in patients with neutropenia. Lancet 345:1607–1609

Peterson L J. Contemporary management of deep neck infections. J Oral Maxillofac Surg 51:226–231

Richard P, Del Valle G A, Moreau P et al 1995 Viridans streptococcal bacteraemia in patients with neutropenia. Lancet 345:1607–1609

Scully C, de Almeida O 1992 Orofacial manifestations of the systemic mycoses. J Oral Pathol Med 21:289–294

Shroyer J V, Lew D, Abreo F, Unhold G P 1991 Osteomyelitis of the mandible as a result of sickle cell disease. Report and literature review. Oral Surg Oral Med Oral Pathol 72:25–28

Smithe O P, Prentice H G, Madden G M, Nazareth B 1990 Lingual cellulitis causing upper airways obstruction in neutropenic patients. BMJ 300:24

Sposto M R, Scully C, de Almeida O P, Jorge J, Graner E, Bozzo L 1993 Oral paracoccidioidomycosis. A study of 36 South American patients. Oral Surg Oral Med Oral Pathol 75:461–465

Sposto M R, Mendes-Giannini, Moraes M J, Branco F C, Scully C 1994 Paracoccidioidomycosis manifesting as oral lesions: clinical, cytological and serological investigation. J Oral Pathol Med 23:85–87

Tibbles P M, Edelsberg J S 1996 Hyperbaric oxygen therapy. New Engl J Med 334: 1642–1648

Van Merkensteyn J P R, Balm A J M, Bakker A J M, Borgmeyer-Hoelen A M M J 1994 Hyperbaric oxygen treatment of osteoradionecrosis of the mandible with repeated pathological fracture. Report of a case. Oral Surg Oral Med Oral Pathol 77:461–464

Cysts of the jaws

Cysts are the most common cause of chronic swellings of the jaws. They are more common in the jaws than in any other bone because of the many rests of odontogenic epithelium remaining in the tissues. Cysts formed from this epithelium (odontogenic cysts) account for most cysts of the jaws. By far the most common is the radicular (periodontal or 'dental') cyst.

> Cysts are pathological fluid-filled cavities lined by epithelium

Typical features of jaw cysts

Most jaw cysts behave similarly and usually grow slowly and expansively. They differ mainly in their relationship to a tooth, and the radiographic features are usually a good guide as to their nature (Table 7.1). Even when it is not possible to decide the nature of a cyst, this rarely affects treatment. However, it is particularly important to distinguish keratocysts and unicystic ameloblastomas from common types. These occasionally have identical radiographic appearances, and diagnosis ultimately depends on histopathology.

Table 7.1 Jaw cysts — key features

- Form sharply-defined radiolucencies with smooth borders
- Fluid may be aspirated and thin-walled cysts may be transilluminated
- Grow slowly, displacing rather than resorbing teeth
- Symptomless unless infected and are frequently chance radiographic findings
- Rarely large enough to cause pathological fracture
- Form compressible and fluctuant swellings if extending into soft tissues
- Appear bluish when close to the mucosal surface

The classification of cysts is summarised in Table 7.2. Odontogenic cysts (not surprisingly) affect the tooth-bearing region of the jaws. Most non-odontogenic, true cysts are devel-

opmental, and form in the region of the anterior maxilla. Their relative frequency is shown in Table 7.3, though figures in the different surveys vary as a result of differences in categorisation, what kinds of cysts are included, and other factors.

Table 7.2 Classification of cysts of the jaws

Odontogenic cysts
Developmental
  Dentigerous
  Eruption
  Odontogenic keratocysts
  Gingival
  Lateral periodontal
    Botryoid
Inflammatory
  Radicular
  Paradental
Neoplastic
  Cystic ameloblastomas
  Calcifying odontogenic
  (ghost cell) cyst

Non-odontogenic cysts
Nasopalatine duct cyst
Nasolabial cyst

Cysts without epithelial lining (Pseudocysts)
Solitary (simple) bone cyst
Aneurysmal bone cyst

Table 7.3 Relative frequency of different types of jaw cyst

Cysts	Frequency (%)
Radicular (periodontal)	65–70
Dentigerous	15–18
Keratocysts	3–5
Nasopalatine	5–10
Lateral periodontal	<1
Paradental	<1

Radicular cysts are discussed first, being the most common type, the treatment of which forms the basis for that of most other jaw cysts.

RADICULAR CYSTS

Clinical features

Radicular cysts are the most common cause of major, chronic swellings and the most common type of cyst of the jaws. They are rarely seen before the age of 10 and are most frequent between the ages of 20 and 60 years. They are more common in males than females, roughly in the proportion of 3 to 2. The maxilla is affected more than three times as frequently as the mandible.

Radicular cysts, like other cysts of the jaws, cause slowly progressive painless swellings, with no symptoms until they become large enough to be conspicuous (Fig. 7.1). If infection enters, the swelling becomes painful and may rapidly expand, partly due to inflammatory oedema. The swelling is rounded and at first hard. Later, when the bone has been reduced to eggshell thickness, a crackling sensation may be felt on pressure. Finally, part of the wall is entirely resorbed, leaving a soft fluctuant swelling, bluish in colour, beneath the mucous membrane. The dead tooth from which the cyst has originated is (by definition) present, and its relationship to the cyst will be apparent in a radiograph (Fig. 7.2).

> *Practical point* Always determine the vitality of teeth associated with a jaw cyst

Pathogenesis and pathology

The main factors responsible for cyst development are summarised in Table 7.4.

Fig. 7.1 Typical clinical appearance of a cyst. This radicular cyst in the right maxillary alveolar process forms a rounded swelling with a bluish colour.

Fig. 7.2 A radicular cyst on a grossly carious and non-vital first permanent molar. A rounded and sharply defined area of radiolucency is associated with the apices of the roots.

Table 7.4 **Major factors in the pathogenesis of cyst formation**

- Proliferation of epithelial lining and fibrous capsule
- Hydrostatic pressure of cyst fluid
- Resorption of surrounding bone

Epithelial proliferation

Infection from the pulp chamber induces inflammation and proliferation of the epithelial rests of Malassez. If infection can be eliminated from the root canal, small radicular cysts (up to 1 or 2 cm diameter) may regress without surgery.

Hydrostatic effects of cyst fluids

That radicular and many other cysts expand in balloon-like fashion, wherever the local anatomy permits, indicates that internal pressure is a factor in their growth. The hydrostatic pressure within cysts is about 70 cm of water and therefore higher than the capillary blood pressure. Cyst fluid is largely inflammatory exudate and contains high concentrations of proteins, some of high molecular weight which can exert osmotic pressure.

Consistent with the inflammation usually present in cyst walls, cyst fluid may contain cholesterol, breakdown products of blood cells, exfoliated epithelial cells, and fibrin.

The cyst wall does not seem to act entirely as a simple semipermeable membrane. Low molecular weight proteins are present in similar concentrations to those in the plasma but there are smaller amounts of high molecular weight proteins. The capillaries in the cyst wall are more permeable as a result of inflammation and contribute varying amounts of immunoglobulins and other proteins. The net effect is that pressure is created by osmotic tension within the cyst cavity.

CHAPTER 7

Bone-resorbing factors

Experimentally, cyst tissues in culture release bone-resorbing factors. These are predominantly prostaglandins E_2 and E_3. Different types of cysts and tumours may produce different quantities of prostaglandins but, if so, it is unclear whether this affects the mode of growth of the cyst. Collagenases are present in the walls of keratocysts, but their contribution to cyst growth is also unclear.

Pathology

All stages can be seen, from a periapical granuloma containing a few strands of proliferating epithelium derived from the epithelial rests of Malassez (Figs 7.3 and 7.4) to an enlarging cyst with a hyperplastic epithelial lining and dense inflammatory infiltrate. Epithelial proliferation results from irritant products leaking from an infected root canal to cause chronic periapical inflammation.

The epithelial lining consists of stratified squamous epithelium of variable thickness, but lacks a defined basal cell layer and is sometimes incomplete. Early, active epithelial proliferation is associated with obvious chronic inflammation and may then be thick, irregular and hyperplastic (Fig. 7.5) or appear net-like, forming rings and arcades (Fig. 7.6). Hyaline bodies may be seen in the epithelium (Fig. 7.7) and mucous cells are often present as a result of metaplasia (Fig. 7.8). Long-standing cysts typically have a thin flattened epithelial lining, a thick fibrous wall and minimal inflammatory infiltrate.

Fig. 7.4 A developing radicular cyst. An epithelium-lined cavity has formed in this large periapical granuloma. There is a thick fibrous capsule infiltrated by chronic inflammatory cells and containing a group of cholesterol clefts. The alveolar bone has been resorbed and remodelled to accommodate the slowly expanding swelling.

Fig. 7.5 Radicular cyst. At this early stage the epithelial lining is hyperplastic and there is a relatively dense inflammatory infiltrate.

Fig. 7.3 The earliest stages of formation of a radicular cyst. Some periapical granulomas, such as this, contain proliferating strands of odontogenic epithelium. In places the epithelium has broken down centrally to form small epithelium-lined spaces.

The cyst capsule and wall. The capsule consists of collagenous fibrous connective tissue. During active growth the capsule is vascular and infiltrated by chronic inflammatory cells adjacent to the proliferating epithelium. Plasma cells are often prominent or predominant, and are a response to antigens leaking through the tooth apex. In larger, more mature cysts the epithelial lining becomes flattened and inflammatory cells become progressively fewer. In the bony wall there is osteoclastic activity and resorption. Beyond the zone of resorption

Fig. 7.6 Higher power of the lining of a radicular cyst. The arcaded epithelium contains numerous neutrophils emigrating into the lumen and there are pale staining areas of foamy macrophages in the inner wall.

Fig. 7.7 Hyaline or Rushton bodies. These translucent or pink staining lamellar bodies are formed by the cyst lining epithelium and indicate the odontogenic origin of a cyst.

Fig. 7.8 Mucous metaplasia in a radicular cyst. In less inflamed cysts the lining epithelium may undergo metaplasia to a respiratory type of epithelium with goblet cells and cilia.

there is usually active bone formation. The net effect is that a cyst expands but retains a bony wall, even after it has extended beyond the normal bony contours. This bony wall nevertheless becomes progressively thinner, as repair is slower than resorption, until it forms a mere eggshell, then ultimately disappears altogether and the cyst starts to distend the soft tissues.

Clefts. Within the cyst capsule there are often areas split up by fine needle-shaped clefts (Figs 7.9 and 7.10). These are left by cholesterol dissolved out during preparation for sectioning. The cholesterol is derived from breakdown of blood cells. Small clefts are enclosed by foreign body giant cells, and extravasated red cells and blood pigment are associated. Clefts may also be seen extending into the cyst contents but are formed in the cyst wall.

Cyst fluid. The fluid is usually watery and opalescent or sometimes more viscid and yellowish, and sometimes shimmers with cholesterol crystals. A smear of this fluid may show typical notched cholesterol crystals microscopically (Fig. 7.11). Histologically, the protein content of the fluid is usually seen as amorphous eosinophilic material, often containing broken-down leukocytes and cells distended with fat globules.

Radiography

A radicular cyst appears as a rounded, radiolucent area with a

Fig. 7.9 Cholesterol clefts in a cyst wall. This low power view shows the relationship of cholesterol clefts to the cyst. Cholesterol crystals are formed in the fibrous wall. The epithelium overlying this focus has broken down and the cholesterol leaks into the cyst contents. Elsewhere the lumen is lined by a flattened layer of squamous epithelium.

Fig. 7.10 Cholesterol clefts. Cholesterol has been dissolved out during preparation of the slide, leaving clefts. The crystals are treated as foreign bodies and flattened multinucleate foreign body giant cells are seen along the edges of several clefts.

Fig. 7.11 Cholesterol crystals from a cyst aspirate indicating the presence of inflammation. The rectangular shape with a notched corner is characteristic.

Table 7.5   Radicular cysts — key features

- Form in bone in relation to the root of a non-vital tooth
- Arise by epithelial proliferation in an apical granuloma
- Are usually asymptomatic unless infected
- Diagnosis is by the combination of radiographic appearances, a non-vital tooth and appropriate histological appearances
- Clinical and radiographic features are usually adequate for planning treatment
- Do not recur after competent enucleation
- Residual cysts can remain after the causative tooth has been extracted and diagnosis is then less obvious
- Cholesterol crystals often seen in the cyst fluid but not specific to radicular cysts

Fig. 7.12   Residual cyst. The causative tooth has been extracted leaving the cyst in situ. See also Figure 7.13.

Fig. 7.13   Radiographic appearance of the residual cyst shown in Figure 7.12. Note the thin bulging periosteal new bone layer which can give rise to the clinical sign of eggshell crackling. (Figures 7.12 and 7.13 kindly lent by Mr P Robinson.)

sharply defined outline. A condensed radiopaque periphery is present only if growth is unusually slow and is usually more prominent in older patients. The dead tooth from which the cyst has arisen can be seen and often has a large carious cavity. Adjacent teeth may be tilted or displaced a little or occasionally become slightly mobile. Very large cysts in the maxilla may extend in any available direction and become irregular. Infection of a cyst causes the outline to become hazy as a result of greater vascularity and resorption of the surrounding bone. Key features of radicular cysts are summarised in Table 7.5.

Residual cysts

A radicular cyst may persist after extraction of the causative tooth. Residual cysts are a common cause of swelling of the edentulous jaw in older persons (Figs 7.12 and 7.13). Residual cysts may interfere with the fit of dentures, but may slowly regress spontaneously. This is suggested by the progressive thinning of the lining (Fig. 7.14).

Lateral radicular cysts

Lateral radicular cysts rarely form at the side of a non-vital tooth as a result of the opening of a lateral branch of the root canal.

Fig. 7.14 Lining of a residual cyst. There is only a minor degree of inflammation and the epithelium forms a thin regular layer.

Differential diagnosis

There are many causes of circumscribed areas of radiolucency in the jaws (Table 7.6).

Table 7.6 Differential diagnosis of cyst-like areas of radiolucency
• Anatomical structures (maxillary antrum and foramina) • Cysts of other types and pseudocysts • Neoplasms, particularly ameloblastoma (Ch. 8) • Giant cell granuloma of the jaws (Ch. 9) • Hyperparathyroidism (Ch. 10) • Cherubism (Ch. 10)

Radicular cysts are usually readily recognised by their clinical and radiographic features. The cystic nature of a lesion can be confirmed by aspirating its contents via a needle inserted through the wall under aseptic conditions. The presence of fluid does not distinguish one cyst from another or a cystic neoplasm from a true cyst. The presence of cholesterol crystals is not of diagnostic significance.

Histologically, the lining of simple stratified squamous epithelium with an inflammatory infiltrate confirms the diagnosis. Distinguishing features of other types of cysts are discussed below.

Neoplasms. Benign (odontogenic) tumours, or occasionally an ameloblastoma, may appear radiographically as a simple cyst. It is essential that the whole of a cyst lining be available for examination, since part of the lining, even though neoplastic, may appear as a thin layer of flattened stratified squamous epithelium like that of a simple cyst. Resorption of adjacent teeth suggests a neoplasm rather than a cyst but is not diagnostic in itself. Rarely a secondary tumour of the jaw may cause a sharply-defined area of radiolucency. More often it causes a lesion with a hazy outline and irregular shape. Tumours also tend to be painful and to grow more rapidly than cysts. Nevertheless, it may be difficult or impossible to distinguish

them from infected cysts radiographically, but at operation the solid nature of a tumour will be obvious and histological examination will confirm the diagnosis.

Treatment

Enucleation and primary closure

Enucleation is the usual method and is generally entirely effective (Table 7.7). The affected (dead) tooth may be extracted or root-filled and preserved. A mucoperiosteal flap over the cyst is raised and a window is opened in the bone to give adequate access. The cyst is then carefully separated from its bony wall. The entire cyst is removed intact and should be sent in fixative for histological examination. The edges of the bone cavity are smoothed off, free bleeding is controlled and the cavity is irrigated to remove debris. The mucoperiosteal flap is replaced and sutured in place. The sutures should be left for at least 10 days.

Table 7.7 Advantages and limitations of enucleation of cysts	
Advantages	*Possible disadvantages*
• The cavity usually heals without complications • Little aftercare is necessary • A complete lining is available for histological examination	• Infection of the clot filling the cavity • Recurrence due to incomplete removal of the lining • Serious haemorrhage (primary or secondary) • Damage to apices of vital teeth projecting into the cyst cavity • Damage to the inferior dental nerve • Opening the antrum when enucleating a large maxillary cyst • Fracture of the jaw if an exceptionally large mandibular cyst is enucleated

The disadvantages are largely theoretical and in competent hands even very large cysts can be enucleated safely. Recurrence is remarkably rare. There are few contraindications: they are relative rather than absolute.

Marsupialisation

Marsupialisation is a largely outmoded treatment. The cyst is opened essentially as for enucleation but the lining is sutured to the mucous membrane at the margins of the opening. The aim is to produce a self-cleansing cavity which becomes, in effect, an invagination of the oral tissues. However, considerable aftercare is needed to keep the cavity clean. The cavity is initially packed with ribbon gauze, and after the margins have healed a plug or extension to a denture is made to close the opening. Food debris has to be regularly washed out, but once the cavity has filled up from the base and sides sufficiently to become self-cleansing the plug can be removed. The cavity usually becomes closed by regrowth of the surrounding tissue and restoration of the normal contour of the part. However, the orifice may close and the cyst reforms. Also the complete lining is not available for histological examination.

The main application of marsupialisation is for temporary decompression of exceptionally large cysts where fracture of the jaw is a risk. When enough new bone has formed, the cyst can be enucleated. Occasionally the tooth in a dentigerous cyst is needed and marsupialisation may allow it to erupt.

PARADENTAL CYSTS

Paradental cysts occasionally result from inflammation round partially erupted teeth, particularly mandibular third molars. They affect males predominantly, usually between the ages of 20 and 25 years. The affected tooth is vital but typically shows pericoronitis. Histologically the cyst resembles a radicular cyst, but for an intense inflammatory infiltrate in the wall.

Enucleation is effective.

DENTIGEROUS CYSTS

A dentigerous cyst surrounds the crown of a tooth and is a dilatation of the follicle (Figs 7.15 and 7.16). The cyst is attached to the neck of the tooth, prevents its eruption and may displace it for a considerable distance.

Clinical features

Dentigerous cysts are more than twice as common in males as females. They are uncommon in children and are most often found in patients between the ages of 20 and 50.

Fig. 7.16 An enucleated dentigerous cyst. The tooth lies with its crown within the cyst cavity and with the cyst wall attached round its neck. The fibrous wall of the cyst is thick and has shelled out cleanly from the surrounding tissues.

Like other cysts, uncomplicated dentigerous cysts cause no symptoms until the swelling becomes noticeable. Alternatively a dentigerous cyst may be a chance radiographic finding or may be found when the cause of a missing tooth is sought. Infection of a dentigerous cyst causes the usual symptoms of pain and accelerated swelling.

Radiography

The cavity is well circumscribed, rounded and unilocular and contains the crown of a tooth displaced from its normal position (Fig. 7.17). Occasionally there may be pseudoloculation as a result of trabeculation or ridging of the bony wall. The slow growth of dentigerous cysts usually results in a sclerotic bony outline and a well-defined cortex. The affected tooth is often displaced a considerable distance, and a third molar, for instance, may be pushed to the lower border of the mandible. Rarely, if the cyst remains unrecognised for a long period, the enclosed tooth may become resorbed (Fig. 7.18).

These features readily distinguish a dentigerous cyst from a radicular cyst. However, a keratocyst or ameloblastoma may occasionally envelop the crown of the tooth, and either of these may create the radiographic appearance of a dentigerous cyst.

Fig. 7.15 Dentigerous cyst. This cyst has been removed together with its associated tooth. The cyst surrounds the crown and is attached at the cementoenamel junction.

Fig. 7.17 Dentigerous cyst. The cyst has developed around the crown of the buried third molar (left), but has extended forward to involve the root of a vital second molar. It should not, however, be confused with a radicular cyst arising from the latter.

Fig. 7.18   Resorption of tooth associated with a dentigerous cyst. The crown of this buried canine within the cyst shows resorption. This is unusual and is seen only in long-neglected cysts, as in this otherwise edentulous patient.

The diagnosis ultimately therefore depends on histological examination.

> Dentigerous cysts contain the crown of an unerupted tooth and have an epithelial lining, derived from enamel epithelium, attached to the tooth at the amelodentinal junction

Pathogenesis and pathology

Attachment of the cyst lining at or near the amelocemental junction suggests that dentigerous cysts arise as a result of cystic change in the remains of the enamel organ after enamel formation is complete. Division between the remnants of the internal enamel epithelium covering the enamel and the external enamel epithelium, forming the greater part of the cyst lining, can occasionally be seen at the attachment of the cyst to the neck of the tooth (Figs 7.19 and 7.20).

Progressive growth of the cyst leads to dilatation of the dental follicle. Factors triggering these changes are not known. However, there is a strong association between failure of eruption of teeth and formation of dentigerous cysts, which predominantly affect teeth that are particularly prone to failure of eruption, namely, maxillary canines and mandibular third molars in particular.

Fig. 7.19   Dentigerous cyst. The cyst surrounds the crown of this molar and the wall is attached to its cementoenamel junction. There is a uniform, thin epithelial lining with minimal inflammatory infiltrate. Cholesterol clefts are numerous in the lumen, a result of the formation of cholesterol crystals in the wall.

Fig. 7.20   Dentigerous cyst. To the left is the dentine (D). E is the enamel space left after decalcification and is separated from the cyst cavity (C) by a thin layer left by the inner enamel epithelium. The cyst itself appears to have formed as a result of accumulation of fluid between the inner and outer enamel epithelium and by continued proliferation of the latter to form the cyst lining, which joins the tooth at the epithelial attachment.

The lining of dentigerous cysts typically consists of thin, sometimes bilaminar, stratified epithelial cells and, frequently, numerous mucous cells (Fig. 7.21). This epithelium may occasionally keratinise by metaplasia. The fibrous wall is similar to

Fig. 7.21 Section through the full thickness of the wall of a dentigerous cyst. There is minimal inflammation and the epithelium is only two or three cells thick. Beyond the fibrous tissue the outermost layer of the wall is formed by woven bone, a feature common to most types of intraosseous cyst.

Fig. 7.22 Dentigerous cyst. In this uncomplicated cyst there is no inflammation and the wall comprises a layer of fibrous tissue lined by a thin layer of stratified squamous epithelium.

that of radicular cysts but inflammatory changes are typically absent (Fig. 7.22).

Treatment principles

If the tooth is in a favourable position and space is available, it may occasionally be possible to marsupialise a dentigerous cyst to allow the tooth to erupt. Alternatively the tooth can be transplanted to the alveolar ridge or extracted, as appropriate, and the cyst enucleated. Key features of dentigerous cysts are summarised in Table 7.8.

Table 7.8 Dentigerous cysts — key features

- Arise in bone and contain the crown of an unerupted tooth which is usually displaced
- Are most frequently associated with unerupted third molars and canines
- Clinical and radiographic features usually provide an accurate preoperative diagnosis but confirmation is histological
- May be mistaken radiographically for an odontogenic keratocyst or ameloblastoma
- Respond to enucleation or marsupialisation and do not recur after treatment

ERUPTION CYST

An eruption cyst occasionally forms over a tooth about to erupt. Strictly speaking an eruption cyst is a soft-tissue cyst but probably arises from enamel organ epithelium after enamel formation is complete, and is, in effect, a superficial dentigerous cyst.

Clinical features

Eruption cysts affect children and involve teeth having no predecessors (deciduous teeth or permanent molars). The cyst lies superficially in the gingiva overlying the unerupted tooth and appears as a soft, rounded, bluish swelling (Fig. 7.23). The epithelial lining is separated from the alveolar mucosa by a thin layer of fibrous tissue (Fig. 7.24).

Management

The cyst roof may be removed to allow the tooth to erupt, but most eruption cysts probably burst spontaneously and never come to surgery.

Fig. 7.23 An eruption cyst over an erupting upper molar. There has been bleeding into the cyst cavity as a result of trauma.

Fig. 7.24 Roof of an eruption cyst. At the upper surface is the keratinised epithelium of the alveolar ridge and, below, separated by a thin layer of relatively uninflamed fibrous tissue, the lining of an eruption cyst.

Fig. 7.25 Odontogenic keratocyst. Part of a panoramic tomogram showing typical appearances. The cyst is multilocular and has extended a considerable distance along the medullary cavity without appreciable expansion or displacement of the teeth.

ODONTOGENIC KERATOCYSTS

Keratocysts are uncommon but important because of their strong tendency — unlike other cysts — to recur after removal.

Clinical features

Most series have recorded a peak incidence between ages 20 to 30 but other large series have shown additional peaks between 50 and 70 years. The mandible is usually affected. At least 50% of keratocysts form in the angle of the mandible, extending forwards into the body and upwards into the ramus. Keratocysts, like other jaw cysts, are symptomless until the bone is expanded or they become infected. The main difference is that expansion of the jaw is much less than the radiographic extent of the cyst. Hence clinical signs often fail to appear until the cyst is well advanced, and relatively extensive cysts are occasionally found by chance on radiography.

Radiography

Keratocysts appear as well-defined radiolucent areas, either more or less rounded with a scalloped margin or multiloculated and simulating an ameloblastoma (Fig. 7.25). The bony wall appears sharply demarcated. Occasionally, a keratocyst may envelop an unerupted tooth and be indistinguishable radiographically from a dentigerous cyst. Roots of adjacent teeth may become displaced.

Key features of keratocysts are summarised in Table 7.9.

Pathogenesis and pathology

Keratocysts probably arise from any of the primordial epithelia (the dental lamina or its remains) or, as originally believed, from the enamel organ before tooth formation. However, it is difficult to reconcile such origins with the appearance of kera-

Table 7.9 Odontogenic keratocysts — key features

- Usually multilocular
- Form intraosseously, most frequently in the posterior alveolar ridge or angle of mandible
- May grow round a tooth
- Spread extensively along marrow spaces before expanding the jaw
- Frequently recur after enucleation
- Do not respond to marsupialisation
- Definitive diagnosis only by histopathology, although clinical and radiographic features may allow fairly accurate preoperative diagnosis
- May be easily confused with ameloblastoma or, less likely, with dentigerous cysts
- May be part of the jaw cyst/basal cell naevus syndrome

tocysts in middle age and their relatively rapid epithelial turnover. The aetiology of keratocysts is therefore speculative.

Radioactive labelling used to estimate mitotic activity suggests that keratocyst lining may be proliferating more actively than mucosal epithelium. Mural growth therefore appears to be more important in the enlargement of keratocysts than osmotic pressure exerted by the cyst's contents. This active mural growth and epithelial proliferation is probably a factor determining the frequency with which keratocysts recur.

Two types of keratocyst are recognised. They have slightly different demographic characteristics (Table 7.10) but the important difference is that parakeratotic cysts are far more likely to recur than orthokeratotic cysts. The histological appearances of the lining of keratocysts are characteristic (Table 7.11). If inflammation becomes superimposed the epithelial lining can lose its characteristic features and come to resemble that of a radicular cyst (Fig. 7.29).

Growth of keratocysts is by extension of finger-like processes into marrow spaces rather than by expansion. Growth of the

Table 7.10 Important features of keratocysts

Feature	Parakeratotic	Orthokeratotic
Relative frequency (%) (approximate)	88	12
Sex (%)		
Male (overall 61.5%)	62%	57%
Female (overall 38.5%)	38%	43%
Age at presentation (years)	34	40
Association with impacted tooth (%)	48	76
Midline location (%)	6	16
Pain (%)	15	9
Radiographic appearance	Usually multilocular	Frequently monolocular
Recurrence rate (%)	43	4

Table 7.11 Typical histological features of keratocysts

- Epithelial lining of uniform thickness
- Flat lower border of epithelium
- Clearly-defined basal layer of tall cells in parakeratinised cysts (Fig. 7.26)
- Thin eosinophilic layer of prekeratin in parakeratinised cysts
- Cyst lining typically much folded (Fig. 7.27)
- Epithelial lining weakly attached to the fibrous wall
- Abundant orthokeratin formation and well-defined granular cell layer in orthokeratinised cysts (Fig. 7.28)
- Thin fibrous wall
- Inflammatory cells typically absent or scanty

Fig. 7.26 Odontogenic keratocyst. High power showing the typical features of the epithelial lining: a flat basement membrane; elongated palisaded basal cells; 10–20 cells in thickness and with a corrugated parakeratotic surface.

wall, being greater than expansion of the cyst cavity, causes the lining to become much folded.

Management

The diagnosis should preferably be confirmed before operation, both to exclude an ameloblastoma and also because of the problem of removing keratocysts entirely.

Aspiration is unlikely to be helpful. Squames in the cyst fluid

Fig. 7.27 Odontogenic keratocyst. Folding of the wall and separation of the epithelium from the connective tissue wall are characteristic features.

Fig. 7.28 Odontogenic keratocyst. In this orthokeratinised variant there is a thick layer of keratin at the epithelial surface and filling the lumen.

Fig. 7.29 Inflamed odontogenic keratocyst. Around the periphery the cyst shows the typical features of a thin, uninflamed fibrous wall and regular epithelium with a flat basement membrane but, centrally, inflammation in a mural nodule has resulted in loss of typical features and hyperplastic strands of non-keratinised epithelium have formed.

Table 7.12 Possible reasons for recurrence of keratocysts

- Thin, fragile linings, difficult to enucleate intact
- Finger-like cyst extensions into cancellous bone
- Daughter cysts sometimes present in the wall
- More rapid proliferation of keratocyst epithelium
- Other dental lamina remnants may produce another keratocyst (pseudorecurrence)
- Inferior standard of surgical treatment

are not in themselves diagnostic as other cysts can form keratin and, very rarely, a carcinoma with cystic change may shed squames into its interior.

Keratocyst fluid has a low soluble protein content but, in practice, biopsy confirms the diagnosis more reliably and quickly.

On confirmation of the diagnosis, treatment should be by complete enucleation. This is usually difficult as the lining is friable (particularly if inflamed) but treatment should be thorough, to try to be certain that every fragment of lining has been removed.

Recurrence

Recurrence rates of up to 60% have been reported, but are affected by various factors (Table 7.12).

A major factor leading to recurrence is the difficulty in removing every trace of the epithelial lining. Its more vigorous proliferative activity compared with that of other cyst linings may allow a few remaining epithelial cells to readily form another cyst. Formation of another cyst from other dental lamina remnants is not strictly a recurrence but the fact that recurrences can appear up to 40 years after enucleation suggests this may happen. Otherwise recurrence is often within the first 5 years after treatment. Vigorous treatment is likely to reduce the risk of recurrence, but there is no absolute certainty of a cure and patients should be followed up with regular radiographic examinations.

The syndrome of multiple jaw cysts and basal cell carcinomas

This syndrome, often called the Gorlin–Goltz syndrome, is heritable as an autosomal dominant trait (Table 7.13).

Table 7.13 Gorlin–Goltz syndrome — key features

- Characteristic facies with frontal and parietal bossing and broad nasal root (Fig. 7.30)
- Multiple keratocysts of the jaws (Figs 7.31 and 7.32)
- Multiple, naevoid basal cell carcinomas of the skin
- Skeletal anomalies (usually of a minor nature) such as bifid ribs and abnormalities of the vertebrae
- Intracranial anomalies may include calcification of the falx cerebri and abnormally-shaped sella turcica

A great variety of other abnormalities may be present, and effects on the patient depend on the predominant manifestation.

Fig. 7.30 Basal cell naevus (Gorlin's syndrome). The typical facies with a broad nasal root and mild frontal bossing.

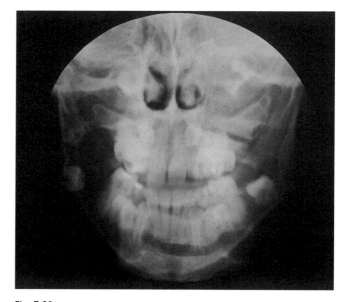

Fig. 7.31 PA jaws of the same patient with the basal cell naevus (Gorlin's) syndrome shown in Figure 7.30. Odontogenic keratocysts are present in the ramus and angle of the mandible on both sides, that on the right causing significant expansion.

Thus in some cases there are innumerable basal cell carcinomas. Though termed 'naevoid', these tumours differ from typical basal carcinomas only in their early onset. Other patients have many jaw cysts, necessitating repeated operations. The importance of this syndrome, from the dental viewpoint, is to warn the patient of the likelihood of development of further cysts, which must be dealt with by orthodox means as they arise. If neglected, these cysts can cause complications, like

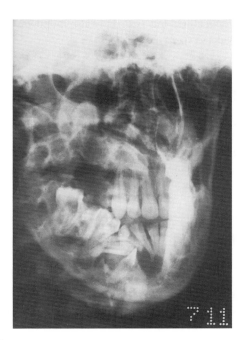

Fig. 7.32   Oblique lateral radiograph of a patient with the basal cell naevus (Gorlin's) syndrome. A very large odontogenic keratocyst involves the whole ramus and body, causing considerable expansion, especially at the lower border.

Fig. 7.34   Gingival cyst of the new born (Bohn's nodules). This section from an embryo shows cyst formation in the rests of Serres superficial to the developing teeth. The cysts are lined by keratinising epithelium.

Fig. 7.33   Odontogenic keratocyst in the basal cell naevus syndrome. Although the cysts in syndrome patients are often indistinguishable from typical odontogenic keratocysts, there may be extensive islands of epithelium in the cyst wall and many daughter cysts.

Fig. 7.35   Gingival cyst of adult. Typical presentation as a superficial cyst in the attached gingiva of a premolar tooth.

other jaw cysts. Structurally the cysts, like other keratocysts, are more common in the body or ramus of the mandible. Otherwise they are rarely distinguishable but may have many daughter cysts in the walls (Fig. 7.33).

GINGIVAL CYSTS

Dental lamina cyst of the newborn (Bohn's nodules)

Up to 80% of newborn infants have small nodules or cysts in the gingivae, due to proliferation of the epithelial rests of Serres (Fig. 7.34).

Cysts (Epstein's pearls) may also arise from non-odontogenic epithelium along the midpalatine raphe. These may enlarge sufficiently to appear as creamy-coloured swellings a few millimetres in diameter, but they also resolve spontaneously in a matter of months.

Gingival cysts of adults

Gingival cysts are exceedingly rare. They usually form after the age of approximately 40. Clinically, they form dome-shaped swellings less than 1 cm in diameter and sometimes erode the underlying bone (Fig. 7.35). They are lined by very thin, flat, stratified squamous epithelium and may con-

Fig. 7.36 Lateral periodontal cyst. Typical radiographic appearance showing a well-demarcated rounded radiolucency between the roots of the lateral incisor and canine, the roots of which have been displaced.

tain fluid or layers of keratin. They do not recur after enucleation.

LATERAL PERIODONTAL CYSTS

These uncommon intraosseous cysts form beside a vital tooth. They are usually seen by chance in routine radiographs and resemble other odontogenic cysts, apart from their position beside a tooth (Fig. 7.36), near the crest of the ridge. They cause no symptoms unless they erode through the bone to extend into the gingiva.

Microscopically, the lining is squamous or cuboidal epithelium, frequently only one or two cells thick, but sometimes with focal thickenings. Some of the cells may have clear cytoplasm and resemble those seen in the dental lamina.

The cyst should be enucleated and the related tooth can be retained if healthy.

Botryoid odontogenic cyst

The botryoid odontogenic cyst is probably a variant of, and even more rare than, the lateral periodontal cyst. It typically affects the mandibular premolar to canine region in adults over 50.

Microscopically, it is typically multilocular with fine fibrous septa. The lining consists of flattened non-keratinised epithelium interspersed with clear, glycogen-containing cells and sporadic bud-like proliferations protruding into the cyst. It should be enucleated or conservatively excised as it has a strong tendency to recur.

Glandular odontogenic cyst

The glandular odontogenic cyst is another rare entity with many features in common with botryoid odontogenic cysts but there are pools of mucin and mucous cells in variable numbers

within the epithelium. It is frequently also multilocular and has a strong tendency to recur.

UNICYSTIC AMELOBLASTOMA

Most ameloblastomas contain microcysts but the unicystic variant has a lining of flattened tumour cells, which resemble those of non-neoplastic cysts, and a nodule of tumour in the wall or bulging into the lumen. Unicystic ameloblastomas frequently mimic dentigerous cysts radiographically (Ch. 8).

CALCIFYING ODONTOGENIC CYST

This uncommon lesion is probably a cystic neoplasm: solid variants are rare (Ch. 8). The cyst lining consists of epithelium, often with palisading of the basal cells which may resemble ameloblasts. The most striking feature is areas of abnormal keratinisation producing swollen cells whose outlines and nuclei become progressively paler (ghost cells).

NASOPALATINE DUCT CYSTS

Nasopalatine cysts are uncommon. They form in the midline of the anterior maxilla. The nasopalatine, incisive canal, median palatine, palatine papilla and median alveolar cysts are variants of the same lesion, varying slightly in position in relation to the postulated line of the incisive canal.

Clinical features

Nasopalatine duct cysts are slow growing and resemble other cysts of the jaws clinically, apart from their site. Occasionally they cause intermittent discharge with a salty taste. If allowed to grow sufficiently large, nasopalatine cysts may cause a swelling in the midline of the anterior part of the palate (Fig. 7.37), particularly when superficial (so-called palatine papilla cyst).

Radiography shows a rounded radiolucent area with a well-defined, often sclerotic margin in the anterior part of the midline of the maxilla (Fig. 7.38). They occasionally appear heart-shaped because of radiographic superimposition of the nasal spine. They are usually symmetrical but may be slightly larger to one side. The anterior palatine fossa must be distinguished from a small nasopalatine cyst. The maximum size of a normal fossa is up to 6 or 7 mm.

Key features of nasopalatine duct cysts are summarised in Table 7.14.

Pathogenesis and pathology

Nasopalatine cysts arise from the epithelium of the nasopalatine duct in the incisive canal. In humans, vestiges of a primi-

Fig. 7.37 Nasopalatine cyst. Typical presentation with a dome-shaped bluish enlargement overlying the incisive canal.

Fig. 7.39 Nasopalatine cyst. The lining, in part at least, may consist of respiratory (ciliated columnar) epithelium, as here.

Fig. 7.38 Nasopalatine cyst. The usual appearance is a rounded or pear-shaped area of radiolucency, mainly in the midline.

Fig. 7.40 Nasopalatine cyst. The cyst wall contains nerves and blood vessels of the incisive canal.

Table 7.14 Nasopalatine duct cysts — key features

- Often asymptomatic, chance radiographic findings
- Form in the incisive canal region
- Arise from vestiges of the nasopalatine duct and may be lined by columnar respiratory epithelium
- The long sphenopalatine nerve and vessels may be present in the wall
- Can usually be recognised radiographically
- Histological examination necessary to exclude other cyst types arising at this site
- Do not recur after enucleation

Treatment

Nasopalatine duct cysts should be enucleated. Recurrence is unlikely.

NASOLABIAL CYST

This very uncommon cyst forms outside the bone in the soft tissues, deep to the nasolabial fold. It probably arises from remnants of the nasolacrimal duct and is occasionally bilateral.

The lining is pseudostratified columnar epithelium, with or

tive organ of smell in the incisive canal can be found in the form of incomplete epithelium-lined ducts, cords of epithelial cells, or merely epithelial rests.

The epithelial lining is usually either stratified squamous epithelium or ciliated columnar (respiratory) epithelium, or both together (Fig. 7.39). Mucous glands are often, and neurovascular bundles are sometimes, present in the wall (Fig. 7.40). These are the long sphenopalatine nerve and vessels which pass through the incisive canal and are often removed with the cyst.

without some stratified columnar epithelium. If allowed to grow sufficiently large, the cyst produces a swelling of the upper lip and distorts the nostril. Treatment is usually by simple excision but occasionally may be complicated if the cyst has perforated the nasal mucosa and discharged into the nose.

So-called globulomaxillary cysts

These exceedingly rare cysts have been traditionally ascribed to proliferation of sequestered epithelium along the line of fusion of embryonic processes. It is now accepted that this view of embryological development is incorrect and there is no evidence that epithelium becomes buried in this fashion. Most so-called globulomaxillary cysts are usually found to be odontogenic cysts of various types.

CYSTS WITHOUT EPITHELIAL LINING

Solitary (simple) bone cyst

Solitary bone cysts are mostly seen in teenagers, and are uncommon after the age of 25. They form painless swellings or are chance radiographic findings. The mandible is mainly affected. Females are affected more often, in a ratio of about 3 to 2.

Radiographically, these cavities form rounded, radiolucent areas which generally tend to be less sharply defined than odontogenic cysts and have two unusual features. First, the area of radiolucency is typically much larger than the size of the swelling suggests. Second, the cavity arches up between the roots of the teeth and may as a consequence be first seen on a bite-wing radiograph (Fig. 7.41 and 7.42).

Fig. 7.41   Solitary bone cyst. Typical appearance showing a moderately well-defined but non-corticated radiolucency extending up between the roots of the teeth.

Fig. 7.42   Solitary bone cyst. Oblique lateral view showing a large rounded expansile radiolucent lesion extending from the first premolar to the angle. This cyst is more expansile than is usual and shows the variability of presentation of a solitary bone cyst.

Fig. 7.43   Solitary bone cyst. The scanty cyst lining comprises bone and a thin layer of fibrous tissue. Epithelium is not present and in some cases even the fibrous lining is lacking.

Pathogenesis and pathology

Solitary bone cysts used to be known as 'haemorrhagic' or 'traumatic' bone cysts and were postulated to result from injury to, and haemorrhage within, the bone of the jaw. This was then supposed to be followed by failure of organisation of the clot and of repair of the bone. However, there is little evidence to support this theory. Blood-filled bone cavities form in the jaws as a consequence of enucleation of true cysts, but solitary bone cysts do not arise as a result. Further, a common form of treatment is to open solitary bone cysts to allow bleeding into the cavity. Normal healing then follows. It seems hardly likely that intrabony haemorrhage can both cause and cure these lesions. Futile speculation about these lesions should not obscure the fact that their cause remains unknown.

The cavity has a rough bony wall. There may be a thin connective tissue lining or only a few red cells, blood pigment or giant cells adhering to the bone surface (Fig. 7.43). There are often no cyst contents but there may sometimes be a little fluid.

Key features of solitary bone cysts are summarised in Table 7.15.

> **Table 7.15** Solitary bone cysts — key features
>
> - Often chance radiographic findings. Rarely expand the jaw
> - Are of unknown aetiology
> - Have no epithelial lining. Appear empty at operation or contain pale fluid
> - Diagnosis suggested by radiographic features (especially extension between tooth roots) and findings at operation
> - Histology confirms the lack of epithelial lining
> - Resolve after surgical opening and closure, or occasionally spontaneously

Management

Solitary bone cysts are not seen in elderly patients, or in those that have refused surgery, so that it is apparent that these lesions resolve spontaneously. It may be necessary, however, to open the cavity, if only to confirm the diagnosis. The characteristic lack of cyst fluid and the unlined bony wall are usually enough to provide a diagnosis, but it is preferable, if possible, to remove any connective tissue lining for histological examination. Opening of the cavity is followed by healing, probably as a result of bleeding. Alternatively, healing after opening of the cavity is merely coincidental and due to natural regression of the lesion.

Aneurysmal bone cyst

Aneurysmal bone cysts are exceedingly rare in the jaws. Little is known of their pathogenesis and the most likely possibility is that they are vascular malformations.

Clinical features

Most patients are between 10 and 20 years of age, and there appears to be no strong predilection for either sex. The mandible is usually affected.

The main manifestation is usually a painless swelling and a radiolucent area, which may be balloon-like or occasionally show a suggestion of trabeculation or loculation.

Key features of aneurysmal bone cysts are summarised in Table 7.16.

Pathology

The aneurysmal bone cyst is in no sense a cyst except in its radiographic appearance. Histologically there is a highly cellular mass of blood-filled spaces which has been likened to a blood-filled sponge (Fig. 7.44). The extreme cellularity, mitotic activity and frequent presence of many giant cells may lead to

> **Table 7.16** Aneurysmal bone cysts—key features
>
> - Rare in the jaws
> - Jaw lesions are usually in the mandibular ramus and angle
> - Affect patients usually between 10 and 20 years of age
> - Are of unknown aetiology
> - Form very expansile soap-bubble radiolucencies which may be mistaken clinically and radiographically for ameloblastoma or odontogenic keratocyst
> - Histologically consist of a mass of blood-filled spaces with scattered giant cells
> - Are treated by curettage but sometimes recur

Fig. 7.44 Aneurysmal bone cyst. Cyst wall composed of loose fibrous tissue containing occasional giant cells and large blood-filled spaces.

confusion with a sarcoma. It is essential that this mistake should not be made and the patient subjected, as a consequence, to unnecessarily radical and possibly hazardous treatment. Treatment consists of thorough curettage which may need to be repeated, as the lesion occasionally recurs.

NEOPLASTIC CHANGE WITHIN CYSTS

Neoplasms, either ameloblastomas or carcinomas, could conceivably arise from the epithelial lining of cysts. There is scant evidence that ameloblastomas arise in this way, and the idea almost certainly results from incorrect radiographic interpretation or faulty histological diagnosis.

There are a few well-authenticated cases of carcinomas arising from cyst linings but it is exceedingly rare. It is essential to exclude other possibilities before such a diagnosis is made. Since cysts of the jaws are common, a neoplasm might develop coincidentally nearby and grow until it involves and fuses with the cyst wall.

CYSTS OF THE SOFT TISSUES

Some cysts described earlier form in or extend into the soft tis-

Fig. 7.45 Sublingual dermoid cyst. This is an unusually large specimen but appears even larger because the patient is raising and protruding her tongue. This cyst, unlike a ranula, can be seen to have a thick wall because it has arisen in the deeper tissues of the floor of the mouth.

sues overlying the jaws. However, most soft-tissue cysts are non-odontogenic. The most common soft-tissue cysts are mucoceles (extravasation or retention cysts) and the ranula which originate in minor salivary glands (Ch. 18), but the sublingual dermoid is a developmental anomaly.

Sublingual dermoid

These cysts probably form as a result of some abnormality of development of the branchial arches or pharyngeal pouches.

Clinical features

Dermoid cysts develop between the hyoid and jaw or may form immediately beneath the tongue (Fig. 7.45). They are sometimes filled with desquamated keratin, giving them a semisolid, putty-like consistency. A sublingual dermoid is more deeply placed than a ranula; the latter is obviously superficial, having a thin wall and a bluish appearance. A dermoid causes no symptoms until large enough to interfere with speech or eating. Nevertheless, a large swelling can be accommodated in the floor of the mouth without disability and can be completely concealed by the tongue in its normal resting position.

Pathology

The lining of *epidermoid* cysts is keratinising stratified squamous epithelium alone. Less often, cysts also have dermal appendages in the wall and are then referred to as *dermoid* cysts. Still others are lined partly by keratinising stratified squamous epithelium and partly by respiratory (ciliated columnar stratified) epithelium.

These cysts should be dissected out.

SUGGESTED FURTHER READING

Ackerman G L, Cohen M, Altini M 1987 The paradental cyst: a clinicopathological study of 57 cases. Oral Surg Oral Med Oral Pathol 64:308–312

Altini M, Shear M 1992 The lateral periodontal cyst: an update. J Oral Pathol Med 21:245–250

Browne R M (ed) 1991 Investigative pathology of odontogenic cysts. CRC Press, Boca Raton

Cawson R A, Binnie W H, Eveson J W 1994 Color atlas of oral disease, 2nd edn. Mosby-Wolfe, London

Cawson R A, Langdon J D, Eveson J W 1996 Surgical pathology of the mouth and jaws. Wright, Oxford

Craig G T 1976 The paradental cyst. A specific inflammatory odontogenic cyst. Br Dent J 141:9–14

Crowley T E, Kaugars G E, Gunsolley J C 1992 Odontogenic keratocysts: a clinical and histologic comparison of the parakeratin and orthokeratin variants. J Oral Maxillofac Surg 50:22–26

Friedrichsen S W 1993 Long-term progression of a traumatic bone cyst. A case report. Oral Surg Oral Med Oral Pathol 76:421–424

Gurol M, Burkes J, Jacoway J 1995 Botryoid odontogenic cyst: analysis of 33 cases. J Periodontol 66:1069–1073

Hernandez G A, Castro A, Castro G, Amador E 1993 Aneurysmal bone cyst versus hemangioma of the mandible. Report of a long-term follow-up of a self-limiting case. Oral Surg Oral Med Oral Pathol 76:790–796

Hussain K, Edmondson H D, Browne R M 1995 Glandular odontogenic cysts. Diagnosis and treatment. Oral Surg Oral Med Oral Pathol 79:593–603

Kuroi M 1980 Simple bone cyst of the jaw: review of the literature and report of a case. J Oral Surg 38:456–459

Li T–J, Browne R M, Matthews J B 1994 Quantification of PCNA cells within odontogenic jaw cyst epithelium. J Oral Pathol Med 23:184–189

Lombardi T, Odell E W, Morgan P R 1995 p53 immunohistochemistry of odontogenic keratocysts in relation to recurrence, basal cell budding and basal-cell naevus syndrome. Arch Oral Biol 40:1081–1084

Meiselman F 1994 Surgical management of the odontogenic keratocyst: conservative approach. J Oral Maxillofac Surg 520:960–963

Motamedi M H K, Yazdi E 1994 Aneurysmal bone cyst of the jaws: analysis of 11 cases. J Oral Maxillofac Surg 52:471–475

Saito Y, Hoshina Y, Nagamine T, Nakajima T, Suzuki M, Hayashi T 1992 Simple bone cyst. A clinical and histopathologic study of fifteen cases. Oral Surg Oral Med Oral Pathol 74:487–491

Semba I, Kitano M, Mimura T, Sonoda S, Miyawaki A 1994 Glandular odontogenic cyst: analysis of cytokeratin expression and clinicopathological features. J Oral Pathol Med 23:377–382

Shear M 1992 Cysts of the oral regions, 3rd edn. Wright, Bristol

Shear M 1994 Developmental odontogenic cysts. An update. J Oral Pathol Med 23:1–11

Swanson K S, Kaugars G E, Gunsolley J C 1991 Nasopalatine duct cyst: an analysis of 334 cases. J Oral Maxillofac Surg 49:268–271

Szerlip L 1966 Traumatic bone cysts. Resolution without surgery. Oral Surg 21:201–204

Vergel A M, Bond J R, Shives T C, McLeod R A, Unni K K 1992 Aneurysmal bone cyst. A clinicopathologic study of 228 cases. Cancer 69:2921–2931

Weathers D R, Waldron C A 1973 Unusual multilocular cysts of the jaws (botryoid odontogenic cysts). Oral Surg Oral Med Oral Pathol 36:235–241

Williams T P, Connor F A 1994 Surgical management of the odontogenic keratocyst: aggressive approach. J Oral Maxillofac Surg 520:964–966

Woolgar J A, Rippin J W, Browne R M 1987 A comparative histological study of odontogenic keratocysts in basal cell naevus syndrome and control patients. J Oral Pathol 16:75–80

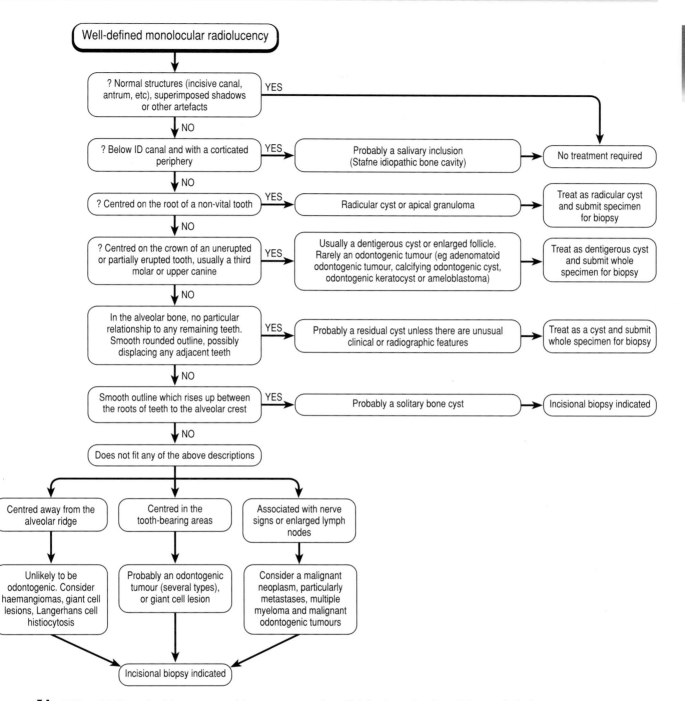

Well-defined monolocular radiolucency

? Normal structures (incisive canal, antrum, etc), superimposed shadows or other artefacts — **YES** → No treatment required

NO

? Below ID canal and with a corticated periphery — **YES** → Probably a salivary inclusion (Stafne idiopathic bone cavity) → No treatment required

NO

? Centred on the root of a non-vital tooth — **YES** → Radicular cyst or apical granuloma → Treat as radicular cyst and submit specimen for biopsy

NO

? Centred on the crown of an unerupted or partially erupted tooth, usually a third molar or upper canine — **YES** → Usually a dentigerous cyst or enlarged follicle. Rarely an odontogenic tumour (eg adenomatoid odontogenic tumour, calcifying odontogenic cyst, odontogenic keratocyst or ameloblastoma) → Treat as dentigerous cyst and submit whole specimen for biopsy

NO

In the alveolar bone, no particular relationship to any remaining teeth. Smooth rounded outline, possibly displacing any adjacent teeth — **YES** → Probably a residual cyst unless there are unusual clinical or radiographic features → Treat as a cyst and submit whole specimen for biopsy

NO

Smooth outline which rises up between the roots of teeth to the alveolar crest — **YES** → Probably a solitary bone cyst → Incisional biopsy indicated

NO

Does not fit any of the above descriptions

- Centred away from the alveolar ridge → Unlikely to be odontogenic. Consider haemangiomas, giant cell lesions, Langerhans cell histiocytosis
- Centred in the tooth-bearing areas → Probably an odontogenic tumour (several types), or giant cell lesion
- Associated with nerve signs or enlarged lymph nodes → Consider a malignant neoplasm, particularly metastases, multiple myeloma and malignant odontogenic tumours

→ Incisional biopsy indicated

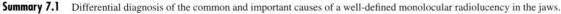

Summary 7.1 Differential diagnosis of the common and important causes of a well-defined monolocular radiolucency in the jaws.

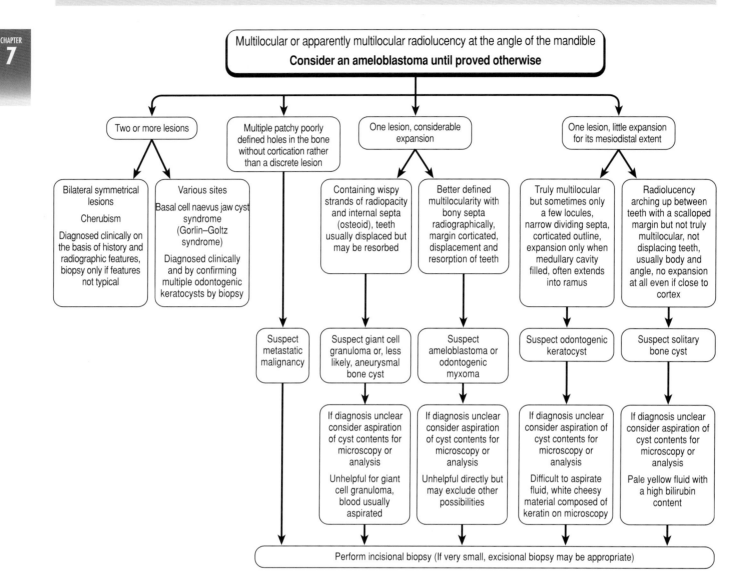

Summary 7.2 Differential diagnosis of a multilocular radiolucency at the angle of the mandible.

Odontogenic tumours and tumour-like lesions of the jaws

Tumours or tumour-like swellings of the jaws can be odontogenic or non-odontogenic (Table 8.1).

Table 8.1 Important causes of tumours (swellings) of the jaws

- Cysts, predominantly odontogenic cysts
- Odontogenic tumours
- Giant cell lesions
- Fibro-osseous lesions
- Primary (non-odontogenic) neoplasms of bone
- Metastatic neoplasms
- Chronic osteomyelitis

The most common neoplasms of the jaws are odontogenic (Table 8.2).

Table 8.2 Important types of odontogenic tumour

- Benign epithelial neoplasms
  Ameloblastoma
  Adenomatoid odontogenic tumour
  Calcifying epithelial odontogenic tumour
  Calcifying odontogenic cyst
  Squamous odontogenic tumour
- Benign mixed
  Ameloblastic fibroma
- Benign connective tissue
  Odontogenic fibroma
  Odontogenic myxoma
  Cementoblastoma
- Hamartomas
  Odontomas
- Malignant epithelial neoplasms
  Odontogenic carcinomas
- Malignant connective tissue neoplasms
  Odontogenic sarcomas

AMELOBLASTOMA

Ameloblastomas are the most common neoplasms of the jaws. They are usually first recognised between the ages of 30 and 50.

They are rare in children and old people. Eighty per cent form in the mandible; of these, 70% develop in the posterior molar region, and often involve the ramus. They are symptomless until the swelling becomes obtrusive (Fig. 8.1).

Radiographically, ameloblastomas typically form rounded, cyst-like, radiolucent areas with moderately well-defined margins and characteristically appear multilocular (Fig. 8.2). Lingual expansion may sometimes be seen but is not pathognomonic of ameloblastoma. Other variants are a honeycomb pattern or a single well-defined cavity indistinguishable from a radicular or, rarely, a dentigerous cyst (Fig. 8.3). However, differentiation from non-neoplastic cysts and other tumours or tumour-like lesions of the jaws is not possible by radiography alone.

Pathology

Follicular ameloblastomas are the most common and most readily recognisable type, with islands and trabeculae of epithelial cells in a connective tissue stroma (Fig. 8.4). These epithelial processes consist of a well-organised single layer of tall, columnar, ameloblast-like cells, which have nuclei at the opposite pole to the basement membrane (reversed polarity) and sur-

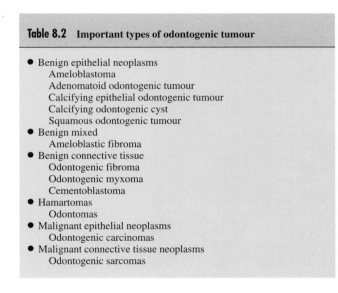

Fig. 8.1 Ameloblastoma. Typical presentation. There is a rounded, bony swelling of the posterior alveolar bone, body and angle of the mandible. There is no ulceration, a feature only seen in very large tumours which have perforated the cortex.

Fig. 8.2 Ameloblastoma. The typical radiological appearance of ameloblastoma is a multilocular cyst or multiple cyst cavities of different sizes, as shown here.

Fig. 8.3 Ameloblastoma. This ameloblastoma forms a monolocular radiolucency enveloping the crown of an unerupted tooth. The radiological appearance mimics a dentigerous cyst, reinforcing the maxim that ameloblastoma should be considered in the differential diagnosis of every radiolucency at the angle of the mandible.

round a core of loosely arranged polyhedral or angular cells, resembling stellate reticulum (Figs 8.5 and 8.6).

Cyst formation is common and varies from microcysts within a predominantly solid tumour to a cyst which may envelop the main tumour mass. Cysts may develop either within the epithelial islands or result from cystic degeneration of the connective tissue stroma (Fig. 8.7). When a cystic area of an ameloblastoma envelops the remainder of the tumour, the neoplastic epithelial cyst lining often becomes flattened and resembles that of a non-neoplastic cyst. Biopsy of the cyst wall alone may, therefore, lead to its being mistaken for a simple cyst.

Plexiform ameloblastomas consist mainly of thin trabeculae of small, darkly staining epithelial cells in a sparsely cellular connective tissue stroma (Fig. 8.8).

Acanthomatous ameloblastomas show squamous metaplasia of the central cores of neoplastic epithelium (Fig. 8.9).

Basal cell ameloblastomas are rare but consist of more darkly-staining cells predominantly in a trabecular pattern with little evidence of palisading at the periphery. They have been mistaken for basal cell carcinomas.

Granular cell ameloblastomas are also rare. They usually resemble the follicular type, but the epithelium, particularly in the central areas of the tumour islands, forms sheets of large eosinophilic granular cells (Fig. 8.10).

Fig. 8.4 Ameloblastoma. At low power the multicystic nature of the ameloblastoma is apparent and a large cyst cavity is just visible in the upper part of the picture. Towards the lower edge the tumour is separated from the cortex of the mandible by a well-defined zone of connective tissue infiltrated by cords and islands of the tumour.

Fig. 8.5 Ameloblastoma. Islands of follicular ameloblastoma comprising stellate reticulum and a peripheral layer of elongated ameloblast-like cells.

Fig. 8.7 Ameloblastoma. Plexiform ameloblastoma composed of interconnecting strands of epithelium surrounding islands of connective tissue. Several of the stromal islands have degenerated to form small cystic cavities.

Fig. 8.6 Ameloblastoma. At high power in this follicular ameloblastoma the palisaded, elongated peripheral cells with reversed polarity are seen to be very similar in appearance to ameloblasts.

Fig. 8.8 Ameloblastoma, plexiform type. There are thin, interlacing strands of epithelium but typical ameloblasts are not seen.

These varied histological appearances have not been convincingly shown to affect the tumour's behaviour.

Management

The diagnosis must be confirmed by biopsy. Treatment is by wide excision, preferably taking up to 2 cm of apparently normal bone around the margin. Complete excision is curative but anything less is followed by recurrence (Fig. 8.11).

Complete excision of a large ameloblastoma may mean total resection of the jaw and bone grafting. However, ameloblastomas only gradually erode compact bone and the lower border may be spared. An extensive operation can therefore be avoided by leaving the lower border of the jaw intact and extending the resection

Fig. 8.9 Squamous metaplasia in an ameloblastoma. Stellate reticulum-like cells have undergone squamous metaplasia to form keratin.

Fig. 8.10 Ameloblastoma. Granular cell change in an ameloblastoma. Ameloblast and stellate reticulum-like cells have undergone degenerative change to form large pink granular cells. In some tumours this change is extensive and the term 'granular cell ameloblastoma' is applied.

Fig. 8.11 Ameloblastoma. Islands of ameloblastoma penetrating surrounding bone at the periphery of the lesion. Such bony infiltration demands that ameloblastoma is excised with a margin rather than curetted.

subperiosteally. Bony repair causes much of the jaw to reform. Regular radiographic follow-up is essential as any recurrence may not appear for several years. Limited reoperation can be performed if necessary. The patient must be warned of the necessity of regular follow-up and, possibly, of a further operation.

Maxillary ameloblastomas are less common but readily spread through the thin bones of the base of the skull, are difficult to excise completely and are potentially lethal.

Plexiform unicystic ameloblastoma

This is a distinct entity. Persons between the ages of 10 and 19

Fig. 8.12 Ameloblastoma. Part of the lining of a large cyst within an ameloblastoma showing how the epithelium has become flatened and lost its typical features. Histological diagnosis may not be possible unless solid tumour is included in the specimen.

years are predominantly affected. In over 80% of cases the cyst encloses the crown of a tooth and mimics a dentigerous cyst radiographically.

Histologically, the tumour forms a mass in the cyst wall and consists of slender trabeculae of nondescript epithelial cells and no ameloblast-like cells. The cyst wall is lined by tumour cells but they are flattened and easily mistaken for those of a non-neoplastic cyst (Fig. 8.12).

Unicystic plexiform ameloblastomas differ from the solid types in that they can be enucleated with a low risk of recurrence. A 10% recurrence rate 10 years after enucleation can be expected. However, not all unicystic ameloblastomas respond in this way. Other types of ameloblastoma can become cystic, and even plexiform unicystic ameloblastomas can sometimes extend into the surrounding tissues, with a higher risk of recurrence after enucleation.

> The possibility that any radiolucency at the angle of the mandible might be an ameloblastoma should not be dismissed until the diagnosis is confirmed by biopsy

Key features of ameloblastomas are summarised in Table 8.3.

Table 8.3   Ameloblastoma — key features

- Neoplasm of odontogenic epithelium
- The most common odontogenic neoplasm
- Usually presents between ages 30 and 50 years
- Locally invasive but does not metastasise
- Typically appears as a multilocular cyst radiographically
- Most commonly forms in posterior mandible
- Treated by excision with a margin of normal tissue

Malignant ameloblastoma and ameloblastic carcinoma

Both of these exceptionally rare tumours are little more than pathological curiosities — though not to the patient of course.

Malignant ameloblastoma is a histologically typical ameloblastoma, which nevertheless gives rise to pulmonary metastases that retain the microscopic appearances of the primary. Few reported cases have been authenticated, and some, at least, have resulted from aspiration implantation. If so, local excision of the secondary deposit should be curative.

Ameloblastic carcinoma is a tumour which initially resembles an ameloblastoma histologically, but loses differentiation and behaves malignantly. It spreads to lymph nodes or beyond. Later, the microscopic appearances become similar to a squamous cell carcinoma. Rarely the progressive loss of differentiation can be seen in successive specimens from the same patient and confirms the diagnosis (Fig. 8.13). The treatment is that of an intraosseous carcinoma but the prognosis is poor if metastases are present.

ADENOMATOID ODONTOGENIC TUMOUR

Adenomatoid odontogenic tumour is uncommon, completely benign and probably a hamartoma.

Clinically, adenomatoid odontogenic tumours are found either in late adolescence or young adulthood. Females are twice as frequently affected as males. The tumour is most often sited in the anterior maxilla and forms a very slow-growing swelling. Alternatively, it may be noticed by chance on a radiograph where it frequently simulates a radicular or dentigerous cyst. Most specimens are only a few centimetres in diameter.

Pathology

A well-defined capsule encloses whorls and strands of epitheli-

Fig. 8.13 Ameloblastic carcinoma. Very rarely a malignant variant of the ameloblastoma is encountered. Histologically they may be indistinguishable from other carcinomas, but in some cases, as here, a peripheral layer of palisaded ameloblast-like cells remains, indicating the tumour's odontogenic origin.

Fig. 8.14 Adenomatoid odontogenic tumour. The epithelial cells form compact whorls and among them are several rounded cysts lined by columnar cells. The tumour is surrounded by a fibrous capsule.

Fig. 8.15 Adenomatoid odontogenic tumour. At higher power the duct-like spaces which give the tumour its name are seen.

um, among which are microcysts, resembling ducts cut in cross-section and lined by columnar cells similar to ameloblasts (Figs 8.14 and 8.15). These microcysts may contain homogeneous eosinophilic material. Microcysts have led to the tumours being called adenomatoid, but they are not ducts and are never seen cut longitudinally. Fragments of amorphous or crystalline calcification may also be seen among the sheets of epithelial cells.

These lesions shell out readily, enucleation is curative and recurrence is almost unknown.

Key features of adenomatoid odontogenic tumour are summarised in Table 8.4.

Table 8.4	Adenomatoid odontogenic tumour — key features

- Rare
- Hamartoma of odontogenic epithelium
- Usually presents between ages 15 and 20 years
- Most common in the anterior maxilla
- Often appears as a unilocular dentigerous cyst
- Responds to enucleation

CALCIFYING EPITHELIAL ODONTOGENIC TUMOUR

This tumour, with bizarre microscopic features, is often termed a Pindborg tumour, after its discoverer. Though rare, it is important because it could be mistaken for a poorly differentiated carcinoma microscopically.

Clinically, adults are mainly affected at an average age of about 40. The typical site is the posterior body of the mandible, which is twice as frequently involved as the maxilla. Symptoms are usually lacking until a swelling appears. Radiographs show a translucent area with poorly-defined margins and, usually, increasing radiopacities within the tumour as it matures.

Pathology

Calcifying epithelial odontogenic tumours consist of sheets or strands of epithelial cells in a connective tissue stroma (Fig. 8.16). The epithelial cells are polyhedral and typically have distinct outlines and intercellular bridges. Gross variation in nuclear size, including giant nuclei, is frequently striking (Fig. 8.17). These nuclei are usually hyperchromatic and, though mitoses are rare, produce an alarming resemblance to a poorly-differentiated carcinoma. However, unlike most carcinomas, a stromal inflammatory reaction is typically absent. Within the tumour, there are typically homogeneous hyaline

Fig. 8.17 Calcifying epithelial odontogenic tumour. At higher power the epithelial cells are seen to have sharply defined cell membranes resembling squamous epithelium and pleomorphic hyperchromatic nuclei. The pale pink material is amyloid-like.

areas, with the staining characteristics of amyloid. These may calcify and form concentric masses in and around degenerating epithelial cells and may form large masses.

Calcifying epithelial odontogenic tumours are not encapsulated, are locally invasive and behave similarly to ameloblastomas. Diagnosis depends on histological examination. It is particularly important to distinguish this pleomorphic tumour from a poorly-differentiated carcinoma to avoid overtreatment. Complete excision of the tumour with a border of normal bone should be curative, but recurrence follows incomplete excision.

Key features of calcifying epithelial odontogenic tumour are summarised in Table 8.5.

Fig. 8.16 Calcifying epithelial odontogenic tumour (Pindborg tumour). The tumour is composed of strands and sheets of polyhedral epithelial cells lying in pale pink staining amyloid-like material. Some of this material has mineralised, stains a darker blue colour and gives rise to radiopacities within the lesion.

Table 8.5	Calcifying epithelial odontogenic tumour — key features

- Rare neoplasm of odontogenic epithelium
- Usually presents between ages 30 and 50 years
- Many bizarre pleomorphic and hyperchromatic nuclei and formation of amyloid-like material
- Solid tumour, mixed radiolucency
- Most commonly forms in posterior mandible
- Locally invasive but does not metastasise
- Treated by excision with a small margin

CLEAR CELL ODONTOGENIC CARCINOMA

This very rare neoplasm affects elderly patients (60–74 years).

Symptoms include mild pain or tenderness, or loosening of teeth of either jaw associated with expansion of the jaw and a ragged area of radiolucency.

Pathology

Clear cell odontogenic carcinoma is poorly circumscribed and consists mainly of clear cells with a central nucleus and a well-defined cell membrane. They form large sheets, separated by thin fibrous septa (Fig. 8.18). Inflammatory cells are scanty but areas of haemorrhage may be seen. Nervous tissue may be enveloped and the tumour invades surrounding tissues. Important differences from calcifying epithelial odontogenic tumour are the lesser degree of nuclear pleomorphism and the lack of calcifications or amyloid-like material.

Treatment

This tumour is capable of metastasising to regional nodes and distant organs and has occasionally been fatal. Wide excision followed by radiotherapy is required.

CALCIFYING (GHOST CELL) ODONTOGENIC CYST

The calcifying odontogenic cyst is rare and the solid form is even less common. It is a benign neoplasm but has a malignant variant.

Clinically, almost any age and either jaw can be affected. The site is most often anterior to the first molar, but occasionally it is the gingival mucosa and the underlying bone is merely indented. On radiographs, the appearance is usually cystic but it may be multilocular or contain flecks of calcification. Occasionally roots of adjacent teeth are eroded.

Pathology

The lining of cystic areas consists of squamous epithelium with cuboidal or ameloblast-like basal cells (Figs 8.19 and 8.20). This epithelium is sometimes thick and can contain areas resembling stellate reticulum. Solid variants of this tumour may therefore resemble an ameloblastoma.

The most conspicuous feature is abnormal keratinisation producing areas of swollen, eosinophilic cells which become progressively paler, leaving only their outlines (ghost cells) or

Fig. 8.19 Calcifying odontogenic cyst. Ameloblast-like basal cells can be seen. In addition there is a small patch of abnormal keratinisation.

Fig. 8.18 Clear cell odontogenic carcinoma. This rare epithelial odontogenic tumour is composed of pale-staining clear cells.

Fig. 8.20 Calcifying odontogenic cyst. There is a thin lining of epithelium with a basal layer of columnar cells and the lumen is filled by ghost cells shed into the cyst cavity.

Fig. 8.21 Calcifying odontogenic cyst. In another part of the specimen there is extensive abnormal keratinisation forming a mass of ghost cells with prominent cell membranes and a few fragments of degenerated nuclei centrally.

Fig. 8.22 Squamous odontogenic tumour. The lesion is composed of islands of squamous epithelium without peripheral palisaded cells.

hyaline masses (Fig. 8.21). The ghost cells typically calcify in patchy fashion, and where this keratin-like material comes into contact with connective tissue it excites a foreign body reaction. Approximately 10% of calcifying odontogenic cysts are associated with odontomas or other odontogenic tumours.

The behaviour of a calcifying odontogenic cyst is similar to that of a non-neoplastic cyst; overlying bone is only occasionally eroded and enucleation is usually effective. Key features are summarised in Table 8.6.

Table 8.6 Calcifying odontogenic cyst — key features

- Rare
- Probably a neoplasm of odontogenic epithelium
- Wide age range
- Radiographically unilocular, often undistinguishable from non-neoplastic jaw cysts
- Calcifications in the cyst wall may suggest the diagnosis
- Forms at any site in alveolar ridge, usually posteriorly
- Occasionally forms in soft tissue of the gingiva
- Diagnosis by finding ghost and ameloblast-like cells histologically
- Usually responds to enucleation like a non-neoplastic cyst
- Solid lesions may be more aggressive

SQUAMOUS ODONTOGENIC TUMOUR

This rare tumour mainly affects young adults and involves the alveolar process of either jaw, close to the roots of erupted teeth.

Radiographically, the squamous odontogenic tumour can mimic severe bone loss from periodontitis or produce a cyst-like area.

Pathology

Circumscribed, rounded or more irregular islands of squamous epithelium with flattened peripheral cells are set in a fibrous stroma (Fig. 8.22). Foci of keratin or parakeratin may form in the epithelium, which may also contain laminated calcifications or globular eosinophilic structures.

This tumour is benign, though there may occasionally be invasion of adjacent structures by maxillary lesions. However, curettage and extraction of any teeth involved usually appears to be effective.

AMELOBLASTIC FIBROMA

This tumour, though rare, is important in the differential diagnosis of ameloblastoma.

Clinically, ameloblastic fibromas usually affect young adults or adolescents. They are slow growing and usually asymptomatic, but eventually expand the jaw. Radiographically, they can appear as multi- or unilocular cysts in the posterior body of the mandible.

Pathology

Both the epithelium and connective tissue are neoplastic. The epithelium consists of ameloblast-like or more cuboidal cells surrounding others resembling stellate reticulum or more com-

Fig. 8.23 Ameloblastic fibroma. The appearance is somewhat similar to that of ameloblastoma but the pattern of budding strands is distinctive and the connective tissue resembles the undifferentiated mesenchyme of the dental papilla.

Fig. 8.24 Ameloblastic fibroma. At higher power the resemblance to dental papilla, ameloblasts and stellate reticulum is seen more clearly.

pact epithelium. The epithelium is sharply circumscribed by a basal membrane and forms islands, strands or mushroom-like proliferations in a loose but cellular, fibromyxoid connective tissue, which resembles the immature dentine papilla (Figs 8.23 and 8.24).

An ameloblastic fibroma may rarely be combined with mixed calcifying dental tissues (ameloblastic fibro-odontoma), and radiographs typically show the densely opaque dental tissues in the otherwise radiolucent area.

Ameloblastic fibromas and fibro-odontomas are benign. They do not infiltrate bone and they separate readily from their bony walls. Conservative resection is effective, but, if incomplete, recurrence follows. Key features are summarised in Table 8.7.

Ameloblastic sarcoma (ameloblastic fibrosarcoma)

This is the rare malignant counterpart of ameloblastic fibroma. It is invasive and destructive but has little tendency to metastasise.

Table 8.7 Ameloblastic fibroma — key features

- Rare
- Neoplasm of both odontogenic epithelium and mesenchyme
- Usually seen in children or young adults
- Solid lesion but appears as unilocular or multilocular radiolucency
- Treated by excision with a small margin

ODONTOGENIC MYXOMA

The odontogenic myxoma is peculiar to the jaws and consists of dental mesenchyme.

Clinically, young people are predominantly affected. The tumour gives rise to a fusiform swelling and a radiolucent area with scalloped margins or a soap-bubble appearance (Fig. 8.25).

Pathology

Myxomas consist of scanty, spindle-shaped or angular cells with long, fine, anastomosing processes, distributed in loose mucoid material (Figs 8.26 and 8.27). A few collagen fibres may also form, and there may be small, scattered epithelial rests. The margins of the tumour are ill defined and peripheral bone is progressively resorbed.

Myxomas are benign, but can infiltrate widely. Wide excision is required but, in spite of vigorous treatment, some tumours persist and have been seen over 30 years after the original operations. By this time they appear inactive and are symptomless.

Rare variants with a more cellular and pleomorphic microscopic picture may be categorised as myxosarcomas but appear to have little or no potential for metastasis. Key features are summarised in Table 8.8

Table 8.8 Odontogenic myxoma — key features

- Rare
- Neoplasm of odontogenic mesenchyme
- Usually seen in young adults
- Benign but prone to recurrence
- Forms a multilocular, sometimes soap-bubble radiolucency
- Most common site is posterior mandible
- Treated by excision

ODONTOGENIC FIBROMA

The odontogenic origin of this rare endosteal tumour is suggested by its site and the presence of epithelial rests.

Clinically, an odontogenic fibroma more frequently affects the mandible. It forms a slow-growing asymptomatic mass which may eventually expand the jaw. If found by chance in a

Fig. 8.25 Odontogenic myxoma of the mandible. An occlusal view showing the finely trabeculated, soap-bubble appearance and gross expansion of the mandible. Evidence of residual tumour was still present after 35 years in spite of vigorous treatment, both surgery and radiotherapy, in its earlier stages.

Fig. 8.26 Odontogenic myxoma. This cross-section of the mandible through a myxoma shows extensive bony resorption and gross expansion. The pale staining myxoid lesion gives the tumour an empty appearance.

Fig. 8.27 Odontogenic myxoma. High power view showing the typical appearance of sparse fibroblasts lying in a myxoid or ground substance-rich matrix.

Fig. 8.28 Odontogenic fibroma. This rare mesenchymal odontogenic tumour consists of fibrous tissue containing rests and strands of odontogenic epithelium resembling those found in the periodontal ligament.

radiograph, it appears as a sharply defined, rounded lucent area in a tooth-bearing region.

Pathology

Odontogenic fibromas consist of spindle-shaped fibroblasts and bundles of whorled collagen fibres (Fig. 8.28), and may contain strands of odontogenic epithelium.

Odontogenic fibromas are benign and shell out from their surroundings.

CEMENTOBLASTOMA

Cementoblastoma is the only neoplasm of cementum. Other lesions formerly categorised as cementomas or cemental dysplasias are now categorised as fibro-osseous lesions (Ch. 10)

A cementoblastoma is a benign neoplasm and forms a mass of cementum-like tissue as an irregular or rounded mass attached to the root of a tooth, usually a mandibular first molar.

Clinically, cementoblastomas mainly affect young adults, particularly males, typically below the age of 25. They are slow-growing and the jaw is not usually expanded. Rarely a cementoblastoma can cause gross bony swelling and pain.

Radiographically, there is typically a radiopaque mass, with a thin radiolucent margin, attached to the roots of a tooth (Fig. 8.29). The mass may be rounded or irregular in shape and mottled in texture. Resorption of related roots is common, but the tooth remains vital.

Pathology

The mass consists of cementum which often contains many reversal lines, resembling Paget's disease. Cells are enclosed within the cementum, and in the irregular spaces are many osteoclasts and osteoblast-like cells (Figs 8.30 and 8.31). The cellular appearance may sometimes be so active as to be mistaken for an osteosarcoma.

Peripherally, there is a broad zone of unmineralised tissue and a surrounding connective tissue capsule. These appearances are essentially the same as those of an osteoblastoma, a rare bone tumour. They are only distinguishable by the cementoblastoma's relationship to a tooth (Fig. 8.32).

Fig. 8.30 Cementoblastoma. A dense mass of interconnected trabeculae of osteoid is fused to the resorbed roots of the first permanent molar.

Cementoblastomas are benign and, if completely excised and the tooth extracted, there should be no recurrence. Incomplete removal leads to continued growth. Key features are summarised in Table 8.9.

ODONTOMAS (ODONTOMES)

Odontomas are developmental malformations (hamartomas) of

Fig. 8.29 Periapical radiograph showing the typical appearances of a cementoblastoma, a radiopaque mass with a radiolucent rim attached to the root apex. (By kind permission of Mr E Whaites.)

Table 8.9 Cementoblastoma — key features

- Neoplasm of cementoblasts (odontogenic mesenchyme)
- Usually seen in young adults
- Benign
- Radiopaque with a narrow lucent rim
- Most common site is at the apex of a vital lower first molar
- Treated by enucleation

Fig. 8.31 Cementoblastoma. At high power at the periphery of the lesion there are radiating seams of osteoid with a thick layer of atypical cementoblasts on their surface.

Fig. 8.32 Resorbed root at the centre of a cementoblastoma showing continuity of cementum with the mineralised tissue of the lesion.

Fig. 8.33 Compound odontoma. The mass consists of many denticles which overlap each other in the radiograph but are nevertheless just visible as individual tooth-like structures.

Fig. 8.34 Compound odontoma. A denticle of dentine surrounded by enamel matrix lying within more irregular calcified tissues.

enamel and cementum are in normal anatomical relationships with one another, and, also like teeth, odontomas may erupt.

Odontomas affect the maxilla slightly more frequently than the mandible and are often recognised in early adolescence by the dense opacity of the enamel component in routine radiographs. When odontomas have erupted, infection develops in one of the many stagnation areas, and abscess formation commonly follows. In other cases, odontomas displace teeth or block their eruption or become involved in cyst formation.

Compound odontomas

These consist of many separate, small, tooth-like structures (denticles), probably produced by localised, multiple bud-

dental tissues, not neoplasms. Like teeth, once fully calcified they do not develop further. Even when the morphology is grossly distorted (as in complex odontomas), the pulp, dentine,

Fig. 8.35 Compound odontoma. Sections from various areas of the odontoma, seen in the radiograph shown in Figure 8.33, show denticles of dentine and enamel cut in various planes, and more irregular calcified tissues, within a connective tissue capsule.

ding-off from the dental lamina and formation of many tooth germs.

Clinically, a compound odontoma usually forms in the anterior part of the jaws and gives rise to a painless swelling. The denticles may be seen radiographically as separate calcified bodies (Fig. 8.33).

Histologically, the denticles are embedded in fibrous connective tissue, and have a fibrous capsule (Figs 8.34 and 8.35).

The mass should be enucleated as a potential obstruction to tooth eruption or cyst formation.

Complex odontoma

Complex odontomas consist of an irregular mass of hard and soft dental tissues, having no morphological resemblance to a tooth and frequently forming a cauliflower-like mass.

Clinically, complex odontomas are usually seen in young persons, but may escape diagnosis until late in life. Typically, a hard painless swelling is present but the mass may start to erupt and infection follows. The mass may also undergo cystic change or resorption. Radiographically, when calcification is complete, an irregular radiopaque mass containing areas of densely radiopaque enamel is seen (Fig. 8.36).

Histologically, the mass consists of all the dental tissues in a disordered arrangement, but frequently with a radial pattern. The pulp is usually finely branched so that the mass is perforated, like a sponge, by small branches of pulp (Fig. 8.37). Key features are summarised in Table 8.10.

The mass should be removed by conservative surgery.

Table 8.10   Odontomas — key features

- Hamartomas of odontogenic epithelium and mesenchyme
- Usually found between ages 10 and 20 years
- Benign
- Develop in sequence, like surrounding teeth, with initial (crypt-like) radiolucent phase, intermediate stage of mixed radiolucency, finally densely radiopaque
- May be compound (many small teeth) or complex (disordered mass of dental hard tissue)
- Most common sites are anterior maxilla and posterior mandible
- Respond to enucleation

Other types of odontomas

In the past, complex classifications have been devised to

Fig. 8.36 Complex odontoma. In this radiograph the odontoma overlies the crown of a buried molar and shows the typical dense amorphous area of radiopacity.

Fig. 8.37 Complex odontoma. A disorganised mass of dentine, enamel and cementum penetrated by fine divisions of pulp.

include such developmental anomalies as *dilated*, *invaginated* and *geminated* odontomas. These abnormalities are, in part, obviously tooth-like. Dilated and gestant odontomas arise by invagination of cells of the enamel organ or of the epithelial sheath of Hertwig, which actively proliferate until they expand the developing tooth. Gestant odontomas range in severity from a cingular pit in an otherwise normal upper lateral incisor to the so-called *dens in dente*. Minor morphological anomalies such as these have been discussed in Chapter 2.

Dentinoma. Calcified masses called 'dentinomas' have rarely been described. However, dentine forms only under the inductive effect of ameloblasts and the existence of dentinomas is no longer accepted.

Mixed odontogenic tumours. Very occasionally odontomas and odontogenic tumours are combined.

SUGGESTED FURTHER READING

Baden E, Doyle J, Mesa M, Fabie M, Lederman D, Eichen M 1993 Squamous odontogenic tumour. Report of three cases including the first extraosseous case. Oral Surg Oral Med Oral Pathol 75:733–738

Bang G, Koppang H S, Hansen L S et al 1989 Clear cell odontogenic carcinoma: report of three cases with pulmonary and lymph node metastases. J Oral Pathol Med 18:113–118

Bredenkamp J K, Zimmerman M C, Mickel R A 1989 Maxillary ameloblastoma. A potentially lethal neoplasm. Arch Otolaryngol Head Neck Surg 115:99–104

Bruce R A, Jackson I T 1991 Ameloblastic carcinoma. Report of an aggressive case and review of the literature. J Craniomaxillofac Surg 19:267–271

Buchner A 1991 The central (intraosseous) calcifying odontogenic cyst: an analysis of 215 cases. J Oral Maxillofac Surg 49:330–339

Buchner A, Merrell P W, Hansen L S, Leider A S 1991 Peripheral (extraosseous) calcifying odontogenic cyst. A review of forty-five cases. Oral Surg Oral Med Oral Pathol 72:65–70

Cawson R A. Myxoma of the mandible with a 35 year follow-up. Br J Oral Surg 10:59–63

Daley T D, Wysocki G P 1994 Peripheral odontogenic fibroma. Oral Surg Oral Med Oral Pathol 78:329–336

Franklin C D, Pindborg J J 1976 The calcifying epithelial odontogenic tumor. A review and analysis of 113 cases. Oral Surg 42:753–765

Gardner D G, Corio R L 1984 Plexiform unicystic ameloblastoma. A variant of ameloblastoma with low-recurrence rate after enucleation. Cancer 53:1730–1735

Gerol M, Burkes E J 1995 Peripheral ameloblastoma. J Periodontol 66:1065–1068

Gorlin R J, Pindborg J J, Redman R S, Williamson J J, Hansen L S 1964 The calcifying odontogenic cyst — a new entity and possible analogue of the cutaneous epithelioma of Malherbe. Cancer 17:723–729

Handlers J P, Abrams A M, Melrose R J, Danforth R 1991 Central odontogenic fibroma: clinicopathologic features of 19 cases and review of the literature. J Oral Maxillofac Surg 49:46–54

Holmlund A, Anneroth G, Lundquist G, Nordenram A 1991 Ameloblastomas orginating from odontogenic cysts. J Oral Pathol Med 20:318–321

Hong S P, Ellis G L, Hartman K S 1991 Calcifying odontogenic cyst: a review of ninety-two cases with re-evaluation of their nature as neoplasms, the nature of ghost cells, and subclassification. Oral Surg Oral Med Oral Pathol 72:56–64

Kaugars G E, Miller M E, Abbey L M 1989 Odontomas. Oral Surg Oral Med Oral Pathol 67:172–176

Keszler A, Dominguez F V, Giannunzio G 1995 Myxoma in childhood: an analysis of 10 cases. J Oral Maxillofac Surg 53:518–521

McCoy B P, Carroll M K O, Hall J M 1992 Carcinoma arising in a dentinogenic ghost cell tumor. Oral Surg Oral Med Oral Pathol 74:371–378

Muller S, Parker D C, Kapadia S B, Budnick S D, Barnes E L 1995 Ameloblastic fibrosarcoma of the jaws. A clinicopathologic and DNA analysis of five cases and review of the literature. Oral Surg Oral Med Oral Pathol 79:469–477

Peltola J, Magnusson B, Hopponen R-P, Borrman H 1994 Odontogenic myxoma — a radiographic study of 21 tumours. Br J Oral Maxillofac Surg 32:298–301

Philipsen H P, Reichert P A, Zhang K J, Nikai H, Yu Q X 1991 Adenomatoid odontogenic tumor: biologic profile base on 499 cases. J Oral Pathol Med 20:149–158

Pindborg J J, Kramer I R H, Shear M 1992 Histological typing of odontogenic tumours, 2nd edn. World Health Organization/Springer Verlag, Berlin

Reichart P A, Philipsen H P, Sonner S 1995 Ameloblastoma: biological profile of 3677 cases. Oral Oncol Eur J Cancer 31B:86–99

Ulmansky M, Hjorting-Hansen E, Praetorius F, Haque M F 1994 Benign cementoblastoma. a review and five new cases. Oral Surg Oral Med Oral Pathol 77:48–55

Williams T P 1993 Management of ameloblastoma: a changing perspective. J Oral Maxillofac Surg 51:1064–1070

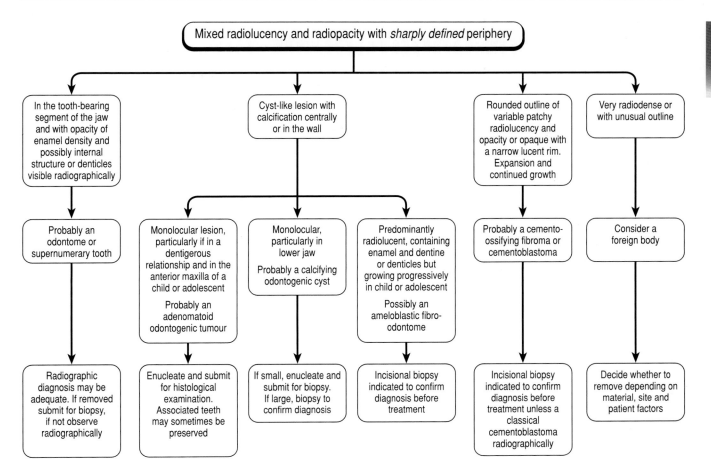

Summary 8.1 Differential diagnosis and management of sharply defined mixed radiolucencies in the jaws.

Non-odontogenic tumours of the jaws

Almost any type of tumour can arise in the jaws but most of them are considerably more common in other parts of the skeleton. Only the more important examples (Table 9.1) are considered here.

Table 9.1 Non-odontogenic tumours of bone

Primary—Benign
Osteoma
Osteochondroma
Cemento-ossifying fibroma
Central giant cell granuloma
Haemangioma
Melanotic neuroectodermal
   tumour

Primary — malignant
Osteosarcoma
Chondrosarcoma
Multifocal or potentially multifocal:
   Myeloma
   Langerhans' cell histiocytosis

Metastatic
Carcinoma

OSTEOMA AND OTHER BONY OVERGROWTHS

True tumours consisting of bone (either compact or cancellous) are occasionally seen, but localised overgrowths of bone (exostoses) are more common. They consist of lamellae of compact bone, but large specimens may have a core of cancellous bone. Small exostoses may form irregularly on the surface of the alveolar processes (Fig. 9.1) and specific variants are *torus palatinus* and *torus mandibularis*. They differ from other exostoses only in that they develop in characteristic sites and are symmetrical.

Torus palatinus commonly forms towards the posterior of the midline of the hard palate (Fig. 9.2). The swelling is rounded and symmetrical, sometimes with a midline groove. It is not usually noticed until middle age and, if it interferes with the fitting of a denture, should be removed.

Tori mandibularis form on the lingual aspect of the mandible

Fig. 9.1 Exostoses. Bony exostoses, aside from tori, are found most frequently buccally on the alveolar bone and are often symmetrically arranged.

Fig. 9.2 Torus palatinus. Palatal tori range from small smooth elevations to lobular swellings such as this. The bone is covered by only a thin mucosa which is prone to trauma.

opposite the mental foramen. They are typically bilateral, forming hard, rounded swellings (Fig. 9.3). The management is the same as that of torus palatinus.

Compact and cancellous osteoma

Compact osteomas consist of lamellae of bone, sometimes in layers like an onion but not in haversian systems (Fig. 9.4). This dense bone contains occasional vascular spaces, and

Fig. 9.3 Mandibular tori. The typical appearance of bilateral tori lingual to the lower premolars.

Fig. 9.5 Cancellous osteoma of the mandible. The tumour has arisen from a relatively narrow base lingually to the molars but has been moulded forward during growth by pressure of the tongue. The trabecular pattern of cancellous bone can be seen. A torus mandibularis arises further forward on the jaw, arises from a broad base and is usually bilateral.

abnormalities such as dental defects and epidermal cysts or fibromas. It is inherited as an autosomal dominant trait but penetrance is weak.

OSTEOCHONDROMA (CARTILAGE-CAPPED OSTEOMA)

This bony overgrowth grows by ossification beneath a cartilaginous cap. Most cases arise from the region of the coronoid or condylar process and form a hard bony protuberance which can interfere with joint function. The cartilaginous cap may not be visible in radiographs. Almost any age can be affected.

Pathology

The lesion is subperiosteal and has a cap of hyaline cartilage where the cartilage cells are sometimes regularly aligned or irregular and contain minute foci of ossification (Fig. 9.6). As age advances, the mass progressively ossifies.

These tumours are benign and usually cease to grow after skeletal maturation. Removal is therefore curative.

Fig. 9.4 Compact osteoma. Dense bone is laid down in lamellae with occasional vascular spaces, but there is no attempt to form Haversian systems.

grows very slowly. Cancellous osteomas consist of slender trabeculae of bone, with interstitial marrow spaces and a lamellated cortex (Fig. 9.5).

Osteomas should be excised only if they become large enough to cause symptoms or interfere with the fitting of a denture.

Gardner's syndrome

Gardner's syndrome comprises multiple osteomas of the jaws, polyposis coli with a high malignant potential, and often other

CEMENTO-OSSIFYING FIBROMA

No practical distinction can be made between so-called cementifying and ossifying fibromas.

Clinically, cemento-ossifying fibromas are uncommon. They usually form in the mandibular premolar or molar region. The most common complaint is a painless swelling, unless seen by chance in a radiograph. They are most common between 20 and 40 years. Females may be twice as frequently affected as males.

Radiographically, cemento-ossifying fibromas are radiolucent with varying degrees of calcification, particularly near their centre (Fig. 9.7). They have well-defined margins and

Fig. 9.6 Osteochondroma. There is a superficial cap of hyaline cartilage which undergoes endochondral ossification to form normal trabeculae of lamellar bone. The marrow spaces contain normal marrow continuous with those in the underlying bone.

Fig. 9.8 Cemento-ossifying fibroma. This example contains densely mineralised and darkly staining islands of cementum-like bone lying in cellular fibrous tissue. Towards the actively growing margin of the lesion (upper part) the fibrous tissue is more cellular and is forming woven bone.

Fig. 9.7 Cemento-ossifying fibroma. The tumour forms a characteristic rounded well-circumscribed lesion radiographically, cloudily radiolucent in its earlier and radiopaque in its later stages. It is slow-growing, as can be seen by the displacement of the teeth.

sometimes a radiolucent rim. Roots may be displaced or occasionally resorbed. Large mandibular tumours are rare but can cause a characteristic downward bowing of the lower border of the jaw.

Pathology

Cemento-ossifying fibromas consist of stellate or spindle-shaped fibroblasts, with a widely variable degree and many patterns of cellularity, and of collagen formation (Fig. 9.8).

The types of calcifications within the tumour also vary widely. Trabeculae of woven bone with osteoblastic rimming are often prominent and may form a reticular pattern. Sometimes

Fig. 9.9 Cemento-ossifying fibroma. In this mature lesion there are large coalescing islands of dense bone and little fibrous tissue. Note the well-demarcated periphery of fibrous tissue which has shelled away from the adjacent bone during removal.

acellular calcifications resembling cementicles predominate. These nodules are minute at first, but gradually grow, fuse and ultimately form a dense mass (Fig. 9.9).

Cemento-ossifying fibromas may sometimes be indistinguishable histologically from fibrous dysplasia except by the clinical and radiographic findings. Important differences are that a cemento-ossifying fibroma more frequently affects the mandible, is well circumscribed and can have a fibrous capsule. Fibrous dysplasia, by contrast, merges with normal bone at its margins. It can also extend to the alveolar margin but does not fuse with or otherwise distort the roots of teeth.

Some areas of a cemento-ossifying fibroma may resemble other fibro-osseous lesions, but it is better circumscribed and can be readily enucleated.

Cemento-ossifying fibromas are slow growing, may have a definable capsule and can be enucleated. Occasionally, large tumours which have distorted the jaw require local resection and bone grafting. Recurrence is exceptional. Rarely also, a densely calcified cemento-ossifying fibroma has to be widely excised as a focus of chronic osteomyelitis if infected by extraction of an associated tooth. Key features are summarised in Table 9.2.

Fig. 9.10 Giant cell granuloma. This maxillary lesion has perforated the cortex and formed an ulcerated bluish soft-tissue mass on the alveolar ridge. The underlying alveolar bone is considerably expanded.

Table 9.2 Cemento-ossifying fibroma — key features

- Forms in the premolar/molar region of the mandible
- Females probably affected twice as frequently as males
- Slow-growing, well circumscribed, sometimes encapsulated
- Histologically, variable patterns and degrees of cellularity and collagen formation
- Calcifications may be trabeculae of woven bone or cementicle-like
- Responds to enucleation

GIANT CELL ('REPARATIVE') GRANULOMA

Giant cell granulomas are hyperplastic rather than neoplastic. The giant cell tumour (osteoclastoma), by contrast, is an aggressive neoplasm which chiefly affects the limbs but virtually never the jaws.

Pathogenesis. The earlier name 'giant cell reparative granuloma' derives from the unconvincing idea (also applied to solitary bone cysts) that they were reactions to trauma which caused intramedullary haemorrhage (Ch. 7). They are probably developmental.

Giant cell granuloma is usually seen in young people under 20, and in females twice as frequently as males. The mandible, anterior to the first molars, where the teeth have had deciduous predecessors, is the usual site. There is frequently only a painless swelling but growth is sometimes rapid and the mass can rarely erode through the bone, particularly of the alveolar ridge, to produce a purplish soft-tissue swelling (Fig. 9.10).

Radiographs show a rounded cyst-like radiolucent area, often faintly loculated or with a soap-bubble appearance (Fig. 9.11). Roots of teeth can be displaced or, occasionally, resorbed.

Fig. 9.11 Giant cell granuloma. Characteristic radiographic appearance of an expansile radiolucency with scalloped margins containing numerous thin internal septa of wispy bone and osteoid.

Pathology

Giant cell granuloma forms a lobulated mass of proliferating vascular connective tissue packed with giant cells (osteoclasts) (Fig. 9.12). Signs of bleeding into the mass and deposits of haemosiderin are frequently seen (Fig. 9.13). Fibroblastic proliferation or prominent osteoid and bone formation are common. There are no changes in blood chemistry,

Curettage of giant cell granulomas is usually adequate and wide excision unnecessary; small fragments that may be left behind may cause little trouble, rarely require further treatment and may resolve spontaneously. Recurrence follows incomplete

Fig. 9.12 Giant cell granuloma. High power showing the osteoclast-like giant cells with numerous, evenly dispersed nuclei.

Fig. 9.13 Giant cell granuloma. The tissue is vascular and contains much extravasated blood, around which giant cells are clustered.

removal and a further limited operation may become necessary. Key features are summarised in Table 9.3.

Table 9.3 Central giant cell granuloma — key features

- Benign hyperplastic lesion of unknown aetiology
- More common in young females but seen over a wide age range
- Very expansile and may be destructive. May penetrate cortical bone and periosteum
- Solid but appears as unilocular or multilocular cyst-like radiolucency
- Forms in alveolar ridge, anterior to 6s, more frequently in the mandible but often in the maxilla
- No changes in blood chemistry
- Treated by curettage but second operation sometimes required

---

Other giant cell lesions of the jaws

Several other jaw lesions (Table 9.4) can resemble a giant cell granuloma microscopically, and must be considered in the differential diagnosis.

Table 9.4 Differential diagnosis of giant cell lesions of the jaws

- *Hyperparathyroidism*. Histologically indistinguishable from giant cell granuloma but serum calcium levels are raised (Ch. 10)
- *Cherubism*. May be indistinguishable from giant cell granuloma histologically, but lesions are symmetrical, near the angles of the mandible (Ch. 10)
- *Giant cell tumour (osteoclastoma)*. Aggressive tumour of long bones.
  Broadly similar histologically to giant cell granuloma but a distinct entity in terms of behaviour
- *Aneurysmal bone cysts*. May contain many giant cells but consist predominantly of multiple blood-filled spaces (Ch. 7)
- *Fibrous dysplasia*. Only limited foci of giant cells. No defined margins radiographically. Growth ceases with skeletal maturity (Ch. 10)

HAEMANGIOMA OF BONE

Haemangiomas are rare tumours of bone, but a relatively high proportion are in the mandible, particularly in women.

Clinically, haemangiomas cause progressive painless swellings which, when the overlying bone is resorbed, may become pulsatile. Teeth may be loosened and there may be bleeding, particularly from the gingival margins involved by the tumour.

Radiographically, there is a rounded or pseudoloculated radiolucent area with ill-defined margins or a soap-bubble appearance.

Pathology

Haemangiomas of bone are essentially similar to those in soft tissues. They are usually cavernous (Fig. 9.14), but there is also an arteriovenous type (fast-flow angioma) which has large feeder arteries and, as a consequence, tends to expand rapidly and is likely to bleed severely if opened.

Management

A haemangioma may be unsuspected if its vascularity is not obvious. Opening it or extracting a related tooth may therefore release torrents of blood, occasionally with fatal results. However, once the diagnosis has been made, wide en bloc resection is the only practical treatment. If there are identifiable feeder vessels selective arterial embolisation makes surgery considerably safer.

Fig. 9.14 Haemangioma of bone. The marrow spaces contain very large blood-filled sinuses with thin walls and the lesion is poorly localised and permeates between the bony trabeculae.

Fig. 9.15 Melanotic neuroectodermal tumour of infancy. The anterior maxilla of this neonate contains an expansile radiolucency which has displaced tooth germs and eroded the alveolar bone.

MELANOTIC NEUROECTODERMAL TUMOUR OF INFANCY (PROGONOMA)

This rare tumour, which arises from the neural crest, may appear in the anterior maxilla in the first few months of life. It is usually painless and slowly expansive, but occasionally grows rapidly.

Radiographically, there is an area of bone destruction, frequently with ragged margins, and displacement of the developing teeth (Fig. 9.15). However, the lesion is benign.

Pathology

There are pigmented and non-pigmented cells in a fibrous stroma. The pigmented cells have large pale nuclei and are filled with coarse melanin-containing cytoplasmic granules (Fig. 9.16). They form solid groups or line small spaces. The non-pigmented cells have large, densely hyperchromatic nuclei and form small groups, either in the stroma or in the spaces lined by the pigmented cells (Fig. 9.17).

Management

The tumour is non-encapsulated but usually separates easily from the bone at operation. Conservative treatment is usually curative but, even when excision is incomplete, recurrence is rare. Irradiation is contraindicated. Key features are summarised in Table 9.5.

Fig. 9.16 Melanotic neuroectodermal tumour of infancy. Pale pink staining epithelial cells, some of which are pigmented (centrally), arranged in clusters and surrounded by small, round, darkly staining tumour cells.

Fig. 9.17 Melanotic neuroectodermal tumour of infancy. Higher power showing the melanin pigment granules within a strand of epithelium

137

Fig. 9.18 Osteosarcoma. The pictures show the progress of the tumour over a period of 3 months. The patient died with metastases in the lungs, about a month after the second picture was taken.

Table 9.5 Melanotic neuroectodermal tumour of infancy — key features

- Very rare
- Congenital or appears in first few months
- Presents as expansion of anterior maxilla, typically bluish in colour
- Benign but destroys bone
- Responds to conservative excision or curettage

MALIGNANT NEOPLASMS OF BONE

Osteosarcoma

Osteosarcoma is highly malignant and the most common *primary* (nonodontogenic) neoplasm of bone, but overall is rare, especially in the jaws.

Osteosarcomas rarely have identifiable causes. A few develop late in life after irradiation or Paget's disease of bone, but the latter type virtually never affects jaws.

Osteosarcoma of the jaws is typically seen between the ages of 30 and 40. Males are slightly more frequently affected, and the body of the mandible is a common site. There is typically a firm swelling which grows noticeably in a few months and becomes painful (Fig. 9.18). Teeth may be loosened and there may be paraesthesia or loss of sensation in the mental nerve area. Metastases to the lungs may develop early.

Radiographically, appearances are variable but irregular bone destruction usually predominates over bone formation. Bone formation in a soft-tissue mass is highly characteristic (Fig. 9.19). A sun-ray appearance or Codman's triangles at the margins, due to lifting of the periosteum and new bone forma-

Fig. 9.19 Osteosarcoma. Radiograph of the jaw removed from the patient seen in Figure 9.18 shows the irregular bone destruction and pattern of new bone formation which replaces the normal structure.

tion, are rarely seen and not specific to osteosarcoma. Radiographs of the chest should also be taken, as secondary deposits may already be present.

Pathology

The neoplastic osteoblasts vary in size and shape; they may be small and angular or large and hyperchromatic (Fig. 9.20). Mitoses may be seen, particularly in the more highly cellular areas. Giant cells may be conspicuous, but many cells are nondescript. Bone formation does not necessarily predominate and osteoid formation is the main diagnostic criterion and is seen in

Fig. 9.20 Osteosarcoma. Trabeculae of abnormal woven bone surrounded by atypical cells in which mitoses are frequent and pleomorphism is conspicuous.

Fig. 9.21 Osteosarcoma. A post-mortem specimen of lung from the same patient shown in Figure 9.18. Malignant cells infiltrate the alveoli and are forming woven bone.

metastases (Fig. 9.21). Cartilage and fibrous tissue are usually also present and sometimes predominate but usually only in part of the tumour. A small biopsy may, therefore, show only a single tissue, such as cartilage, and be mistaken for a chondrosarcoma.

Key features are summarised in Table 9.6.

Table 9.6   Osteosarcoma of the jaws — key features
● Rare
● Patients' mean age is about 35
● Occasionally follows irradiation
● Usually affects the mandible
● Radiographically, bone formation is seen in a soft-tissue mass
● Treated by radical surgery, sometimes with additional chemotherapy
● Slightly better prognosis than osteosarcoma of the long bones

Management

Osteosarcoma is rapidly invasive and can metastasise early. Treatment is by early mandibulectomy or maxillectomy together with wide excision of any soft-tissue extensions of the tumour. This may be combined with radiotherapy and/or chemotherapy. The prognosis depends mainly on the extent of the tumour at operation and deteriorates with spread to the soft tissues, to lymph nodes (in about 10% of cases) or to the base of the skull. In approximately 50% there is local recurrence within a year of treatment and a sharp deterioration in prognosis. The 5-year survival rate may range from 40% for tumours less than 5 cm in diameter to zero for tumours over 15 cm.

CHONDROMA AND CHONDROSARCOMA

The diagnosis of chondroma of the jaws should generally be avoided as most prove to be chondrosarcomas. They are rare tumours of the maxillary bones.

Histologically, chondromas consist of hyaline cartilage but the cells are irregular in size and distribution. Calcification or ossification may develop. However, about 20% of chondrosarcomas in the maxillofacial area were originally thought to have been chondromas.

Management. Excision should include a wide margin of normal tissue because of the difficulty in distinguishing benign from malignant tumours.

Chondrosarcoma

Chondrosarcomas of the jaws affect adults at an average age of about 45. The anterior maxilla is the site in 60% of cases.

Pain, swelling or loosening of teeth associated with a radiolucent area are typical. The radiolucency can be well or poorly circumscribed, or may appear multilocular. Calcifications are frequently present and may be widespread and dense.

Pathology

The cartilage in jaw tumours is usually comparatively well formed or, less often, poorly differentiated or myxoid (Fig. 9.22). The chondrocytes are pleomorphic, often binucleate and may show mitotic activity (Fig. 9.23).

Fig. 9.22 Chondrosarcoma. Lobules of abnormal hyaline cartilage are formed in a disorganised fashion by sheets of malignant cells.

Fig. 9.23 Chondrosarcoma. Higher power of cartilage within a chondrosarcoma showing the abnormal chondrocytes and disorganised mineralisation.

Maxillofacial chondrosarcomas are aggressive, and local recurrence or persistent tumour is the main cause of death. Lungs or other bones are the usual sites of distant spread but fewer than 10% of these tumours metastasise.

Chondrosarcomas must be widely excised as early as possible, but this can be difficult in the maxillofacial region. Inadequate excision usually leads to recurrences beyond the original site and deterioration of the prognosis. The response to radiotherapy is usually poor.

Mesenchymal chondrosarcoma is an uncommon but highly malignant variant. It is a highly cellular tumour in which there are only small foci of tissue recognisable as poorly-formed cartilage. It is sometimes very vascular.

EWING'S SARCOMA

Ewing's sarcoma is rare but, when it affects the head and neck region, has a predilection for the body of the mandible.

Clinically, patients are usually children or young adults. Typical symptoms are bone swelling and often pain, progressing over a period of months. Teeth may loosen and the overlying mucosa ulcerate. Fever, leucocytosis, a raised ESR and anaemia may be associated and indicate a poor prognosis.

Pathology

Ewing's sarcoma cells resemble lymphocytes but are about twice their size and are of neuroectodermal origin. They have darkly-staining nuclei and a rim of cytoplasm, which is typically vacuolated and stains for glycogen. The cells form diffuse sheets or loose lobules, separated by septa. Distant spread is usually to the lungs and other bones. Lymph nodes are occasionally involved.

The initial treatment is wide excision or, if not possible, megavoltage irradiation. Combination chemotherapy should also be given and appears to have improved the survival rate but increases the risk of lymphoid tumours later.

MULTIPLE MYELOMA

Multiple myeloma is a neoplasm of plasma cells which produce a monoclonal immunoglobulin. It causes multiple foci of bone destruction, bone pain and tenderness. Rarely a jaw lesion or a complication such as oral amyloidosis may be the first symptoms. Proliferation of myeloma cells in the marrow frequently causes anaemia and sometimes thrombocytopenia. Infections may result from depressed production of normal immunoglobulins. Occasionally myeloma is detected before symptoms appear, by the chance finding, in a routine examination, of a greatly raised ESR as a result of overproduction of immunoglobulin (usually IgG).

Skeletal radiographs typically show multiple punched-out areas of radiolucency, particularly in the vault of the skull.

Pathology

Myeloma appears as sheets of neoplastic plasma cells which may be well or poorly differentiated (Figs 9.24 and 9.25). Diagnosis depends on marrow biopsy and confirmation by serum electrophoresis showing a monoclonal band (Fig. 9.26). Light-chain overproduction is common and leads to Bence Jones proteinuria and often amyloidosis.

There is frequently an initial response with combination chemotherapy, but fewer than 20% of patients survive for 5 or more years. Dental treatment may be complicated by anaemia, haemorrhagic tendencies or increased susceptibility to infection.

Fig. 9.24 Multiple myeloma. The lesion is composed of a uniform and dense infiltrate of neoplastic plasma cells with darker than normal staining nuclei.

Fig. 9.25 Multiple myeloma. Immunocytochemistry for λ light chain results in a brown positive stain in all cells, indicating a monoclonal and therefore neoplastic proliferation of plasma cells.

Fig. 9.26 Immunoelectrophoresis comparing patient's and control serum for their content of κ and λ light chains. The patient has a raised level of κ light chain.

Table 9.7   Multiple myeloma — key features
• Myeloma is a malignant bone-seeking neoplasm of plasma cells
• Radiographically, punched-out lesions appear, particularly in the skull
• Similar lesions may appear in the jaws
• Malignant plasma cells show varying degrees of dedifferentiation
• Monoclonal immunoglobulin (usually IgG) produced
• Anaemia, purpura or immunodeficiency may be associated
• Light-chain production can lead to amyloidosis causing macroglossia in 20%
• Short-term benefit only from combination chemotherapy
• Solitary (soft-tissue or intraosseous) myelomas rare but may affect maxillofacial region. They progress to multiple myeloma

SOLITARY (EXTRAMEDULLARY) PLASMACYTOMA

Approximately 80% of these rare tumours form in the soft tissues of the head and neck region. Multiple myeloma develops in up to 50% of patients within 2 years.

Solitary plasmacytoma of bone occasionally affects the jaw. Bone pain, tenderness or a swelling and a sharply defined area of radiolucency are typical. Treatment is by radiotherapy. The prognosis is significantly better than for soft-tissue plasmacytoma. Over 65% of patients survive for 10 or more years, but the majority eventually develop multiple myeloma.

Histologically the appearances of solitary and multiple myeloma are the same. Key features are summarised in Table 9.7.

AMYLOIDOSIS

Amyloidosis is the deposition in the tissues of an abnormal pro-tein with characteristic staining properties. It can result from overproduction of immunoglobulin light chains, usually by multiple myeloma. In over 20% of such cases amyloid is deposited in the mouth, particularly the tongue, to cause macroglossia or localised swellings, or both (Fig. 9.27). Macroglossia due to amyloid can be so gross as to protrude from the mouth. Purpura and anaemia may be associated.

Pathology

Amyloid appears as weakly eosinophilic, hyaline homogeneous material. It is typically perivascular and stains with Congo red, which also shows a characteristic apple-green birefringence under polarised light (Fig. 9.28). There is also fluorescence with thioflavine T and a characteristic fibrillary structure by electron microscopy.

Widespread amyloidosis can cause fatal renal failure but

Fig. 9.27 Amyloidosis. These slightly yellow nodules on the lateral border of an enlarged tongue are characteristic of amyloidosis.

Fig. 9.29 Langerhans' cell histiocytosis. This localised lesion (eosinophilic granuloma) has produced an ulcerated mass on the maxillary alveolar ridge. The clinical appearances are non-specific.

Fig. 9.28 Amyloidosis. Amyloid identified in the tissues by its green birefringence under polarised light when stained with Congo red.

Fig. 9.30 Langerhans' cell histiocytosis. This localised lesion (eosinophilic granuloma) shows the characteristic appearance of a well-defined radiolucency scooped out of the alveolar bone. The margin is corticated in places, but less well-defined elsewhere.

progress of the disease may be delayed by chemotherapy. Alternatively the patient may die from myeloma when it is the cause of amyloidosis.

LANGERHANS' CELL HISTIOCYTOSIS (HISTIOCYTOSIS X)

Langerhans' cells are dendritic, macrophage-like cells within epithelia. They act as antigen-presenting cells, but occasionally give rise to bone tumours. Three forms are recognised:

1. Solitary eosinophilic granuloma
2. Multifocal eosinophilic granuloma (including Hand–Schüller–Christian disease)
3. Letterer–Siwe syndrome.

In these tumours, both the surface markers of Langerhans' cells and, by electron microscopy, the characteristic Birbeck granules may be recognisable.

Solitary eosinophilic granuloma

Solitary eosinophilic granuloma of the jaw causes localised bone destruction with swelling and often pain (Fig. 9.29). Occasionally, gross periodontal destruction exposes the roots of the teeth. A rounded area of radiolucency with indistinct margins (Fig. 9.30) and an appearance of teeth 'floating in air' are typical.

Pathology. There are varying proportions of histiocyte-like Langerhans' cells and eosinophils, sometimes with other types of granulocytes (Fig. 9.31). The Langerhans' cells have pale,

Fig. 9.31 Langerhans' cell histiocytosis. Clusters of eosinophils in a background of paler staining Langerhans' cells.

Fig. 9.32 Langerhans' cell histiocytosis. Higher power showing the pale staining Langerhans' cells with their characteristic folded, bilobed (coffee bean) nuclei.

vesiculated and often lobulated nuclei, and weakly eosinophilic cytoplasm (Fig. 9.32).

The response to curettage is often good.

Hand–Schüller–Christian disease

This term refers to histiocytosis causing exophthalmos, diabetes insipidus and lytic skull lesions, but this triad is present in only a minority. Usually the skull, axial skeleton and femora, and also sometimes the viscera (hepatosplenomegaly) or the skin, may be involved.

Letterer–Siwe syndrome

This aggressive form of histiocytosis affects infants or young children. Progression to widespread disease, with involvement of skin, viscera and bones, can be rapidly fatal despite treatment by irradiation and/or chemotherapy.

Overall, the behaviour of Langerhans' cell histiocytosis is

unpredictable, but the younger the patient and the greater the number of organ systems affected, the worse the prognosis. Key features are summarised in Table 9.8.

Table 9.8 Langerhans' cell histiocytosis — key features

- Isolated or multifocal tumours of Langerhans' (histiocyte-like) cells
- In adults can give rise to benign chronic tumour (eosinophilic granuloma)
- Eosinophilic granulomas form sharply-demarcated radiolucencies
- Alveolar bone around teeth may be destroyed (teeth 'floating in air' appearance)
- May mimic juvenile periodontitis
- In childhood is frequently a disseminated malignant disease
- Diagnosis is by biopsy
- Solitary lesions respond to curettage or resection
- Children may require chemotherapy. Significant mortality in infants

METASTATIC TUMOURS

Carcinomas of various organs (Table 9.9) are common tumours and the most frequent metastases reaching the jaw by the bloodstream.

Fig. 9.33 Metastatic carcinoma of the mandible. Swelling developed in the ramus quite suddenly in this apparently fit patient. Investigations showed a deposit of poorly differentiated carcinoma in the jaw and signs of a bronchial carcinoma.

143

Fig. 9.34 Metastatic bronchogenic carcinoma. This small metastasis in the alveolar bone has produced a poorly-demarcated, patchy radiolucency and destroyed the lamina dura around the root apex. Such small lesions have been mistaken for periapical granulomas radiographically.

Table 9.9 Important sites of primary tumours metastasising to the jaws
● Breast
● Bronchus
● Prostate
● Thyroid
● Kidney

Fig. 9.36 Metastatic carcinoma in the jaw. Section across a mandible shows a deposit of carcinoma which has destroyed the cortex of the bone and is extending into the medulla.

Rarely a malignant deposit in the jaw causes the first symptoms and can lead to diagnosis of the primary. More often the growth has been treated earlier. In either case a metastasis in the jaw is indicative of life-threatening disease. Patients are usually middle-aged or elderly.

Common symptoms are pain or swelling of the jaw (Fig. 9.33) and there may be paraesthesia or anaesthesia of the lip. There is typically an area of radiolucency with a hazy outline (Figs 9.34

Fig. 9.35 Metastatic carcinoma in the mandible. A large and poorly defined radiolucent metastasis has destroyed most of the posterior body of the mandible, resulting in a pathological fracture.

and 9.35). It sometimes simulates an infected cyst or may be quite irregular and simulate osteomyelitis. Sometimes the entire mandible may have a motheaten appearance. Bone sclerosis is a typical result of prostatic carcinoma.

Pathology

Secondary deposits are usually adenocarcinomas but depend on the nature of the primary growth. Osteoclastic bone destruction at the periphery of the deposit is the most common

effect (Fig. 9.36). After histological confirmation of the diagnosis, a careful history, especially of previous operations, may be required.

General and blood examinations and a skeletal survey will show the extent of the disease. The primary growth should be treated if still feasible. In most cases bony metastases imply that palliative treatment is the best that can be achieved. Irradiation may sometimes make the lesion in the jaw regress for a time and lessen pain.

SUGGESTED FURTHER READING

Auclair P L, Cuenin P, Kratochvil F J, Slater L J, Ellis G L 1988 A clinical and histomorphologic comparison of the central giant cell granuloma and the giant cell tumor. Oral Surg Oral Med Oral Pathol 66:197–208

Barrera-Franco J L, Flores-Flores G, Mosquedo-Taylor A 1993 Mandibular metastasis as the first manifestation of hepatocellular carcinoma: report of a case and review of the literature. J Oral Maxillofac Surg 51:318–321

Bunel K, Sindet-Pedersen S 1993 Central hemangioma of the mandible. Oral Surg Oral Med Oral Pathol 75:565–570

Cawson R A, Binnie W H, Eveson J W 1994 Color atlas of oral disease, 2nd edn. Mosby-Wolfe, London

Cawson R A, Langdon J D, Eveson J W 1996 Surgical pathology of the mouth and jaws. Wright, Oxford

Dagenais M, Pharoah M J, Sikorski P A 1992 The radiographic characteristics of histiocytosis X. A study of 29 cases that involve the jaws. Oral Surg Oral Med Oral Pathol 74:230–236

Emile J-F, Wechsler J, Brousse N et al 1995 Langerhans cell histiocytosis. Definitive diagnosis with the use of monoclonal antibody O10 on routinely paraffin-embedded samples. Am J Surg Pathol 19:636–641

Epstein J B, Voss N J S, Stevenson-Moore P 1984 Maxillofacial manifestations of multiple myeloma. An unusual case and review of the literature. Oral Surg Oral Med Oral Pathol 57:267–271

Favara B E, Jaffe R 1994 The histopathology of Langerhans cell histiocytosis. Br J Cancer 70 (suppl. XXIII): S17–S23

Fechner R E, Mills S E 1992 Tumors of the bones and joints. Atlas of tumor pathology, third series, fascicle 8. Armed Forces Institute of Pathology, Washington DC

Flick W G, Lawrence F R 1980 Oral amyloidosis as initial symptom of multiple myeloma. Oral Surg Oral Med Oral Pathol 49:18–20

Furutani M, Ohnishi M, Tanaka Y 1994 Mandibular involvement in patients with multiple myeloma. J Oral Maxillofac Surg 52:23–25

Garrington G E, Collett W K 1988 Chondrosarcoma. I. A selected literature review. J Oral Pathol 17:1–11

Garrington G E, Collett W K 1988 Chondrosarcoma. II. Chondrosarcoma of the jaws: analysis of 37 cases. J Oral Pathol 17:12–20

Garrington G E, Scofield H H, Cornyn J, Hooker SP 1967 Osteosarcoma of the jaws. Analysis of 56 cases. Cancer 20:377–391

Hackney F L, Aragon S B, Aufdemorte T B, Holt R G, Sickels J E V 1991 Chondrosarcoma of the jaws: clinical findings, histopathology and treatment. Oral Surg Oral Med Oral Pathol 71:139–143

Harris M 1993 Central giant cell granulomas regress with calcitonin therapy. Br J Oral Maxillofac Surg 31:89–94

Hartman K S 1980 Histiocytosis X. A review of 114 cases with oral involvement. Oral Surg Oral Med Oral Pathol 49:38–54

Hawkins P N 1994 Amyloidosis. Medicine Int 22:76–82

Henry C H, Granite E L, Rafetto L K 1992 Osteochondroma of the mandibular condyle: report of a case and review of the literature. J Oral Maxillofac Surg 50:1102–1108

Hirshberg A, Leibovich P, Buchner A 1994 Metastatic tumors to the jaw bones: analysis of 390 cases. J Oral Pathol Med 23:337–341

Kanazawa H, Shoji A, Yokoe H, Midorikawa S, Takamiya Y 1993 Solitary plasmacytoma of the mandible. Case report and review of the literature. J Cranio Maxillofac Surg 21:202–206

Kilpatrick S E, Wenger D E, Gilchrist G S, Shives T C, Woolan P C 1995 Langerhans cell histiocytosis (histiocytosis X) of bone. A clinicopathologic analysis of 263 pediatric and adult cases. Cancer 76:2471–2484

Lambertenghi-Delilliers G, Bruno E, Cortelezzi A, Fumagalli L, Morosini A 1988 Incidence of jaw lesions in 193 patients with multiple myeloma. Oral Surg Oral Med Oral Pathol 65:533–537

Lieberman P H, Jones C R, Steinman R M et al 1996 Langerhans cell (eosinophilic) granulomatosis. A clinicopathologic study encompassing 50 years. Am J Surg Pathol 20:519–552

Lucas D R, Unni K K, Mc Leod R A, O'Connor M I, Sim F H 1994 Osteoblastoma: a clinicopathologic study of 306 cases. Hum Pathol 25:117–134

Millar B G, Browne R M, Flood T R 1990 Juxtacortical osteosarcoma of the jaws. Br J Oral Maxillofac Surg 28:73–79

Mintz G A, Abrams A M, Carlsen G D, Melrose R J, Fister H W 1981 Primary malignant giant cell tumor of the mandible. Report of a case. Oral Surg Oral Med Oral Pathol 51:164–171

Mosby E L, Lowe M W, Cobb C M, Ennis R L 1992 Melanotic neuroectodermal tumor of infancy: review of the literature and report of a case. J Oral Maxillofac Surg 50:886–894

Ormiston I W, Piette E, Tideman H, Wu P C 1994 Chondrosarcoma of the mandible presenting as periodontal lesions: report of 2 cases. J Craniomaxillofac Surg 22:231–235

Regezi J A, Zarbo R J, McClatchey K D, Courtney R M, Crissman J D 1987 Osteosarcomas and chondrosarcomas of the jaws: immunohistochemical correlations. Oral Surg Oral Med Oral Pathol 64:302–307

Reinish E I, Raviv M, Srolovitz, Gornitsky M 1994 Tongue, primary amyloidosis and multiple myeloma. Oral Surg Oral Med Oral Pathol 77:121–125

Whitaker S B, Waldron C A 1993 Central giant cell lesions of the jaws. A clinical, radiologic and histopathologic study. Oral Surg Oral Med Oral Pathol 75:199–208

Willman C L, Busque L, Griffith B B et al 1994 Langerhans' cell histiocytosis (histiocytosis X) — a clonal proliferative disease. N Engl J Med 331:154–160

Wood R E, Nortje C J, Hesseling P, Grotepass F 1990 Ewing's tumor of the jaw. Oral Surg Oral Med Oral pathol 69:120–127

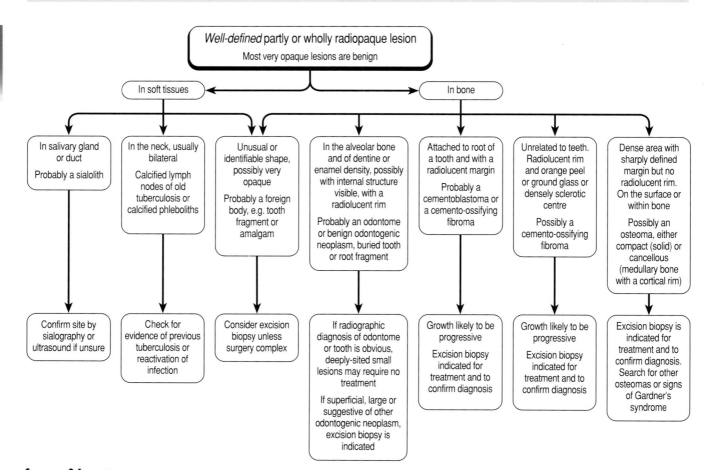

Summary 9.1 Differential diagnosis of a well-defined radio-opaque lesion in the jaws.

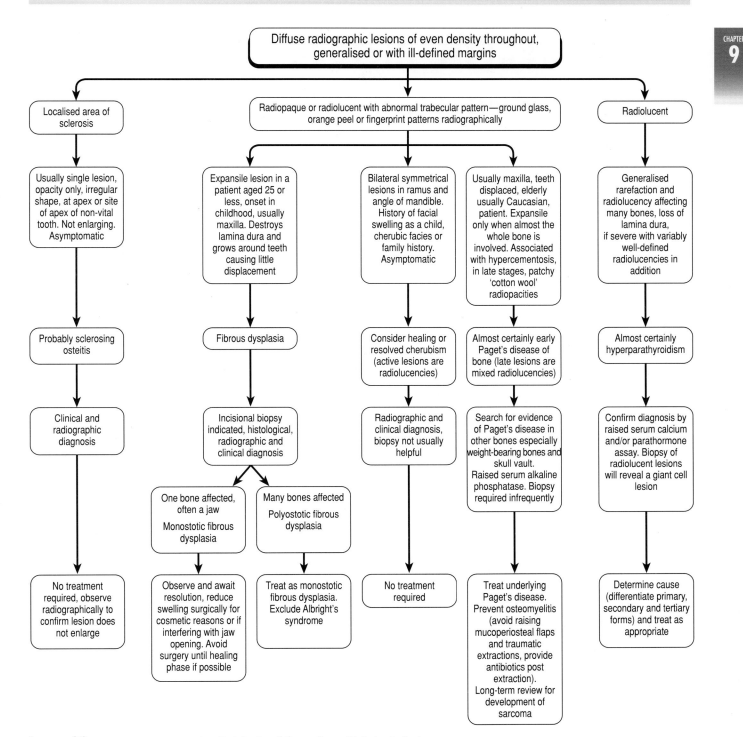

Summary 9.2 Differential diagnosis of an ill-defined or diffuse radiographic lesion in the jaws.

Genetic, metabolic and other non-neoplastic bone diseases

GENETIC DISEASES OF BONE

Osteogenesis imperfecta (brittle bone disease)

In osteogenesis imperfecta, which is usually transmitted as an autosomal dominant trait, the bones are excessively fragile. A defect of biosynthesis of type I collagen causes osteoblasts to fail to form bone in adequate amounts (Fig. 10.1).

The bones are thin and lack the usual cortex of compact bone but development of epiphyseal cartilages is unimpaired so that bones can grow to their normal length but may be so distorted by multiple fractures as to cause dwarfism. The most severe cases (type II) usually die at birth or soon after; mild cases (type V) may have little disability. In the more common form (type I) the many fractures can cause severe deformities (Figs 10.2 and

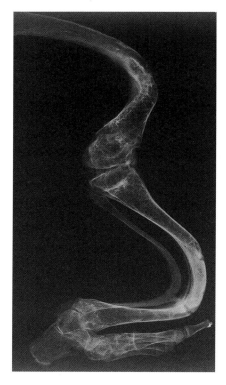

Fig. 10.2 Osteogenesis imperfecta. Leg of an infant with a severe type of osteogenesis imperfecta showing severe bending as a result of multiple fractures under body weight.

10.3). The sclera of the eyes may also appear blue (their thinness allows the pigment layer to show through), deafness also develops and dentinogenesis imperfecta is sometimes associated. There is no effective treatment but it is essential to protect the child from even minor injuries and to minimise deformity by attending to fractures. Care must be taken during dental extractions, but fractures of the jaws are uncommon in this disease.

Key features are summarised in Table 10.1.

Osteopetrosis — marble bone disease

Osteopetrosis is a rare genetic disease in which the bones become solidified and dense (Fig. 10.4) but brittle. There is

Fig. 10.1 Osteogenesis imperfecta. A section from the vault of the skull of a stillborn infant with type III disease; the most severe form of osteogenesis imperfecta shows that the bone is small in amount, primitive (woven) in character and shows no attempt at differentiation into cortical plates and medullary space.

Fig. 10.3 Clinical appearance of a severely affected child with osteogenesis imperfecta type III in which there is progressive deformity.

Table 10.1 Osteogenesis imperfecta — key features

- Thin fragile bones due to inadequate type I collagen formation
- Usually inherited as an autosomal dominant trait
- Multiple fractures typically lead to gross deformities
- Dentinogenesis imperfecta sometimes associated
- Jaw fractures are uncommon

inactivity of osteoclasts and absence of normal modelling resorption. Medullary spaces are minute (Fig. 10.5), and the epiphyseal ends of the bones are club-shaped. Because of the deficiency of marrow space, the liver and spleen take on blood cell formation, but anaemia is common. Osteomyelitis is a recognised complication and prevention of dental infections is important. There is no effective treatment apart from marrow transplantation. Key features are summarised in Table 10.2.

Table 10.2 Osteopetrosis — key features

- Rare genetic defect of osteoclastic activity
- Bones lack medullary cavities but are fragile
- Extramedullary haemopoiesis in liver and spleen but anaemia common
- Osteomyelitis a recognised complication
- Bone marrow transplantation offers the main hope

Fig. 10.4 Osteopetrosis. In contrast with osteogenesis imperfecta the bone is excessively thick and dense as a result of defective resorption.

Fig. 10.5   Osteopetrosis. Almost solid bone with only small lacunae has replaced the medullary space.

Fig. 10.6   Cleidocranial dysplasia. Defective development of the clavicles allows this abnormal mobility of the shoulders. Other members of the family were also affected.

Fig. 10.7   Cleidocranial dysplasia. A radiograph of the jaw of the father of the patient in Figure 10.6. There are many additional teeth but widespread failure of eruption.

Achondroplasia

Achondroplasia is the most common type of genetic skeletal disorder and produces short-limbed dwarfs who traditionally became circus clowns. The essential defect is failure of normal cartilage proliferation in the epiphyses and base of the skull. The limbs are therefore excessively short in relation to the trunk, while the head, which is normal in size, appears disproportionately large. Defective growth at the base of the skull causes the middle third of the face to be retrusive and the profile to be concave. The mandible is often protrusive, and as a result of the disparity of growth of the jaws, there is usually severe malocclusion. There is no effective treatment, but the occlusion may be improved by orthodontic treatment.

Key features are summarised in Table 10.3.

Table 10.3   Achondroplasia — key features
• A common type of genetic dwarfism • Failure of proliferation of cartilage in epiphyses and base of skull • Short limbs but normal-sized skull • Middle third of face retrusive due to deficient growth of skull base • Malocclusion may need correction

Cleidocranial dysplasia

In this rare familial disorder there is defective formation of the clavicles, delayed closure of fontanelles and sometimes retrusion of the maxilla. Partial or complete absence of clavicles allows the patient to bring the shoulders together in front of the chest (Fig. 10.6). This disorder is one of the few recognisable causes of delayed eruption of the permanent dentition. Many permanent teeth may remain embedded in the jaw (Fig. 10.7) and frequently become enveloped in dentigerous cysts (Ch. 2).

Key features are summarised in Table 10.4.

Table 10.4   Cleidocranial dysplasia — key features
• Rare genetic disorder causing defective formation of clavicles, delayed closure of fontanelles and other defects • Many or most permanent teeth typically remain embedded in the jaw • Many additional unerupted teeth also present • Sometimes many dentigerous cysts

Fig. 10.8   Cherubism. The typical 'cherubic' bulging of the cheeks can be seen.

Fig. 10.9   Cherubism. Both rami, much of the body of the mandible and the posterior maxillae are expanded by multilocular radiolucent lesions which have displaced and destroyed developing teeth.

Cherubism

Cherubism is inherited as an autosomal dominant trait, but boys are predominantly affected. Symmetrical swellings appear at the age of 2–4 years in the mandible in the region of the angles and, in severe cases, in the maxillae. The lesions cause fullness of the cheeks (Fig. 10.8), and in severe cases the maxillary swellings cause the eyes to appear turned upwards, producing the so-called cherubic appearance. There is no pain or tenderness, but the regional lymph nodes may be enlarged. Growth is rapid for a few years, then slows down until puberty is reached. There is then slow regression until, by adulthood, normal facial contour may be restored. However, radiolucent areas may persist longer.

Radiographically, there are symmetrical well-defined, apparently multilocular, radiolucent areas with a thin expanded cortex at the angles of the jaws and sometimes also in the maxillae (Fig. 10.9). Teeth are often displaced or buried.

Pathology

The lesions consist of multinucleated giant cells (Fig. 10.10) and resemble giant cell granulomas or hyperparathyroidism. With the passage of time, giant cells become fewer and there is bony repair of the defect (Fig. 10.11).

Fig. 10.10   Cherubism. An early lesion showing multinucleate giant cells lying in haemorrhagic oedematous fibrous tissue. The appearances are indistinguishable histologically from giant cell granuloma.

Fig. 10.11   Cherubism. In a late lesion there is formation of woven bone by the fibrous tissue and giant cells are less numerous. Eventually bone remodelling will restore the contour and quality of the bone.

Management

Because of natural regression of the disease, treatment can usually be avoided. If disfigurement is severe the lesions respond to curettage or to paring down of excessive tissue but, in the early stages particularly, will recur.

Key features are summarised in Table 10.5.

Table 10.5 Cherubism — key features

- Inherited as autosomal dominant trait
- Jaw swellings appear in infancy
- Angle region of mandible affected symmetrically, giving typical chubby face
- Symmetrical involvement of maxillae in more severe cases
- Radiographically, lesions appear as multilocular cyst-like areas
- Histologically, lesions consist of giant cells in vascular connective tissue
- Lesions regress with skeletal maturation and normal facial contour restored

---

Hypophosphatasia

Hypophosphatasia is an uncommon recessive genetic disorder. The early-onset type causes rickets-like skeletal disease with defective mineralisation. Defective cementogenesis results in premature loss of teeth, and this is sometimes the only sign of the disease. Plasma alkaline phosphatase levels are low but urinary phosphoethanolamine excretion is raised. Late-onset hypophosphatasia is sometimes a dominant trait, and its main manifestation is fragility of the bones.

Sickle cell anaemia and thalassaemia major

Bone changes are uncommon but these diseases (Ch. 22), particularly thalassaemia, when severe, can cause bony malformations of the maxillofacial region. In particular, expanded erythropoiesis causes thickening but osteoporosis of the bones of the skull. In sickle cell anaemia infarcts in the jaws are painful. Symptomatically and radiographically they can mimic osteomyelitis. Bone infarcts may appear relatively radiolucent at first, but become sclerotic, and opaque areas in the skull or jaws are left by earlier infarcts.

In thalassaemia the diploic spaces of the skull are enlarged due to marrow expansion and have a hair-on-end appearance radiographically and a thin cortex. The maxillae may also be expanded, causing severe malocclusion. The zygomatic bones are pushed outwards and the nasal bridge is depressed in severe cases.

METABOLIC BONE DISEASE

Rickets

Vitamin D is essential for the absorption and metabolism of cal-

cium and phosphorus. Deficiency during the period of bone development causes rickets, with defective calcification and development of the skeleton, but rarely of the teeth (Ch. 30).

Defective calcium and phosphorus metabolism may also result from chronic renal disease (either hereditary or inflammatory) causing abnormal excretion of these minerals. Defective development of bone (renal rickets) can result.

The onset of rickets is usually in infancy. The main defects are broadening of the growing ends of bones and prominent costochondral junctions due to the epiphyseal defects. The weakened bones bend readily. Typical changes in the skull are wide fontanelles, bossing of the frontal and parietal eminences and thinning of the back of the skull. Radiographs show the wide, thick epiphyses and deformities (Fig. 10.12). There are usually normal serum calcium but low phosphorus levels, or either may be depressed. The alkaline phosphatase level is raised.

Pathology

Throughout the bone but especially at the ends of the shafts, trabeculae become surrounded by newly formed, uncalcified osteoid matrix. In the zone of provisional calcification, mineralisation of cartilage fails, and the cartilage cells continue to proliferate until the epiphyseal plate becomes greatly thickened, wide and highly cellular (Fig. 10.13). Blood vessels invade and branch irregularly among the proliferating cartilage cells. They are accompanied by connective tissue, which further disorganises the epiphysis.

Dental changes. Teeth have a priority over the skeleton for minerals, and dental defects rarely result from rickets. Hypocalcification of dentine, with a wide band of predentine and excessive interglobular spaces, may be seen in unusually severe rickets. Eruption of teeth may be delayed. Rachitic chil-

Fig. 10.12 Rickets. Overgrowth of cartilage (as shown in the section in Figure 10.13) causes the epiphyseal plate to be broad, thick and irregular, and the ends of the bone become splayed. The growing end of the bone is ill-defined and calcification defective.

Fig. 10.13 Rickets. The specimen on the left is from a child of 14 months with rickets due to chronic renal disease. The epiphyseal cartilage shows irregular overgrowth of cartilage cells and absence of calcification; a layer of vascular connective tissue is starting to invade the cartilage in the normal epiphyseal cartilage of a newborn infant (right). The columns of cartilage are short and regular; immediately below them is the zone of provisional calcification with darkly staining trabeculae of calcified osteoid.

dren are not abnormally susceptible to dental caries, and 'shortage of calcium' as a cause of dental caries is a myth.

Treatment

Vitamin D, the equivalent of 2000–3000 iu daily, should be given. The diet should also be adequate in other components. Orthopaedic treatment may be needed to correct deformities.

Scurvy

Scurvy, caused by vitamin C deficiency, leads to defective formation of collagen and osteoid matrix; such matrix as forms is well calcified. Infantile scurvy, with skeletal defects, is largely of historical interest in Britain but has been described, for instance, in an infant whose mother had eccentric ideas about diet. A case has also been described in the USA in 1995.

The amount of osteoid matrix formed is small but highly calcified so that the ends of the long bones are sharply defined radiologically. Weakness of the connective tissue and the haemorrhagic tendency (purpura) cause detachment of the periosteum by bleeding, and bone pain. The haematoma becomes calcified, as shown in the radiograph (Fig. 10.14).

Severe scurvy also causes swollen, bleeding gingivae (Ch. 5) and early tooth loss.

Hyperparathyroidism

Primary hyperparathyroidism is usually caused by hyperplasia or adenoma of the parathyroids but is uncommon.

Fig. 10.14 Scurvy. In contrast to rickets, calcification is unimpeded and there is a thick layer of calcified cartilage at the end of the bone. Osteoid formation, on the other hand, is reduced, so that little bone can be formed. The attachment of the periosteum to the bone is weak, so that it is easily separated; there may be haemorrhage beneath it (as here) due to scorbutic purpura, and this becomes calcified.

Overproduction of parathormone (PTH) mobilises calcium and raises the plasma calcium level.

Postmenopausal women are mainly affected. The major symptoms result from renal damage which leads to hypertension or other cardiovascular disease. Peptic ulcer symptoms or mere malaise are also common. Bone disease is rarely seen now, because of earlier treatment, but small lesions may be detectable radiographically. Among dental patients a cyst-like swelling of the jaw with the histological features of a giant cell lesion is the classical way by which hyperparathyroidism has been detected but is rare. It is essential not to miss this diagnosis because of the risk of irreversible renal damage in the absence of treatment. The possibility of secondary hyperparathyroidism (see below) should also be excluded.

Radiographically, the main effects are thinning of bone trabeculae, subperiosteal resorption of the bone of the fingers and resorption of the terminal phalangeal tufts. In severe disease, radiolucent cyst-like areas (osteitis fibrosa cystica), often with a multiloculated appearance, are a typical but rare finding (Figs 10.15 and 10.16). Alveolar bone may also be resorbed but reforms with treatment (Figs 10.17 and 10.18).

Pathology

Histologically, the cyst-like areas are foci of osteoclasts in a highly vascular stroma (Fig. 10.19). Extensive haemosiderin deposits cause the lesion to appear as a brown tumour.

These foci are indistinguishable from giant cell granulomas of the jaws. Unlike the latter, there are characteristic changes in blood chemistry (Table 10.6) and sometimes multifocal involvement of other bones. Occasionally, bone lesions cause pathological fractures. The increased excretion of calcium leads ultimately to renal calcinosis or stone formation and renal damage. Other clinical features also result from the hypercalcaemia. Blood chemistry examination is essential in patients found to have giant cell lesions of the jaws, especially adults of middle age or over.

Secondary hyperparathyroidism results from prolonged stimulation of the parathyroids by a persistently depressed plasma calcium. The most common cause is chronic renal failure.

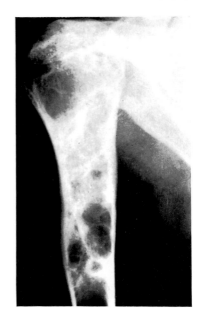

Fig. 10.16 Hyperparathyroidism. Osteitis fibrosa cystica in the humerus of the same patient with a parathyroid adenoma. Note also the loss of trabecular pattern and cortex.

Fig. 10.17 Hyperparathyroidism. A periapical view reveals the relative radiolucency of the bone. There is loss of lamina dura around the roots, loss of trabeculae centrally and coarsening of the trabecular pattern elsewhere.

Secondary hyperparathyroidism is now a more frequent cause of osteolytic bone lesions than primary hyperparathyroidism, but shows the same histological picture of osteoclastic proliferation. Such lesions may also be a sign of rejection of a renal transplant (Fig. 10.20).

Management

In primary hyperparathyroidism, surgical removal of the

Fig. 10.15 Hyperparathyroidism. A patient of 51 with hyperparathyroidism as a result of a parathyroid adenoma. There is an area of bone destruction simulating a multilocular cyst.

Fig. 10.18 Hyperparathyroidism. The same patient after treatment shows improved bone density and reformation of the lamina dura and cortex.

Fig. 10.19 Hyperparathyroidism. Multinucleate osteoclast-like giant cells are lying in a haemorrhagic fibrous tissue. The appearances are indistinguishable from giant cell granuloma histologically.

Table 10.6   Biochemical findings in hyperparathyroidism

- Raised plasma calcium (2.8 mmol/l or more)
- Low plasma phosphorus (less than 0.8 mmol/l)
- Raised plasma parathyroid hormone levels
- Raised plasma alkaline phosphatase (over 100 iu/l).

---

parathyroidism adenoma is curative. For secondary hyperparathyroidism, the renal failure should be treated if possible. Bone lesions may respond to oral administration of vitamin D, whose metabolism is abnormal as a result of the renal disease. If hypercalcaemia is of very long standing, parathyroid hyperplasia may be irreversible (so-called tertiary hyperparathyroidism) and need to be treated by parathyroidectomy.

Fig. 10.20 Hyperparathyroidism. In this patient with hyperparathyroidism as a result of rejection of a kidney graft there is a well-defined area of bone loss.

Key features are summarised in Table 10.7.

Table 10.7   Hyperparathyroidism — key features

- Overproduction of parathyroid hormone due to hyperplasia or adenoma of parathyroid glands leads to mobilisation of bone calcium
- Significant bone disease now uncommon
- Common effects are malaise, hypertension or peptic ulcer
- Jaw lesions are rare, but appear radiographically as multilocular cyst-like areas sometimes with multifocal involvement of other bones
- Histologically, bone lesions consist of vascular foci of giant cells, indistinguishable from giant cell granulomas
- Diagnosis confirmed by raised serum calcium, parathyroid hormone and alkaline phosphatase but low serum phosphorus

---

Gigantism and acromegaly

Overproduction of pituitary growth hormone, usually by an adenoma, before the epiphyses fuse, gives rise to *gigantism*, with overgrowth of the whole skeleton. After fusion of the epiphyses, overproduction of growth hormone gives rise to *acromegaly*. The main features are continued growth at the mandibular condyle, causing gross prognathism, macroglossia, thickening of the facial soft tissues and overgrowth of the hands and feet (Ch. 31).

Fluorosis

Excessive amounts of fluorides in the drinking water, as in certain parts of Northern India, cause severe mottling of the teeth and also sclerosis of the skeleton. The intervertebral ligaments and muscle insertions calcify, causing stiffness (particularly of the back) and pain. Histologically, the bone changes are somewhat similar to those of Paget's disease.

BONE DISEASES OF UNKNOWN CAUSE

Paget's disease of bone (osteitis deformans)

Paget's disease causes bone distortion and weakening, particularly in the elderly.

Patients past middle age are affected most severely. In Britain, up to 3% of people over 40 may have radiographic signs of Paget's disease, but clinical disease is less common. The cause is unknown but intranuclear inclusions compatible with a paramyxo- or other virus have been demonstrated in both osteoblasts and osteoclasts. A genetic factor may also be involved.

Bones most frequently affected are sacrum, spine, skull, femora and pelvis. The disease may be widespread and is usually symmetrical, but sometimes a single bone is affected. In the uncommon severe form, the main features are an enlarged head, thickening of long bones, which bend under stress, and tenderness or aching pain which can be severe and almost intractable. The vault of the skull is more often affected than the facial skeleton, and the maxilla considerably more frequently than the mandible (Fig. 10.21). Narrowing of foramina can occasionally cause cranial nerve deficits.

When the jaws are affected the alveolar process becomes symmetrically and grossly enlarged (Fig. 10.22). There may also be gross and irregular hypercementosis of teeth, which may become fused to sclerotic areas of the bone. Attempts to

Fig. 10.22 Paget's disease of bone. Characteristic features of the involved maxilla are the broadening and deepening of the alveolar process, generalised enlargement and spacing of the teeth.

extract affected teeth may succeed only by tearing away a large mass of bone. Severe bleeding or osteomyelitis of ischaemic bone may follow.

The main radiographic features are lower density of the bone in the early stages and sclerosis in the later stages. Changes are patchily distributed and loss of normal trabeculation causes the bone to have a characteristic cotton-wool appearance.

Pathology

Bone resorption and replacement becomes rapid, irregular, exaggerated and purposeless. The changes progress erratically but the ultimate result is thickening of affected bones without localised swellings.

In the early stages there is typically resorption, which is later followed by sclerosis, but since closely adjacent parts of the bone may show different stages of the disease, a common result is patchy areas of osteoporosis and of sclerosis.

Destruction and new bone formation may alternate rapidly, and the change in bony activity is marked histologically by blue-staining reversal lines. Their irregular pattern characteristically produces a jigsaw puzzle ('mosaic') appearance in the bone (Figs 10.23 and 10.24).

The main histological changes are the irregular pattern of reversal lines, many osteoblasts and osteoclasts (often abnormally large), fibrosis of the marrow spaces and increased vascularity. In the late stages, affected bones are thick, the cortex and medulla are obliterated and the whole bone is spongy in texture.

Serum calcium and phosphorus levels are usually normal, but the alkaline phosphatase level is particularly high and may reach 700 iu/l. The development of osteosarcoma is a recognised but rare complication of Paget's disease and virtually never affects the jaws. Many patients live to an advanced age in spite of their disabilities.

Treatment is with calcitonin or bisphosphonates or both. Calcitonins, such as salcatonin, have to be given by injection and are more effective for reducing bone pain and osteolysis, but can cause nausea and an unpleasant taste. Calcitonin is also

Fig. 10.21 Paget's disease of the skull and maxilla. The thickening of the bone and the irregular areas of sclerosis and resorption, which give it a fluffy appearance, are in striking contrast to the unaffected mandible.

ly and depress bone turnover by slowing both the dissolution and growth of hydroxyapatite crystals.

Key features are summarised in Table 10.8.

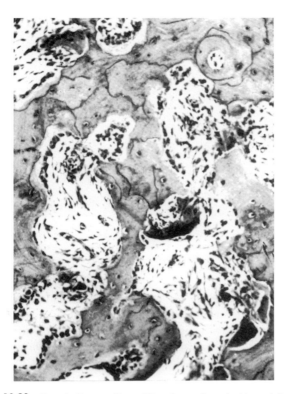

Fig. 10.23 Paget's disease of bone. There is a well-marked 'mosaic' pattern of the bone due to repeated alternation of resorption and apposition. The marrow has been replaced by fibrous tissue and there are many osteoblasts and osteoclasts lining the surface of the bone.

Table 10.8 **Paget's disease — key features**

- Persons past middle age affected.
- Common radiographic finding. Less common as clinical disease
- Enlargement of skull, thickening but weakness of long bones and bone pain are typical of severe disease
- Maxilla occasionally, but mandible rarely affected
- Teeth may show gross irregular hypercementosis
- Radiographically, patchy sclerosis and resorption give a cotton-wool appearance
- Histologically, irregular resorption and apposition leaves jigsaw puzzle ('mosaic') pattern of reversal lines
- Serum alkaline phosphatase up to 700 iu/1

Fibro-osseous lesions

This term is used for disorders ranging from fibrous dysplasia to the circumscribed lesions of ossifying or cementifying fibroma and the cemental dysplasias (Table 10.9). Cherubism is sometimes included but has been described earlier. Behaviour varies but growth in early life with spontaneous arrest and increasing ossification, roughly coinciding with skeletal maturation, is typical of fibrous dysplasia and cherubism. In this difficult area the diagnosis depends greatly on the clinical and radiographic findings.

Table 10.9 **Fibro-osseous lesions**

- Fibrous dysplasia
    Monostotic
    Polyostotic
- Cemento-osseous dysplasias
    Periapical cemental dysplasia
    Focal cemento-osseous dysplasia
    Florid cemento-osseous dysplasia
- Fibro-osseous neoplasms
    Cemento-ossifying fibroma (Ch. 8)

Fig. 10.24 Paget's disease affecting the jaw results in destruction of the lamina dura surrounding the teeth and, at a later stage, involves hypercementosis and sometimes ankylosis.

given preoperatively to reduce bleeding from the highly vascular bone and may help to relieve cranial nerve deficits. Bisphosphonates (such as sodium etidronate) can be given oral-

Fibrous dysplasia

Monostotic fibrous dysplasia gives rise to a bony swelling caused by a poorly-circumscribed area of fibro-osseous proliferation. This typically starts in childhood but usually undergoes arrest in adulthood. The jaws are the most frequent sites in the head and neck region. Males and females are almost equally frequently affected.

Clinically, a painless, smoothly rounded swelling, usually of the maxilla, is typical (Fig. 10.25). The mass may become large enough to disturb function and cause malocclusion by displacing teeth.

Radiographically, there is typically an area of reduced

Fig. 10.25 Fibrous dysplasia. Typical presentation with a poorly-defined, rounded expansion of the maxilla with displacement of teeth and intact overlying mucosa.

Fig. 10.27 Fibrous dysplasia. Slender trabeculae of woven bone, said to resemble Chinese characters in shape, lying in a very cellular fibrous tissue. With maturation there is progressively more bone formation.

Fig. 10.26 Fibrous dysplasia. This is a well-established lesion with a rounded swelling which merges imperceptibly with normal bone surrounding the canine. There is loss of lamina dura and cortex in the affected area and the fine trabecular pattern produces an orange-peel or thumb-print appearance.

radiopacity, with a fine orange-peel texture and an eggshell-thin cortex of expanded bone (Fig. 10.26). The degree of radiopacity depends on the amount of lesional bone, which may give a predominantly radiolucent or more sclerotic appearance. The key feature is that the margins merge imperceptibly with the surrounding normal bone.

Polyostotic fibrous dysplasia is rare but shows histologically similar lesions in several bones, skin pigmentation and endocrine abnormalities. Females are affected in the ratio of 3:1 and the disease may be seen in childhood. *Albright's syndrome* comprises polyostotic fibrous dysplasia, skin pigmentation and sexual precocity.

Polyostotic fibrous dysplasia involves the head and neck region in up to 50% of cases. A jaw lesion may then be the most conspicuous feature and polystotic disease may not be suspect-

ed initially. In a young girl in particular, investigation for other skeletal lesions and pigmentation may therefore be indicated. Skin pigmentation consists of brownish macules which frequently overlie affected bones and appear especially on the back of the neck, trunk, buttocks or thighs, but hardly ever on the oral mucosa.

Pathology

The lesions consist of loose cellular fibrous tissue containing slender trabeculae of woven bone of variable shape which merge imperceptibly into surrounding normal bone (Figs 10.27 and 10.28).

Osteoblasts are scattered throughout the substance of the trabeculae, rather than surrounding them. Some lamellar bone or calcified spherules and occasional loose foci of giant cells can also be seen.

Treatment

The disease is self-limiting, but grossly disfiguring lesions may need to be excised. This should be delayed if possible until the process has become inactive. There is a small risk of sarcomatous change, particularly in the polyostotic variant.

Key features are summarised in Table 10.10.

Cemento-osseous dyplasias

These are probably of periodontal ligament origin and involve the same pathological processes but differ mainly in their extent and radiographic appearances.

Periapical cemental dysplasia

Periapical cemental dysplasia affects women (particularly the

Fig. 10.28 Fibrous dysplasia. There is loss of lamina dura around the teeth and its replacement by lesional bone. These numerous small trabeculae give rise to the ground-glass and orange-peel appearances radiographically.

Table 10.10 Monostotic fibrous dysplasia — key features

- Persons under 20 years mainly affected
- Localised swelling usually of maxilla
- Radiographically, normal bone trabeculation replaced by orange-peel pattern
- Lesions merge imperceptibly with normal bone at the margins
- Histologically, normal bone replaced by fibrous connective tissue containing slender trabeculae of bone
- Usually becomes inactive with skeletal maturation

---

middle-aged) more than 10 times as frequently as men, and is also more common in black individuals. It typically involves the mandibular incisor region, but can affect several sites or be generalised.

It is asymptomatic but can be seen early in radiographs as rounded radiolucent areas related to the apices of the teeth. They simulate periapical granulomas but related teeth are vital. Later, increasing calcification, starting centrally, causes the masses to become densely radiopaque, but all stages of development may be seen in multiple lesions.

Pathology

The lesions resemble cemento-ossifying fibromas histologically and consist, in their early stages, of cellular fibrous tissue containing foci of cementum-like tissue. Progressive calcifi-

Fig. 10.29 Florid cemento-osseous dysplasia. Section of a panoramic tomogram showing the typical appearances of multiple irregular radiopaque masses centred on the roots of the teeth. The periphery of each is radiolucent. Similar lesions were present on the contralateral side of the mandible.

cation leads to the formation of a solid, bone-like mass. Early lesions need to be distinguished from periapical granulomas by dental investigation. Further treatment is unnecessary, as the disorder is self-limiting.

Florid cemento-osseous dysplasia (gigantiform cementoma)

This is probably a florid form of periapical cemental dysplasia and affects a similar group of persons. The sclerotic masses are frequently symmetrical and may involve all four quadrants. They are asymptomatic unless they become infected, but can expand the jaw.

Radiographically, florid cemento-osseous dysplasia appears as radiopaque, somewhat irregular masses without a radiolucent border and in the past has been mistaken for chronic osteomyelitis (Fig. 10.29)

Microscopically, the appearances are generally similar to periapical cemental dysplasia.

Focal cemento-osseous dysplasia

This term is given to changes similar to florid osseous dysplasia but forming a single lesion.

Management of cemento-osseous dysplasias

Prevention of infection of these lesions by unwise extractions or other means must be avoided. Osteomyelitis resulting from such causes is difficult to treat because of the widespread sclerosis in the late stages. Wide excision may then be required to allow resolution. Treatment is otherwise not indicated, except rarely for cosmetic reasons.

SUGGESTED FURTHER READING

Cawson R A, Binnie W H, Eveson J W 1995 Color atlas of oral disease, 2nd edn. Mosby-Wolfe, London

Cawson R A, Langdon J D, Eveson J W 1996 Surgical pathology of the mouth and jaws. Wright, Oxford

Chindia M L, Ocholla T J, Imalingat B 1991 Osteopetrosis presenting with paroxysmal trigeminal neuralgia. A case report. Int J Oral Maxillofac Surg 20:199–200

Droz-Desprez D, Azou C, Bordigoni P, Bonnaure-Mallet M 1992 Infantile osteopetrosis: a case report on dental findings. J Oral Pathol Med 21:422–425

Ebata K, Usami T, Tohnai, Kaneda T 1992 Chondrosarcoma and osteosarcoma arising in polyostotic fibrous dysplasia. J Oral Maxillofac Surg 50:761–764

Freemont A J 1996 The pathology of osteogenesis imperfecta. J Clin Pathol 49:618–619

Frohberg U, Tiner B D 1995 Surgical correction of facial deformities in a patient with cleidocranial dysplasia. J Craniofac Surg 6:49–53

Koury M E, Regezi J A, Perrott D H, Kaban L B 1995 'Atypical' fibro-osseous lesions: diagnostic challenges and treatment concepts. Int J Oral Maxillofac Surg 24:162–169

Melrose R J, Abrams A M, Mills B G 1976 Florid osseous dysplasia. A clinicopathologic study of thirty-four cases. Oral Surg Oral Med Oral Pathol 41:62–68

Ruggieri P, Sim F H, Bond J R, Unni K K 1994 Malignancies in fibrous dysplasia. Cancer 73:1411–1424

Schneider L C, Mesa M L 1990 Differences between florid osseous dysplasia and chronic diffuse sclerosing osteomyelitis. Oral Surg Oral Med Oral Pathol 70:308–312

Shapiro F, Osteopetrosis 1993 Current clinical considerations. Clin Orthop Rel Res 294:34–44

Summerlin D-J, Tomich C E 1994 Focal cemento-osseous dysplasia: a clinicopathological study of 221 cases. Oral Surg Oral Med Oral Pathol 78:611–620

Waldron C A 1993 Fibro-osseous lesions of the jaws. J Oral Maxillofac Surg 51: 828–835

Younai F, Eisenbud L, Sciubba J J 1988 Osteopetrosis: a case report including gross and microscopic findings in the mandible at autopsy. Oral Surg Oral Med Oral Pathol 65:214–221

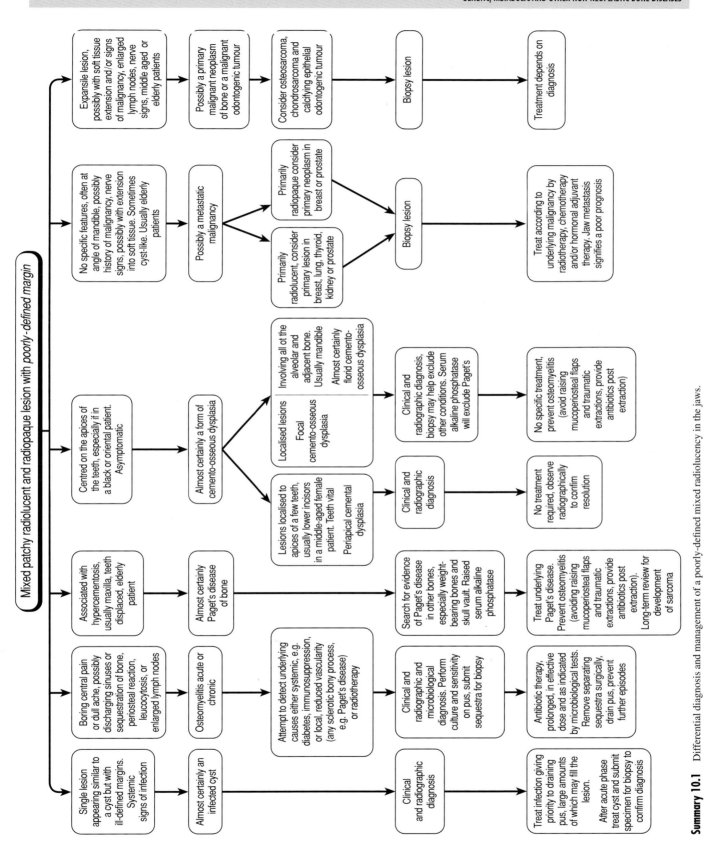

Summary 10.1   Differential diagnosis and management of a poorly-defined mixed radiolucency in the jaws.

The temporomandibular joints and periarticular tissues

Disorders of the temporomandibular joints can cause limitation of movement of the jaw, pain or clicking sounds, alone or in various combinations.

Limitation of movement

Inability to open the mouth fully is usually temporary, and often called *trismus*; occasionally it may be more persistent. Important causes are summarised in Table 11.1.

Table 11.1   **Important causes of trismus**

- Inflammation in or near the joint
- Mandibular block injections
- Injuries
- Tetanus and tetany
- Temporomandibular pain dysfunction syndrome

Pericoronitis is the main inflammatory cause of trismus. Rare causes include suppurative arthritis, osteomyelitis or cellulitis. Mandibular block injections occasionally cause inflammation and oedema of the periarticular tissues, either because of irritation by the local anaesthetic solution or by introducing infection. Rarely, limitation of movement may be more persistent, due to organisation of a haematoma caused by the injection. Operative treatment may then be necessary.

Fracture of the necks of the condyles or dislocation, if untreated, cause an anterior open bite or fixation in the open position, respectively (see Figs 11.3–11.5). Tetanus and tetany are rare causes of spasm of the masticatory muscles. Nevertheless, though rare, it is important to exclude tetanus because of its high mortality. It should be considered whenever a patient develops acute severe limitation of movement of the jaw without local cause.

Pain dysfunction syndrome is a common cause of temporary limitation of movement of the temporomandibular joint, as discussed later.

In all these conditions the essential treatment is to relieve the underlying disorder.

Permanent limitation of movement (ankylosis)

Important causes are summarised in Table 11.2.

Table 11.2   **Important causes of temporomandibular joint ankylosis**

- Extra-articular causes
  - Fibrosis due to burns or irradiation
  - Oral submucous fibrosis
- Intra-articular causes
  - Congenital
  - Trauma
  - Acute pyogenic arthritis
  - Juvenile arthritis
  - Tumours and other abnormalities of the condyle

ORAL SUBMUCOUS FIBROSIS

Oral submucous fibrosis affects those from the Indian subcontinent and many areas of South-east Asia, such as Taiwan. It produces changes similar to those of systemic sclerosis but limited to the oral tissues and without immunological abnormalities.

The aetiology is multifactorial but betel (*pan*) chewing is strongly suspected. Pan typically consists of areca nut, tobacco and lime wrapped in betel leaf. Experimentally, arecoline, a derivative of areca, can induce fibroblast proliferation and collagen synthesis. There is a significant association between areca nut consumption and submucous fibrosis.

Clinically, symmetrical fibrosis of such sites as the buccal mucosa, soft palate or inner aspects of the lips is characteristic. The overlying mucosa may be normal or there may be a vesiculating stomatitis. Fibrosis causes extreme pallor of the affected area (Fig. 11.1), which becomes so hard that it cannot be indented with the finger. Ultimately, opening the mouth may become so limited that eating and dental treatment become increasingly difficult and tube-feeding may become necessary. Alternatively, malignant change can develop (Ch. 16).

Microscopy.   The subepithelial connective tissue becomes thickened, hyaline and avascular, and there may be mild chronic inflammation. The epithelium usually becomes thinned and

Fig. 11.1 Oral submucous fibrosis. Typical appearance in a relatively advanced case with pale fibrotic bands of scarring running across the soft palate and down the anterior pillar of the fauces. Similar fibrous bands were present in the buccal mucosa bilaterally.

Fig. 11.2 Oral submucous fibrosis. There is fibrosis extending from the epithelium down into the underlying muscle, which is replaced by hyalinised fibrous tissue.

may show atypia. Underlying muscle fibres undergo progressive atrophy (Fig. 11.2).

Management

In patients from endemic areas such as India with these lesions, and especially with the characteristic histological changes on biopsy, the diagnosis should be clear.

Treatment is unsatisfactory. Patients must stop betel chewing. Intralesional injections of corticosteroids and muscle-stretching exercises to prevent further limitation of opening may help a little. Plastic surgery is sometimes carried out, but is likely to be followed by relapse. Regular follow-up is important because of the malignant potential of this disease.

Other causes of ankylosis

Systemic sclerosis (scleroderma, Ch. 25) can also cause fixation of the jaw by dense periarticular fibrosis.

Congenital ankylosis is probably due to injury at birth. Later in life, intracapsular fracture of the neck of the condyle disorganises the joint and causes bleeding followed by fibrosis.

However, an effective false joint usually forms and function is little impaired. Acute pyogenic arthritis is rare but, if treated ineffectively, ankylosis of the joint follows. Some types of juvenile arthritis are severe and can lead to ankylosis.

Osteomas, chondromas or hyperplasia of the condyle are rare causes of limitation or loss of movement of the jaw.

Management

When the joint becomes fixed by fibrous adhesions it may be possible to sever them at open operation. If this fails or if there is bony ankylosis, a false joint can sometimes be made by excising the condyle and interposing soft tissue. Alternatively, a wedge resection near the angle may be used for the same purpose.

Dislocation of the jaw

The temporomandibular joint may become fixed in the open position by dislocation; this is usually due to forcible opening of the mouth by a blow on the jaw, or forceful dental extractions under general anaesthesia. It should then be noticed immediately and corrected before the patient recovers consciousness. Downwards and backwards pressure on the lower posterior teeth should be effective.

Occasionally the dislocation remains unnoticed and, surprisingly, a patient may tolerate the disability and discomfort for weeks or even months (Figs 11.3–11.5). In such cases, effusion into the joint becomes organised, forming fibrous adhesions. When this happens, open operation becomes necessary to divide adhesions.

Fig. 11.3 Long-standing dislocation of the jaw: the teeth had been extracted about a month previously; in spite of the patient's inability to close her mouth and the distorted appearance, the dislocation remained unrecognised.

Fig. 11.4   Reduction of the dislocation (performed by open operation because of development of fibrous adhesions) restores the patient's normal appearance and movements of the jaw.

Fig. 11.5   Dislocation of the jaw. Radiography of a temporomandibular joint of the same patient showed complete dislocation of the condyle in front of the eminentia articularis. (Figures 11.3–11.5 by courtesy of Professor I Curson and British Dental Journal 1959 107:351.)

Recurrent dislocation

Recurrent dislocation is a rarity but may be caused by, and is sometimes a typical feature of, some of the floppy joint syndromes, notably Ehlers–Danlos and Marfan's syndromes. In such cases arthroplasty may be needed to improve the stability of the joint.

Tardive dyskinesia

Involuntary, disfiguring grimacing as a result of movements of the jaw and face can be a late ('tardive') complication of treatment with phenothiazine antipsychotics. Metoclopramide, which has phenothiazine-like actions, can cause persistent trismus. There is no reliably effective treatment.

PAIN IN OR AROUND THE JOINT

Pain felt during movements of the temporomandibular joint can come from the joint itself, muscles of mastication or adjacent structures. The main causes are summarised in Table 11.3.

Table 11.3   Important causes of pain felt in the temporomandibular joint region
● Dislocation or fractures of the neck of the condyle
● Infection and inflammation
● Ischaemic pain (cranial arteritis)
● Muscle spasm (pain dysfunction syndrome)
● Salivary gland disease

Dislocation or fractures of the neck of the condyle can cause pain of varying degrees of severity, but, surprisingly often, fractures in this region pass unnoticed. Acute pyogenic arthritis is rare. Other types of arthritis, such as rheumatoid arthritis, can cause temporomandibular joint pain, but not commonly. Cranial arteritis is the main cause of vascular pain as a result of ischaemia of the masticatory muscles. Acute parotitis or malignant neoplasms can be mistaken for temporomandibular joint pain.

PAIN DYSFUNCTION SYNDROME

Pain dysfunction syndrome predominantly affects young women and is characterised by pain, clicking sounds from the joint, or limitation of movement (Table 11.4). The area may be tender to pressure, and a clicking sound, when the mouth is opened or closed, is common. Sometimes pain is felt lower down over the ramus, occasionally at the angle of the jaw and, more rarely still, other sites nearby. Defects of occlusion can often be found, as in any other patients.

Table 11.4   Typical features of pain dysfunction syndrome
● Female to male preponderance of nearly 4 to 1
● Most patients are between 20 and 40 years old
● Onset is usually gradual
● Onset occasionally ascribed to violent yawning, laughing or a similar incident
● Pain usually one-sided, rarely severe
● Typically a dull ache is made worse by mastication
● Pain typically felt in front of the ear
● Frequently also limitation of opening, or 'locking', of the jaw
● Ultimately self-limiting

Aetiology

Abnormalities of occlusion, such as lack of posterior occlusal support from loss of molar teeth, are often blamed but there is no evidence that they are a cause. In spite of the problems created by dentures, for instance, edentulous patients seem rarely, if ever, to be affected. Trauma, particularly minor injuries such as may be caused by violent yawning, laughing, or dental treatment, is occasionally a possible factor but the evidence does not seem strong. Illustrative of some of the difficulties in identifying this complaint and its causes is that its prevalence reported in different surveys ranges from 12% to 86% of adults.

All the evidence suggests that pain dysfunction syndrome is of dubious aetiology that typically affects only a restricted group of the population. It is self-limiting and does not progress to permanent damage or degenerative arthritis later in life. Elderly patients are remarkably free from temporomandibular joint symptoms. Defective neuromuscular coordination, causing areas of spasm of the masticatory muscles, appears to be the main cause.

Investigation

In view of the absence of objective signs, diagnosis is largely by exclusion. Organic causes (as enumerated above) of pain or limitation of movement of the joint should be ruled out by investigation. As in all cases of pain in the region of the jaws, referred pain from the teeth should be carefully excluded.

The temporomandibular joint should be palpated for tenderness or swelling which, if present, suggest organic disease. Crepitus may be felt but is not specific and is not necessarily a sign of significant joint disease. Radiographs of the joints may be taken to make sure that movements are not excessive in either direction and are equal on both sides. However, the main value of radiographs is to exclude such changes as fluid accumulation (widening of the joint space) or damage or deformity of the joint surfaces, indicating organic disease. Trigeminal neuralgia can be occasionally triggered by movement of the jaw and should be suspected in older patients, particularly when the pain is severe and paroxysmal. Response to treatment with carbamazepine is virtually diagnostic of trigeminal neuralgia.

Management

In the USA this complaint has been investigated and treated (often by surgery) so excessively vigorously that the resulting litigation has forced a search for a consensus on management. It is now accepted that the indications for active intervention, particularly surgery or 'occlusal therapy', are of questionable value. Moreover, there is a strong placebo effect in any form of treatment. The main principles of management of pain dysfunction syndrome are summarised in Table 11.5.

Table 11.5 Principles of management of pain dysfunction syndrome

- Reassurance
- Habit management and physical therapy
- Occlusal appliances
- Analgesics

Any abnormal biting habits should be identified and controlled. Faulty neuromuscular control should be dealt with by exercises to correct faulty patterns of activity, as shown by such abnormalities as deviations on closure.

In practice, fitting an acrylic overlay appliance is simple and usually effective. It also tends to relieve abnormal grinding habits. It should cover the occlusal surfaces of the teeth and allow free occlusion without cuspal interference.

Short-term use of simple analgesics may also be helpful.

CRANIAL (GIANT CELL) ARTERITIS

Cranial arteritis occasionally causes ischaemic pain in the masticatory muscles and should be considered in elderly patients who complain of headache and pain on mastication. Its salient features are summarised in Table 11.6.

Table 11.6 Cranial arteritis — key features

- Women, usually over 55 years, predominantly affected
- Weakness, low-grade fever and weight-loss often early features
- Severe throbbing headache is a major symptom
- The temporal artery frequently becomes red, tender, firm, swollen and tortuous
- Ischaemic pain in the masticatory muscles prominent in 20%
- ESR usually greatly raised
- Blindness a common complication
- Good response to early treatment with corticosteroids

Pain on mastication, comparable to and often misnamed jaw claudication (claudication is literally, *limping*), is sometimes the main symptom and present in about 20% of patients. Disturbances of vision or sudden blindness due to involvement of the ophthalmic artery develops in 50% of untreated patients. Polymyalgia rheumatica, with weakness and pain of the shoulder or pelvic girdles, and fever may be associated.

Pathology

Inflammation involves the arterial media and intima. Infiltration by mononuclear cells is typically associated with giant cells (Fig. 11.6). Intimal damage leads to formation of thrombi, which usually become organized and there may be severe dam-

Fig. 11.6   Giant cell (temporal) arteritis. At low power the structure of the artery is seen to be disrupted by inflammatory cells and the lumen is much reduced in size.

Fig. 11.8   Giant cell (temporal) arteritis. At high power multinucleate giant cells, lymphocytes and neutrophils may be seen amongst the remnants of the artery's internal elastic lamina (arrowed).

Fig. 11.7   Giant cell (temporal) arteritis. At higher power the internal elastic lamina of the artery may be seen together with giant cells, lymphocytes and neutrophils in the media.

Fig. 11.9   Osteoarthritis. The fibrocartilage layer is split and the underlying bone shows evidence of resorption and repair centrally.

age to the internal elastic lamina, sometimes going on to complete destruction (Figs 11.7 and 11.8). Healing is by fibrosis, particularly of the media, thickening of the intima, and partial recanalization of the thrombus.

Lesions skip short lengths of an artery and a biopsy should be at least 3 cm long.

Management

The risk of blindness makes it essential to start treatment early. Systemic corticosteroids (starting with 60 mg/day) should be given on the basis of inflamed scalp vessels and a high (>70 mm/h) ESR. Corticosteroids are usually quickly effective and should be continued until the ESR falls to normal.

OSTEOARTHRITIS

Osteoarthritis, though traditionally regarded as a wear and tear disease mainly of the elderly, is a metabolic defect of articular cartilage. There is increased hydration and diminished content of many essential glycosaminoglycans and proteoglycans. Damage to the defective articular cartilage is worsened by physical stresses releasing inflammatory mediators (Fig. 11.9). Hence pain is greatest in heavily-stressed joints, such as the hips in overweight persons. By contrast, there can be gross osteoarthritis and distortion of the joints of the hands without pain.

Key features are summarised in Table 11.7.

Table 11.7 Osteoarthritis — key features

- The elderly most seriously affected
- Predominantly large joint involvement
- Pain mainly in heavily stressed joints
- Articular cartilage destroyed, leading to flattening of joint surfaces
- Osteoarthritis of temporomandibular joints an autopsy finding more frequently than a cause of symptoms

The temporomandibular joint, like most other joints, can be affected by osteoarthritis, but, like other lightly-stressed joints, symptoms may be minimal or absent and the disease only found by chance by radiography.

It is conspicuous that osteoarthritis is predominantly a disease of the elderly who are overall remarkably free from temporomandibular joint symptoms. In their absence, treatment is not indicated, but in the rare cases where pain is associated, anti-inflammatory analgesics can be given. Isolated osteoarthritis of the temporomandibular joints in younger persons is poorly authenticated.

RHEUMATOID ARTHRITIS

This common, multisystem disease causes chronic inflammation of many joints, with pain, progressive limitation of movement and varying degrees of constitutional upset.

Rheumatoid arthritis is the only important inflammatory disease of the temporomandibular joints. Nevertheless it rarely causes significant temporomandibular joint symptoms.

Women are mainly affected, particularly in the fourth and fifth decades. Loss of weight, malaise and depression are common. The smaller joints are mainly affected, and the distribution tends to be symmetrical. The hands are typically affected and show inflammation and swelling of the small joints in active disease. Later there is weakening, wasting and ulnar deviation of the fingers.

The main temporomandibular joint symptoms are crepitus and limitation of movement, but pain itself is surprisingly uncommon. These joints are never involved alone, and other affected joints usually dominate the picture.

The diagnosis depends on the clinical, radiographic and immunological findings. The last includes a raised titre of rheumatoid factor, antinuclear and other antibodies.

Key features are summarised in Table 11.8.

Table 11.8 Rheumatoid arthritis — key features

- Immunologically mediated with multiple autoantibodies
- Women aged 25–40 years mainly affected
- Typically symmetrical joint involvement
- Inflammation and pain lead to weakness and wasting
- Radiographic changes may be seen in temporomandibular joints
- Temporomandibular joint symptoms usually minor

The main radiographic effects are surface and pocket erosions of the bone and flattening of the joint surfaces. Overall, rheumatoid arthritis, despite radiographic changes, is not an important cause of temporomandibular joint pain.

Histologically, there is inflammatory destruction of the condylar surface, which becomes overgrown by granulation tissue (pannus) (Fig. 11.10).

Treatment is predominantly with anti-inflammatory analgesics.

A complication affecting a minority of patients with rheumatoid arthritis is Sjögren's syndrome. This may itself cause pain in the parotid region, which may very occasionally be severe enough to cause confusion with temporomandibular joint pain.

OTHER TYPES OF ARTHRITIS

Most kinds of arthritis can cause pain or limitation of movement of the temporomandibular joint, but rarely do so. They include some of the variants of chronic childhood arthritis, gout, pseudogout (crystalline deposition disease), psoriatic arthropathy and Lyme disease.

TUMOURS OF THE TEMPOROMANDIBULAR JOINT

The most common tumour of the temporomandibular joint is an osteochondroma of the mandibular condyle (Fig. 11.11). It causes progressive limitation of movement.

CONDYLAR HYPERPLASIA

Condylar hyperplasia is an uncommon condition due to greatly increased bone activity, usually in one condyle (Fig. 11.12). It causes facial asymmetry, deviation of the jaw to the opposite

Fig. 11.10 Rheumatoid arthritis. Inflamed villi of pannus growing across the surface of a temporomandibular joint severely affected by rheumatoid arthritis. The condylar surface is destroyed.

Fig. 11.11 Osteochondroma of the condyle. Two cartilage-capped exostoses arising near the condyle have grown progressively to form a distorted condylar head several centimetres across.

Fig. 11.12 Condylar hyperplasia. The condyle retains an immature structure with a thick cartilage layer, calcification and new bone formation, reflecting the continued growth.

side on opening and a cross-bite which usually become conspicuous after puberty.

The condition may stabilise after puberty but, if still active, condylectomy may be required. If condylar overgrowth has ceased, the occlusion and facial symmetry may be restored by surgery.

SUGGESTED FURTHER READING

Bjornland T, Refsum S B 1994 Histopathologic changes in the temporomandibular joint disk in patients with chronic arthritic disease. A comparison with internal derangement. Oral Surg Oral Med Oral Pathol 77:572–578

Borle R M, Borle S R 1991 Management of oral submucous fibrosis: a conservative approach. J Oral Maxillofacial Surg 49:788–791

Buckingham R B, Braun T, Harinstein D et al 1991 Temporomandibular joint dysfunction: a close association with systemic joint laxity (the hypermobile joint syndrome). Oral Surg Oral Med Oral Pathol 72:514–519

Cawson R A, Binnie W H, Eveson J W 1995 Color atlas of oral disease, 2nd edn. Mosby-Wolfe, London

Cawson R A, Langdon J D, Eveson J W 1996 Surgical pathology of the mouth and jaws. Wright, Oxford

Chalmers I M, Blair G S 1973 Rheumatoid arthritis of the temporomandibular joint. A clinical and radiological study using circular tomography. J Med XLII:369–386

Denucci D J, Dionne R A, Dubner R 1996 Identifying a neurobiologic basis for drug therapy in TMDs. J Am Dent Assoc 127:581–593

Goss A N 1992 Toward an international consensus on temporomandibular joint surgery. Report of the Second International Consensus Meeting, April 1992, Buenos Aires, Argentina. Int J Oral Maxillofac Surg 22:78–81

Harris M, Feinmann C, Wise M, Treasure F 1993 Temporomandibular joint and orofacial pain: clinical and medicolegal management problems. Br Dent J 174:129–136

Harris R J 1988 Lyme disease involving the temporomandibular joint. J Oral Maxillofac Surg 46:78–79

Kaban L B, Belfer M L 1981 Temporomandibular joint dysfunction: an occasional manifestation of serious psychopathology. J Oral Surg 39:742–746

Kerscher A, Piette E, Tideman H, Wu P C 1993 Osteochondroma of the coronoid process of the mandible. Oral Surg Oral Med Oral Pathol 75:559–564

Könönen M 1992 Signs and symptoms of craniomandibular disorders in men with Reiter's disease. J Craniomandib Disord Fac Oral Pain 6:247–253

Leighty S M, Spach D H, Myall R W T, Burns J L 1993 Septic arthritis of the temporomandibular joint: review of the literature and report of two cases in children. Int J Oral Maxillofac Surg 22:292–297

Maher R, Lee A J, Warnakulasuriya K A A S, Lewis A J, Johnson N W 1994 Role of areca nut in the causation of oral submucous fibrosis: a case–control study in Pakistan. J Oral Pathol Med 23:65–69

Pillai R, Balaram P, Reddiar K S 1992 Pathogenesis of oral submucous fibrosis. Relationship to risk factors associated with oral cancer. Cancer 69:2011–2020

White R D, Makar J, Steckler R M 1992 Synovial sarcoma of the temporomandibular joint. J Oral Maxillofac Surg 50:1227–1230

SOFT-TISSUE DISEASE

Diseases of the oral mucosa:
Infective stomatitis

A few mucosal diseases such as lupus erythematosus are important indicators of severe underlying systemic disease, and rare conditions such as acanthosis nigricans can be markers of internal malignancy. Pemphigus vulgaris is potentially lethal, as is HIV infection, which can give rise to a variety of mucosal lesions. Biopsy is mandatory, particularly in the bullous diseases, as in such cases the diagnosis can only be confirmed by microscopy. In other cases, microscopic findings can be less definite, but often (as in the case of major aphthae for example) serve to exclude more dangerous diseases. Mucosal ulceration — a break in epithelial continuity — is a frequent feature of stomatitis. Important causes are summarised in Table 12.1. However, ulceration is not a feature of all mucosal diseases, as discussed below.

Table 12.1   **Important causes of oral mucosal ulcers**

Vesiculo-bullous diseases	Ulceration without preceding Nesiculation
Infective	*Infective*
Primary herpetic stomatitis	Cytomegalovirus-associated ulceration
Herpes labialis	Some acute specific fevers
Herpes zoster and chickenpox	Tuberculosis
	Syphilis
Hand-foot-and-mouth disease	
	Non-infective
Non-infective	Traumatic
Pemphigus vulgaris	Aphthous stomatitis
Mucous membrane pemphigoid	Behçet's syndrome
Linear IgA disease	HIV-associated mucosal ulcers
Dermatitis herpetiformis	Lichen planus
Bullous erythema multiforme	Lupus erythematosus
	Eosinophilic ulceration
	Wegener's granulomatosis
	Some mucosal drug reactions
	Carcinoma (Ch. 17)

MUCOSAL INFECTIONS

PRIMARY HERPETIC STOMATITIS

Primary infection is caused by *Herpes simplex* virus, usually

type 1, which, in the non-immune, can cause an acute vesiculating stomatitis. However, most primary infections are subclinical. Thereafter, recurrent (reactivation) infections usually take the form of *Herpes labialis* (cold sores or fever blisters).

Transmission of herpes is by close contact and up to 90% of inhabitants of large, poor, urban communities develop antibodies to herpes virus during early childhood. In many British and US cities, by contrast, approximately 70% of 20-year-olds may be non-immune, because of lack of exposure to the virus. In more affluent countries the incidence of herpetic stomatitis has declined and it is seen in adolescents or adults, rather than children. It is more common in the immunocompromised, such as in HIV infection.

Clinical features

The early lesions are vesicles which can affect any part of the oral mucosa, but the hard palate and dorsum of the tongue are favoured sites (Figs 12.1 and 12.2). The vesicles are dome-shaped and usually 2–3 mm in diameter. Rupture of vesicles leaves circular, sharply defined, shallow ulcers with yellowish or greyish floors and red margins. The ulcers are painful and may interfere with eating.

The gingival margins are frequently swollen and red, particu-

Fig. 12.1   Herpetic stomatitis. Pale vesicles and ulcers are visible on the palate and gingivae, especially anteriorly, and the gingivae are erythematous and swollen.

Fig. 12.2 Herpetic stomatitis. A group of recently ruptured vesicles on the hard palate, a characteristic site. The individual lesions are of remarkably uniform size but several have coalesced to form larger irregular ulcers.

Fig. 12.3 Herpetic vesicle. The vesicle is formed by accumulation of fluid within the prickle cell layer. The virus-infected cells, identifiable by their enlarged nuclei, can be seen in the floor of the vesicle and a few are floating freely in the vesicle fluid.

larly in children, and the regional lymph nodes are enlarged and tender. There is often fever and systemic upset, sometimes severe, particularly in adults.

Oral lesions usually resolve within a week to 10 days, but malaise can persist so long that an adult may not recover fully for several weeks.

Pathology

Vesicles are sharply defined and form in the upper epithelium (Fig. 12.3). Virus-damaged epithelial cells with swollen nuclei and marginated chromatin (ballooning degeneration) are seen in the floor of the vesicle and in direct smears from early lesions (Fig. 12.4). Incomplete division leads to formation of multinucleated cells. Later, the full thickness of the epithelium is destroyed, to produce a sharply defined ulcer (Fig. 12.5).

Diagnosis

The clinical picture is usually distinctive (Table 12.2). A smear showing viral-damaged cells is additional diagnostic evidence. A rising titre of antibodies, reaching a peak after 2–3 weeks, provides absolute but retrospective confirmation of the diagnosis.

Treatment

Acyclovir is a potent antiherpetic drug and is life-saving for potentially lethal herpetic encephalitis or disseminated infection. Acyclovir suspension used as a rinse and then swallowed should accelerate healing of severe herpetic stomatitis if used

Fig. 12.4 A smear from a herpetic vesicle. The distended degenerating nuclei of the epithelial cells cluster together to give the typical mulberry appearance.

sufficiently early. Bed rest, fluids and a soft diet may sometimes be required.

In mild cases, topical tetracycline suspension, rinsed round

Fig. 12.5 Herpetic ulcer. The vesicle has ruptured to form an ulcer (right) and the epithelium at the margin contains enlarged, darkly staining virus-infected cells liberating free virus into the saliva.

Fig. 12.6 Herpes labialis. Typical vesicles (centrally) and bleeding crusted ulcers (patient's left) affecting the vermilion border and skin around the mucocutaneous junction.

Table 12.2 **Typical features of herpetic stomatitis**

- Usually caused by *Herpes simplex* virus type 1
- Transmitted by close contact
- Vesicles, followed by ulcers, affect any part of the oral mucosa
- Gingivitis sometimes associated
- Lymphadenopathy and fever of variable severity
- Smears from vesicles show ballooning degeneration of viral-damaged cells
- Rising titre of antibodies to herpes simplex virus confirms the diagnosis
- Acyclovir is the treatment of choice

the mouth several times a day, relieves soreness and may hasten healing by controlling secondary infection.

Unusually prolonged or severe infections or failure to respond to acyclovir (200–400 mg/day by mouth for 7 days) suggest immunodeficiency, and herpetic ulceration persisting for more than a month is an AIDS-defining illness.

HERPES LABIALIS

After the primary infection, the latent virus can be reactivated in 20–30% of patients to cause cold sores (fever blisters). Triggering factors include the common cold and other febrile infections, exposure to strong sunshine, menstruation or, occasionally, emotional upsets or local irritation, such as dental treatment. Neutralising antibodies produced in response to the primary infection are not protective.

Clinically, changes follow a consistent course with prodromal paraesthesia or burning sensations, then erythema at the site of the attack. Vesicles form after an hour or two, usually in clusters along the mucocutaneous junction of the lips, but can extend on to the adjacent skin (Fig. 12.6).

The vesicles enlarge, coalesce and weep exudate. After 2 or 3 days they rupture and crust over but new vesicles frequently appear for a day or two, only to scab over and finally heal, usu-

Fig. 12.7 Herpetic whitlow. This is a characteristic non-oral site for primary infection as a result of contact with infected vesicle fluid or saliva. The vesiculation and crusting are identical to those seen in herpes labialis.

ally without scarring. The whole cycle may take up to 10 days. Secondary bacterial infection may induce an impetiginous lesion which sometimes leaves scars.

Treatment. In view of the rapidity of the viral damage to the tissues, treatment must start as soon as the premonitory sensations are felt. Acyclovir cream may be effective if applied at this time. This is possible because the course of the disease is consistent and patients can recognise the prodromal symptoms before tissue damage has started.

Herpetic cross-infections

Both primary and secondary herpetic infections are contagious. *Herpetic whitlow* (Fig. 12.7) is a recognised though surprisingly uncommon hazard to dental surgeons and their assistants. Herpetic whitlows, in turn, can infect patients and have led to outbreaks of infection in hospitals and among patients in dental practices. In immunodeficient patients, such infections can be dangerous but acyclovir has dramatically improved the prognosis in such cases and may be given on suspicion.

HERPES ZOSTER OF THE TRIGEMINAL AREA

Zoster (shingles) is characterised by pain, a vesicular rash and stomatitis in the related dermatome. The varicella zoster virus (VZV) causes chickenpox in the non-immune (mainly children), while reactivation of the latent virus causes zoster, mainly in the elderly.

Unlike herpes labialis, repeated recurrences of zoster are very rare. Occasionally there is an underlying immunodeficiency. Herpes zoster is a hazard in organ transplant patients and can be an early complication of some tumours, particularly Hodgkin's disease, or, increasingly, of AIDS, where it is five times more common than in HIV-negative persons and potentially lethal.

Clinical features

Herpes zoster usually affects adults of middle age or over but occasionally attacks even children. The first signs are pain and irritation or tenderness in the dermatome corresponding to the affected ganglion.

Vesicles, often confluent, form on one side of the face and in the mouth up to the midline (Fig. 12.8 and 12.9). The regional lymph nodes are enlarged and tender. The acute phase usually lasts about a week. Pain continues until the lesions crust over and start to heal, but secondary infection may cause suppuration and scarring of the skin. Malaise and fever are usually associated.

Fig. 12.8 Herpes zoster. A severe attack in an older person shows confluent ulceration on the hard and soft palate on one side.

Fig. 12.9 Herpes zoster of the trigeminal nerve. There are vesicles and ulcers on one side of the tongue and facial skin supplied by the first and second divisions.

Patients are sometimes unable to distinguish the pain of trigeminal zoster from severe toothache. This has sometimes led to a demand for a dental extraction. Afterwards, the rash follows as a normal course of events and this has given rise to the myth that dental extractions can precipitate facial zoster.

Pathology

The *Varicella zoster* virus produces similar epithelial lesions to those of herpes simplex, but also inflammation of the related posterior root ganglion.

Management

Herpes zoster is an uncommon cause of stomatitis, but is readily recognisable (Table 12.3).

Table 12.3 Herpes zoster of the trigeminal area — key features

- Recurrence of varicella zoster virus infection typically in the elderly
- Pain precedes the rash
- Facial rash accompanies the stomatitis
- Lesions localised one side, within the distribution of one or more divisions of the trigeminal nerve
- Malaise can be severe and, in AIDS patients, life-threatening
- Treat with systemic acyclovir, intravenously, if necessary
- Sometimes followed by postherpetic neuralgia, particularly in the elderly

According to the severity of the attack, oral acyclovir (200–800 mg 5 times daily, usually for 7 days) should be given at the earliest possible moment, together with analgesics. The addition of prednisone is reported to accelerate relief of pain and healing. In immunodeficient patients, intravenous acyclovir is required and may also be justified for the elderly in whom this infection is debilitating.

Complications. Postherpetic neuralgia mainly affects the elderly and is difficult to relieve (Ch. 35).

CYTOMEGALOVIRUS-ASSOCIATED ULCERATION

Cytomegalovirus (CMV) is a member of the herpes virus group. Up to 80% of adults show serological evidence of CMV infection without clinical effects but it is a common complication of immunodeficiency, particularly AIDS. In the latter it can be life-threatening.

Oral ulcers in which CMV has been identified are sometimes clinically indistinguishable from recurrent aphthae; others have raised, minimally rolled borders. Generally, the ulcers are large, shallow and single, and affect either the masticatory or non-masticatory mucosa. In some cases, oral ulcers may be associated with disseminated CMV infection.

Microscopically, CMV-associated ulcers are non-specific, but cells with typical owl-eye intranuclear inclusions can be seen in the inflammatory infiltrate in the ulcer floor. They are usually recognisable by light microscopy but their nature can be confirmed by immunocytochemistry (see Fig. 1.8), in situ hybridisation or electron microscopy.

The virus present in oral lesions may merely be a passenger, but their causative role is suggested by reports of response to ganciclovir.

HAND-FOOT-AND-MOUTH DISEASE

This common, mild viral infection, which often causes minor epidemics among school children, is characterised by ulceration of the mouth and a vesicular rash on the extremities.

Hand-foot-and-mouth disease is usually caused by strains of Coxsackie A virus. It is highly infectious, frequently spreads through a classroom in schools and may also infect a teacher or parent. The incubation period is probably between 3 and 10 days. *Foot-and-mouth disease* (of cattle) is a quite different rhinovirus infection which rarely affects humans.

Clinical features

The small scattered oral ulcers usually cause little pain. Intact vesicles are rarely seen, and gingivitis is not a feature. Regional lymph nodes are not usually enlarged, and systemic upset is typically mild or absent.

The rash consists of vesicles, sometimes deep seated, or occasionally bullae, mainly seen around the base of fingers or toes, but any part of the limbs may be affected (Fig. 12.10). The rash is often the main feature and such patients are unlikely to be seen by dentists. In some outbreaks either the mouth or the extremities alone may be affected.

Serological confirmation of the diagnosis is possible but rarely necessary, as the history, especially of other cases, and clinical features are usually adequate. The disease typically resolves within a week. No specific treatment is available or needed but myocarditis or encephalitis are rare complications.

Key features are summarised in Table 12.4.

Fig. 12.10 Hand-foot-and-mouth disease. The rash consists of vesicles or bullae on the extremities; in this patient they are relatively inconspicuous.

Table 12.4 Hand-foot-and-mouth disease — key features

- Caused mainly by Coxsackie A viruses
- Highly infectious
- School children predominantly affected
- Occasionally spreads to teacher or parent
- Typically mild vesiculating stomatitis and/or vesiculating rash on extremities
- Rarely severe enough for dental opinion to be sought
- Confirmation of diagnosis (if required) by serology
- No specific treatment available or needed.

THE ACUTE SPECIFIC FEVERS

Fevers which cause oral lesions are rarely seen in dentistry. Those which cause vesicular rashes (smallpox and chickenpox) produce the same lesions in the mouth.

In the prodromal stage of measles, Koplik's spots form on the buccal mucosa and soft palate and are pathognomonic. Palatal petechiae or ulceration, involving the fauces especially, are seen in glandular fever and are accompanied by the characteristic, usually widespread lymphadenopathy.

KAWASAKI'S DISEASE (MUCOCUTANEOUS LYMPH NODE SYNDROME)

Kawasaki's disease is endemic in Japan but uncommon in Britain; it is frequently unrecognised and causes a significant mortality.

Clinical features

Children are affected and have persistent fever, oral mucositis, ocular and cutaneous lesions, and cervical lymphadenopathy (Ch. 26). Oral lesions consist of widespread mucosal erythema with swelling of the lingual papillae (strawberry tongue) but are insignificant compared with the serious cardiac effects (Ch. 27).

TUBERCULOSIS

The recrudescence of tuberculosis in the West is partly a consequence of the AIDS epidemic; moreover, multiply-resistant mycobacteria are becoming widespread. Oral tuberculosis is rare and a complication of pulmonary disease with infected sputum. Those with HIV infection are an important group of victims, but oral tuberculosis is occasionally seen in immuno-competent persons who are usually elderly men with pulmonary tuberculosis that has progressed unrecognised or who have neglected their treatment.

The typical lesion is an ulcer on the mid-dorsum of the tongue; the lip or other parts of the mouth are less often affected. The ulcer is typically angular or stellate, with overhanging edges and a pale floor, but can be ragged and irregular (Fig. 12.11). It is painless in its early stages and regional lymph nodes are usually unaffected.

The diagnosis is rarely suspected until after biopsy.

Pathology

Typical tuberculous granulomas are seen in the floor of the

Fig. 12.11   A tuberculous ulcer of the tongue. The rather angular shape and overhanging edges of the ulcer can be seen. The patient was a man of 56 with advanced but unrecognised pulmonary tuberculosis.

Fig. 12.12   Tuberculous ulcer. At the margin numerous granulomas are present in the ulcer bed. The darkly stained multinucleate Langhans' giant cells are visible even at this low power.

ulcers (Fig. 12.12). Mycobacteria are rarely identifiable in the oral lesion but can be demonstrated in the sputum. Chest radiographs show advanced infection.

Tuberculosis or non-tuberculous mycobacterial infection must be considered in patients with AIDS who develop oral ulceration with histological granuloma formation.

Management

Diagnosis is confirmed by biopsy, chest radiography and a specimen of sputum. Mycobacterial infection is confirmed by culture or PCR.

Oral lesions clear up rapidly if there is effective multidrug chemotherapy for the pulmonary infection. No local treatment is needed.

Tuberculous cervical lymphadenopathy (Ch. 26)

SYPHILIS

As a result of contact tracing and early treatment, only a few hundred cases a year of syphilis are seen in Britain. Oral lesions in each stage of syphilis are clinically quite different from each other. Oral lesions are rarely seen or may pass unrecognised.

Primary syphilis

An oral chancre appears 3–4 weeks after infection and may form on the lip, tip of the tongue or, rarely, other oral sites. It consists initially of a firm nodule about a quarter of an inch (6 mm) across. The surface breaks down after a few days, leaving a rounded ulcer with raised indurated edges. This may resemble a carcinoma, particularly if on the lip. However, the appearances vary. A chancre is typically painless but regional lymph nodes are enlarged, rubbery and discrete. A biopsy may only show non-specific inflammation but sometimes there is conspicuous perivascular infiltration.

Serological reactions are negative at first. Diagnosis therefore depends on finding *Treponema pallidum* by dark-ground illumination of a smear from the chancre, but they must be distinguished from other oral spirochaetes. Clinical recognition of oral chancres is difficult but important. They are highly infective, and treatment is most effective at this stage.

After 8–9 weeks the chancre heals, often without scarring.

Secondary syphilis

The secondary stage develops 1–4 months after infection. It typically causes mild fever with malaise, headache, sore throat and generalised lymphadenopathy, soon followed by a rash and stomatitis.

The rash is variable, but typically consists of asymptomatic pinkish (coppery) macules, symmetrically distributed and starting on the trunk. It may last for a few hours or weeks and its presence or history is a useful aid to diagnosis. Oral lesions, which rarely appear without the rash, mainly affect the tonsils, lateral borders of the tongue and lips. They are usually flat ulcers covered by a greyish membrane and may be irregularly linear (*snail's track ulcers*) or coalesce to form well-defined rounded areas (*mucous patches*).

Discharge from the ulcers contains many spirochaetes, and saliva is highly infective. Serological reactions (see below) are positive and diagnostic at this stage, but biopsy is unlikely to be informative.

Tertiary syphilis

Late-stage syphilis develops in many patients about 3 or more years after infection. The onset is insidious, and during the latent period the patient may appear well. A characteristic lesion is the gumma.

Clinically, a gumma, which may affect the palate, tongue or tonsils, can vary from one to several inches in diameter. It begins as a swelling, sometimes with a yellowish centre which undergoes necrosis, leaving a painless indolent deep ulcer. The ulcer is rounded, with soft, punched-out edges. The floor is depressed and pale (wash-leather) in appearance. It eventually heals, with severe scarring which may distort the soft palate or tongue or perforate the hard palate (Fig. 12.13) or destroy the uvula.

Microscopically, there may be no more than a predominance of plasma cells in the inflammatory infiltrate (a common finding in oral lesions) but associated with peri- or endarteritis. Granuloma formation is rare. Also rarely, there may be diffuse chronic inflammatory infiltration of the lingual muscles or coagulative necrosis mimicking caseation. However, the appearances can be completely non-specific. Diagnosis therefore depends on the serological findings.

Leukoplakia of the tongue may also develop during this late

Fig. 12.13   Tertiary syphilis; gumma of the palate. Necrosis in the centre of the gumma on the palate has caused perforation of the bone and a typical round punched-out hole.

stage (Ch. 16), and other effects of syphilis such as aortitis, tabes or general paralysis of the insane may be associated.

Management

Serological confirmation of the infection is essential (Table 12.5). Tests are either specific (such as the FTA-ABS) or non-specific, as in the VDRL. The VDRL becomes positive 4–6 weeks after infection, and becomes negative only after effective treatment, but false positives can result from several other causes. The FTA-ABS acts as a check against false-positive or false-negative results, but remains positive despite effective treatment for the life of the individual.

Table 12.5   Interpretation of serological tests for syphilis

VDRL	FTA-ABS	Usual interpretation
+	−	False-positive
+	+	Active syphilis
−	+	Treated syphilis

Antibiotics, particularly penicillin, are the mainstay, but tetracycline and erythromycin are also effective. Treatment should be by a specialist and must be continued until non-specific serological reactions (VDRL) are persistently negative.

CANDIDOSIS

Candidal infection can cause a spectrum of lesions (Table 12.6) particularly thrush, chronic white plaques (chronic hyperplastic candidosis) or erythematous areas such as denture stomatitis.

Thrush*

Thrush, a disease recognised in infants by Hippocrates, can also

Table 12.6 Spectrum of oral candidosis

● Acute candidosis
    Thrush
    Acute antibiotic stomatitis
● Chronic candidosis
    Denture-induced stomatitis
    Chronic hyperplastic candidosis (Ch. 16)
    Chronic mucocutaneous candidosis (Ch. 15)
    Erythematous candidosis
● Angular stomatitis (common to all types of oral candidosis)

Fig. 12.14   Thrush. The lesions consist of soft, creamy patches or flecks lying superficially on an erythematous mucosa. This soft palate distribution is particularly frequent in those using steroid inhalers.

affect adults. In the nineteenth century, Trousseau called thrush a 'disease of the diseased', as has been dramatically confirmed by its frequency in HIV infection.

Factors predisposing to candidal infection are shown in Table 12.7.

Table 12.7 Important predisposing factors for oral candidosis
● Immunodeficiency or immunosuppression ● Anaemia ● Suppression of the normal flora of the mouth by antibacterial drugs ● Xerostomia

Neonatal thrush results from immaturity of the immune response, and infection is probably acquired during passage through the birth canal. Any adult male who develops thrush without apparent cause should be suspected of having HIV infection. However, any form of candidosis can be secondary to HIV infection.

Clinical features

Thrush forms soft, friable and creamy-coloured plaques on the mucosa (Fig. 12.14). The distinctive feature is that they can be easily wiped off, to expose an erythematous mucosa. Their extent varies from isolated small flecks to widespread confluent plaque. Angular stomatitis is frequently associated, as it is with any form of intraoral candidosis.

Pathology

A Gram-stained smear shows large masses of tangled hyphae, detached epithelial cells and leukocytes (Fig. 12.15). Biopsy shows hyperplastic epithelium infiltrated by inflammatory oedema and cells, predominantly neutrophils. Staining with

Fig. 12.15   Direct smear from thrush. The tangled mass of Gram-positive hyphae of *Candida albicans* is diagnostic. A few yeast cells may be present as well, but it is the large number of hyphae which is diagnostic.

PAS shows many candidal hyphae growing down through the epithelial cells to the junction of the plaque with the spinous cell layer (Fig. 12.16). At this level there is a concentration of inflammatory exudate and inflammatory cells. More deeply, the epithelium is hyperplastic but attenuated, with long slender processes extending down into the corium, surrounded by a light infiltrate, predominantly lymphoplasmacytic.

The microscopic appearances explain both the friable nature of the plaques of thrush and their ready detachment. Key features are summarised in Table 12.8.

Management

Control of any local cause, such as topical antibiotic treatment, may alone cause thrush to resolve. If not, a course of nystatin or amphotericin lozenges should allow the oral microflora to return to normal. Failure of response to topical antifungals such as nystatin suggests immune deficiency. *HIV infection should always be suspected when thrush is seen in an adult male in*

---

*The term '*thrush*' is not a nickname, as is sometimes thought, but of considerable antiquity. By contrast the pretentious alternative term 'acute pseudomembranous candidosis' is inappropriate as the plaques are not a necrotic slough.

Fig. 12.16 Thrush. At high power the components of a plaque may be clearly seen. The surface layers of the epithelium are separated by inflammatory oedema and are colonised by fungal hyphae and infiltrated by neutrophils.

Table 12.8   Thrush — key features
• Acute candidosis • Secondary to various predisposing factors (Table 12.7) • Common in HIV infection and indicates low immunity • Creamy soft patches, readily wiped off the mucosa • Smear shows many Gram-positive hyphae • Histology shows hyphae invading superficial epithelium with proliferative and inflammatory response • Responds to topical antifungals or itraconazole

whom there is no other detectable cause. In such patients, candidosis may respond to fluconazole or itraconazole, but is typically associated with a low CD4 count and indicates a poor prognosis.

Rarely, persistent thrush is an early sign of chronic mucocutaneous candidosis such as candida-endocrinopathy syndrome (Ch. 15).

Angular stomatitis

Angular stomatitis is typically caused by leakage of candida-infected saliva at the angles of the mouth. It can be seen in infantile thrush, in denture wearers or in association with chronic hyperplastic candidosis. It is a characteristic sign of candidal infection.

Clinically, there is mild inflammation at the angles of the mouth. In elderly patients with denture-induced stomatitis, inflammation frequently extends along folds of the facial skin extending from the angles of the mouth (Fig. 12.17). These folds have frequently but unjustifiably been ascribed to 'closed bite', but in fact are due to sagging of the facial tissues with age. Such folds are difficult to eliminate except by plastic surgery.

Treatment of intraoral candidal infection alone causes angular stomatitis to resolve. If there is coinfection with *Staphylococcus aureus*, local application of fusidic acid cream may be required.

Denture-induced stomatitis

A well-fitting upper denture cuts off the underlying mucosa

Fig. 12.17 Angular stomatitis. Cracking and erythema at the commissure. Some cases, as here, are associated with leakage of saliva, constantly reinfecting the lesion.

Fig. 12.18 Typical denture stomatitis. Clear demarcation between the erythema of the mucosa covered, in this instance, by an orthodontic appliance. The pallor of the palate behind the posterior margin is clearly seen.

from the protective action of saliva. In susceptible patients this can promote candidosis, which is seen as a symptomless area of erythema. The erythema is sharply limited to the area of mucosa occluded by an upper denture or an orthodontic plate (Fig. 12.18). Similar inflammation is not seen under the more mobile lower denture which allows a relatively free flow of saliva beneath it. Angular stomatitis is frequently associated and may form the chief complaint.

In the past, denture-induced stomatitis was ascribed to 'allergy' to denture base material but there is no foundation for this fancy. Methylmethacrylate monomer is mildly sensitising but even the rare individuals sensitised to it can wear the polymerised material without any reaction.

Pathology

Gram-stained smears show candidal hyphae and some yeast forms which have proliferated in the interface between denture base and mucosa. Histologically, there is typically mild acanthosis with prominent blood vessels superficially and a mild chronic inflammatory infiltrate. The inflammation is probably a response to enzymes such as phospholipases produced by this fungus.

Management

The clinical picture is distinctive and the diagnosis is confirmed by finding candidal hyphae in a Gram-stained smear taken from the inflamed mucosa or the fitting surface of the denture. The infection responds to antifungal drugs but topical agents such as nystatin or amphotericin can only gain access to the palate if the patient leaves out the denture while the tablets are allowed to dissolve in the mouth.

Methylmethacrylate denture base also harbours *Candida*

albicans and may therefore form a reservoir which can reinfect the mucosa. Elimination of *C. albicans* from the denture base is important and can be achieved by soaking the denture in 0.1% hypochlorite overnight.

A simpler alternative is to coat the fitting surface of the denture with miconazole gel while it is being worn. The denture should be removed and scrubbed clean at intervals and miconazole reapplied three times a day. This treatment should be continued until the inflammation has cleared and *C. albicans* has been eliminated. This is likely to take 1–2 weeks but patients should be warned not to continue this treatment indefinitely.

Lack of response may be due to poor patient compliance or to an underlying disorder, particularly iron deficiency. If in addition candidal infection is unusually florid or associated with patches of thrush, a blood picture should be requested. Itraconazole or fluconazole orally have a systemic effect and can be used for resistant cases but topical treatment is safer, less expensive and usually satisfactory.

Key features are summarised in Table 12.9.

Table 12.9 Denture-induced stomatitis — key features

- Candidal infection promoted by well-fitting upper denture
- Enclosed mucosa is cut off from protective action of saliva
- Mucosal erythema sharply restricted to area covered by the denture
- Angular stomatitis frequently associated
- Hyphae proliferate in denture–mucosa interface
- Smear shows Gram-positive hyphae
- Resolves after elimination of *C. albicans* by antifungal treatment

---

Acute antibiotic stomatitis

This can follow overuse or topical oral use of antibiotics, especially tetracycline, supressing normal, competing oral flora. It is infrequently seen now. Clinically the whole mucosa is red and sore. Flecks of thrush may be present.

Resolution may follow withdrawal of the antibiotic but is accelerated by topical antifungal treatment.

Generalised candidal erythema, which is clinically similar, can also be a consequence of xerostomia which promotes candidal infection. It is a typical complication of Sjögren's syndrome. Nystatin suspension or miconazole gel held in the mouth is usually effective.

Erythematous candidosis

This term is applied to patchy red mucosal macules due to *C. albicans* infection in HIV-positive patients (see Fig. 24.3). Favoured sites, in order of frequency, are the hard palate, dorsum of the tongue and soft palate.

Treatment with itraconazole is usually effective.

SUGGESTED FURTHER READING

Alrabiah F A, Sacks S L 1996 New antiherpesvirus agents. Their targets and therapeutic potential. Drugs 52:17–32

Cawson R A, Binnie W H, Eveson J W 1994 Color atlas of oral disease, 2nd edn. Mosby-Wolfe, London

Epstein J B, Sherlock C H, Wolber R A 1993 Oral manifestations of cytomegalovirus infection. Oral Surg Oral Med Oral Pathol 75:443–451

Glesby M J, Moore R D, Chaisson RE 1995 Clinical spectrum of herpes zoster in adults infected with human immunodeficiency virus. Clin Infect Dis 21:370–375

Jones A C, Freedman P D, Phelan J A, Baughman R A, Kerpel S M 1993 Cytomegalovirus infections of the oral cavity. Oral Surg Oral Med Oral Pathol 75:76–85

Nachbar F N, Classen V, Nachbar T et al 1996 Orificial tuberculosis detection by polymerase chain reaction. Br J Dermatol 135:106–109

Regezi J A, Eversole R, Barker B F et al 1996 Herpes simplex and cytomegalovirus coinfected ulcers in HIV-positive patients. Oral Surg Oral Med Oral Pathol Oral Radiol Endod 81:55–62

Scully C 1989 Orofacial herpes simplex infections; current concepts in the epidemiology, pathogenesis and treatment, and disorders in which the virus may be implicated. Oral Surg Oral Med Oral Pathol 68:701–710

Whitley R J, Weiss H, Gnann J W 1996 Acyclovir with and without prednisone for the treatment of herpes zoster. A randomized, placebo-controlled trial. Ann Intern Med 125:376–383

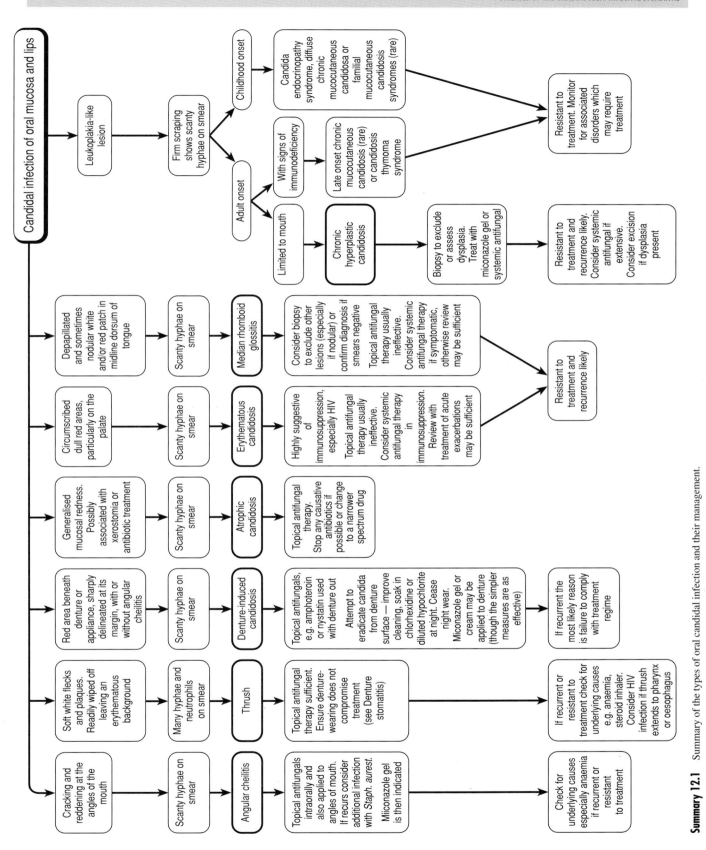

Summary 12.1 Summary of the types of oral candidal infection and their management.

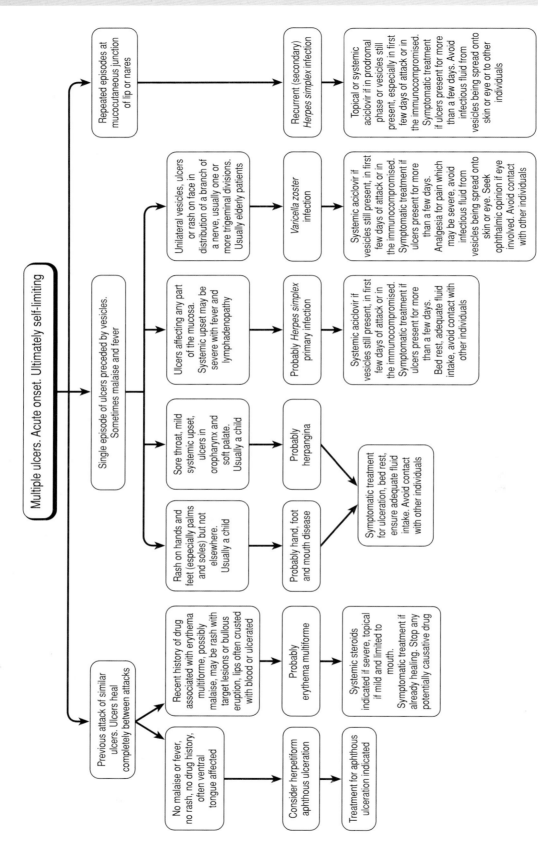

Multiple ulcers. Acute onset. Ultimately self-limiting

Previous attack of similar ulcers. Ulcers heal completely between attacks

No malaise or fever, no rash, no drug history, often ventral tongue affected
→ **Consider herpetiform aphthous ulceration**
→ **Treatment for aphthous ulceration indicated**

Recent history of drug associated with erythema multiforme, possibly malaise, may be rash with target lesions or bullous eruption, lips often crusted with blood or ulcerated
→ **Probably erythema multiforme**
→ **Systemic steroids indicated if severe, topical if mild and limited to mouth. Symptomatic treatment if already healing. Stop any potentially causative drug**

Single episode of ulcers preceded by vesicles. Sometimes malaise and fever

Rash on hands and feet (especially palms and soles) but not elsewhere. Usually a child
→ **Probably hand, foot and mouth disease**

Sore throat, mild systemic upset, ulcers in oropharynx and soft palate. Usually a child
→ **Probably herpangina**

→ **Symptomatic treatment for ulceration, bed rest, ensure adequate fluid intake. Avoid contact with other individuals**

Ulcers affecting any part of the mucosa. Systemic upset may be severe with fever and lymphadenopathy
→ **Probably Herpes simplex primary infection**
→ **Systemic aciclovir if vesicles still present, in first few days of attack or in the immunocompromised. Symptomatic treatment if ulcers present for more than a few days. Bed rest, adequate fluid intake, avoid contact with other individuals**

Unilateral vesicles, ulcers or rash on face in distribution of a branch of a nerve, usually one or more trigeminal divisions. Usually elderly patients
→ **Varicella zoster infection**
→ **Systemic aciclovir if vesicles still present, in first few days of attack or in the immunocompromised. Symptomatic treatment if ulcers present for more than a few days. Analgesia for pain which may be severe, avoid infectious fluid from vesicles being spread onto skin or eye. Seek ophthalmic opinion if eye involved. Avoid contact with other individuals**

Repeated episodes at mucocutaneous junction of lip or nares
→ **Recurrent (secondary) Herpes simplex infection**
→ **Topical or systemic aciclovir if in prodromal phase or vesicles still present, especially in first few days of attack or in the immunocompromised. Symptomatic treatment if ulcers present for more than a few days. Avoid infectious fluid from vesicles being spread onto skin or eye or to other individuals**

Summary 12.2 Differential diagnosis and management of the common and important causes of multiple oral ulcers with acute onset.

Diseases of the oral mucosa:
Non-infective stomatitis

TRAUMATIC ULCERS

Traumatic ulcers are usually caused by a denture and often seen in the buccal of lingual sulcus. They are tender, have a yellowish floor, and red margins; there is no induration. If caused by the sharp edge of a broken-down tooth, they are usually on the tongue or buccal mucosa. Occasionally, a large ulcer may be caused by biting the cheek after a dental local anaesthetic (see Fig. 33.1).

Traumatic ulcers heal a few days after elimination of the cause. If they persist for more than 7–10 days, or there is any other cause for suspicion as to the cause, biopsy should be carried out.

Factitious ulceration (self-inflicted oral lesions)

Factitious ulcers in the mouth are traumatic but considerably less common than the usual type. They are typically a consequence of a disturbed mental state ('a call for attention'). Rarely, factitious oral ulceration has been a prelude to suicide.

The most common type of self-inflicted oral injuries has been so-called self-extraction of teeth. The diagnosis of self-inflicted injuries may be difficult but suspicious features are shown in Table 13.1

Table 13.1   **Features suggestive of factitious oral lesions**

- Lack of correspondence with any recognisable disease
- Bizarre configuration with sharp outlines
- Usually in an otherwise healthy mouth
- Clinical features inconsistent with the history
- In areas accessible to the patient

Investigation may be needed to exclude organic disease. Underlying emotional disturbance is typically well concealed. Frequently the diagnosis can be confirmed only by discreet observation after admission to hospital. The patient's family doctor should be told of the need for specialist psychiatric assessment.

RECURRENT APHTHAE (APHTHOUS STOMATITIS)

Recurrent aphthae constitute the most common oral mucosal disease and affect 10–25% of the population, but many cases are mild and accepted without complaint.

Aetiology

The main factors thought to contribute are shown in Table 13.2.

Table 13.2   **Possible aetiological factors for recurrent aphthae**

- Genetic predisposition
- Exaggerated response to trauma
- Infections
- Immunological abnormalities
- Gastrointestinal disorders
- Haematological deficiencies
- Hormonal disturbances
- Stress

Genetic factors.   There is some evidence for a genetic predisposition. The family history is sometimes positive and the disease appears to affect identical twins more frequently than non-identical. However, this probably applies to a minority. A variety of HLA associations have been reported but no one haplotype seems to be consistently associated. In the possibly related Behçet's disease (see below) the evidence for a genetic predisposition is much stronger.

Trauma.   Some patients think that the ulcers result from trauma because the early symptoms simulate pricking of the mucosa by (for instance) a toothbrush bristle. Trauma may dictate the site of ulcers in patients who already have the disorder, but most aphthae are in relatively protected sites and the masticatory mucosa is generally spared.

Infections.   There is no evidence that aphthae are directly due to any microbes, and there is scanty evidence that cross-reacting antigens from streptococci or L-forms play any significant role. The hypothesis that there may be defective immunoregulation caused by herpes or other viruses is unproven.

Immunological abnormalities. Since the aetiology of recurrent aphthae is unknown, there has been a facile tendency to label them as 'autoimmune'. A great variety of immunological abnormalities have been reported, but there have been almost as many contrary findings and no convincing theory of immunopathogenesis takes into account the clinical features. It is also possible that the immunological abnormalities are as much a consequence of the ulcers as the cause. Evidence of an association with atopic (IgE-mediated) disease is unconfirmed. Circulating antibodies to crude extracts of fetal oral mucosa have been reported, but their titre is unrelated to the severity of the disease and in many patients there are no significant changes in immunoglobulin levels. Antibody-dependent cytotoxic mechanisms have been postulated but not convincingly demonstrated. The histological features of aphthae (see below) have also been invoked to support hypotheses that the disease is either an immune complex-mediated (type III) or a cell-mediated (type IV) reaction, according to taste. However, others have failed to confirm the presence of circulating immune complexes, and in any case the significance of such complexes, which are sometimes detectable in the absence of disease, is notoriously difficult to interpret. Depressed circulating helper/suppressor T lymphocyte ratios have been reported but others have found no difference between active and remittant phases of the disorder. Recurrent aphthae also lack virtually all features of, and any association with, typical autoimmune diseases (Ch. 25). They also fail to respond reliably to immunosuppressive drugs and may become more severe in the immune deficiency state induced by HIV infection.

Gastrointestinal disease. Aphthae were previously known as 'dyspeptic ulcers' but are only rarely associated with gastrointestinal disease. Any association is usually because of a deficiency, particularly of vitamin B_{12} or folate secondary to malabsorption. An association with coeliac disease (sometimes asymptomatic) has been found in approximately 5% of patients with aphthae, but a secondary haematinic deficiency, particularly folate deficiency, is probably the cause.

Haematological deficiencies. Deficiencies of vitamin B_{12}, folate or iron have been reported in up to 20% of patients with aphthae. Such deficiencies are probably more frequent in patients whose aphthae start or worsen in middle age or later. In many such patients, the deficiency is latent, the haemoglobin is within normal limits, and the main sign is micro- or macrocytosis of the red cells. In patients who thus prove to be vitamin B_{12} or folate deficient, remedying the deficiency may bring rapid resolution of the ulcers.

Hormonal factors. In a few women, aphthae are associated with the stressful luteal phase of the menstrual cycle, but there is no strong evidence that hormone treatment is reliably effective.

'Stress'. Some patients relate exacerbations of ulceration to times of stress, and some studies have reported a correlation. However, stress is notoriously difficult to quantify, and a recent study has found no correlation.

In brief, therefore, the aetiology of recurrent aphthae is unclear. There is no evidence that they are a form of autoimmune disease in any accepted sense, and it is uncertain whether many of the reported immunological abnormalities are cause or effect. However, in a minority of patients there is a clear association with haematological deficiencies. The latter in turn may be secondary to disease of the small intestine or other cause of malabsorption.

That speculation about the cause of recurrent aphthae has continued for at least half a century, the variety of current theories and the contradictory findings, indicate how little is known.

Clinical features

Typical features of recurrent aphthae are summarised in Table 13.3.

Table 13.3   Recurrent aphthae — typical features

- Onset frequently in childhood but peak in adolescence or early adult life
- Attacks at variable but sometimes relatively regular intervals
- Most patients are otherwise healthy
- A few have haematological defects
- Most patients are non-smokers
- Usually self-limiting eventually

Females are not significantly more frequently affected than males. The frequency of ulceration typically reaches a peak in early adult life or a little later, then gradually wanes. Recurrent aphthae are rare in the elderly and particularly in the edentulous. However, older persons may be affected if a haematological deficiency develops. The great majority of patients are clerical, semiprofessional or professional workers and are total non-smokers. Occasionally, aphthae start when smoking is abandoned.

The usual history is of painful ulcers recurring at intervals of approximately 3–4 weeks. Occasionally they are continuously present. Unpredictable remissions of several months may be noted. Individual minor aphthae persist for 7–10 days, then heal without scarring.

Aphthae typically affect only the non-keratinised mucosa, such as the buccal mucosa, sulci or lateral borders of the tongue, but major aphthae can affect the masticatory mucosa. Ulcers are of three clinically distinguishable types (Table 13.4).

The pain of major aphthae can interfere with eating. Moreover, major aphthae are sometimes a feature of AIDS and add to such patients' burdens.

Pathology

There is alleged to be initial lymphocytic infiltration followed by destruction of the epithelium and infiltration of the tissues by neutrophils. Mononuclear cells may also surround blood vessels (perivascular cuffing). These changes are said to be

Table 13.4 Types of recurrent aphthae

- *Minor aphthae*
  The most common type
  Non-keratinised mucosa affected
  Ulcers are shallow, rounded, 5–7 mm across, with an
    erythematous margin and yellowish floor (Fig. 13.1)
  One or several ulcers may be present
- *Major aphthae*
  Uncommon
  Ulcers frequently several centimetres across (Fig. 13.2)
  Sometimes mimic a malignant ulcer
  Ulcers persist for several months
  Masticatory mucosa such as the dorsum of the tongue or
    occasionally the gingivae may be involved
  Scarring may follow healing (Fig. 13.3)
- *Herpetiform aphthae*
  Uncommon
  Non-keratinised mucosa affected
  Ulcers are 1–2 mm across
  Dozens or hundreds may be present
  May coalesce to form irregular ulcers (Fig. 13.4)
  Widespread bright erythema round the ulcers

Fig. 13.3 Recurrent aphthous stomatitis, major type. The same ulcer shown in Figure 13.2 but healing. The ulcer is much smaller but there is scarring and puckering of the surrounding mucosa.

Fig. 13.1 Aphthous stomatitis, minor form. A single, relatively large shallow ulcer in a typical site. There is a narrow band of periulcer erythema. These features are non-specific and the diagnosis must be made primarily on the basis of the history.

Fig. 13.4 Recurrent aphthous stomatitis, herpetiform type. There are numerous small, rounded and pinpoint ulcers, some of which are coalescing. The surrounding mucosa is lightly erythematous and the overall picture is highly suggestive of viral infection, but the attacks are recurrent and no virus can be isolated.

Fig. 13.2 Aphthous stomatitis, major type. This large, deep ulcer with considerable surrounding erythema has been present for several weeks.

consistent with either type III or IV reactions, but true vasculitis is not seen. Overall the appearances are non-specific (Fig. 13.5).

Biopsy is of no value in the diagnosis except to exclude carcinoma in the case of major aphthae. Aphthae are not preceded by vesiculation and smears will distinguish herpetiform aphthae from herpetic ulceration.

Diagnosis and management

The most important diagnostic feature is the history of recurrences of self-healing ulcers at fairly regular intervals (Table 13.5). The only other condition with this history is Behçet's disease. Often, increasing frequency of ulcers brings the patient to seek treatment. Otherwise most patients appear well, but haematological investigation is particularly important in older patients. Routine blood indices are informative, and

Fig. 13.5　Recurrent aphtha. Section of an early ulcer showing the break in the epithelium, the inflammatory cells in the floor and the inflammatory changes more deeply where numerous dilated vessels can be seen.

usually the most important finding is an abnormal mean corpuscular volume (MCV). If macro- or microcytosis is present, further investigation is necessary to find and remedy the cause. Treatment of vitamin B_{12} deficiency or folate deficiency is sometimes sufficient to control or abolish aphthae.

Table 13.5	Check-list for diagnosis of recurrent aphthae
History	*The history is all-important* Check for: 　　Recurrences 　　Pattern? Minor, major or herpetiform type? 　　Onset as child or teenager 　　Family history 　　Distribution only on non-keratinised mucosa 　　Signs or symptoms of Behçet's disease 　　(Table 13.6) (ocular, genital, skin, joint lesions)
Examination	Check for: 　　Discrete well-defined ulcers 　　Scarring or soft-palate involvement suggesting 　　　major aphthae 　　Exclude other diseases with specific appearances, 　　　e.g. lichen planus or vesiculobullous disease
Special investigations	*Used to exclude underlying conditions, especially in patients with onset in later life* Check for: 　　Anaemia, iron, folate and vitamin B_{12} status 　　History of diarrhoea, constipation or blood in 　　　stools suggesting gastrointestinal disease, e.g. 　　　coeliac disease or malabsorption

Apart from the minority with underlying systemic disease, treatment is empirical and palliative only. Despite numerous clinical trials, no medication gives completely reliable relief. Patients should therefore be made to understand that the trouble may not be curable but can usually be alleviated and generally resolves eventually of its own accord.

Corticosteroids.　Some patients get relief from Corlan (hydrocortisone hemisuccinate 2.5 mg) pellets allowed to dissolve in the mouth 3 times a day. Corticosteroids are unlikely to hasten healing of existing ulcers, but probably reduce the painful inflammation. The most rational form of treatment is for patients to take these pellets continuously (whether or not ulcers are present) to enable the corticosteroid to act in the very early, asymptomatic stages. This regimen is only applicable to those who have frequent ulcers (at 2- or 3-week intervals or more frequently). This should be tried for 2 months, then stopped for a month to assess any improvement and whether there is any deterioration without treatment.

Triamcinolone dental paste is a corticosteroid in a vehicle which sticks to the moist mucosa. When correctly applied the vehicle absorbs moisture and forms an adhesive gel which can remain in place for one or several hours but it is difficult to apply a fragment of this paste to the ulcer and to get it to adhere firmly. It is only useful for patients with infrequent ulcers, for ulcers near the front of the mouth and for patients dextrous enough to be able to follow the instructions. This gel should form a protective layer over the ulcer to help make it comfortable. The corticosteroid is slowly released and has an anti-inflammatory action. Another alternative is the use of a corticosteroid asthma spray to deposit a potent corticosteroid over the ulcer.

Topical corticosteroids, used as described, have no systemic effect.

Tetracycline mouth rinses.　Controlled trials both in Britain and the USA have shown that tetracycline rinses significantly reduce both the frequency and severity of aphthae. For herpetiform aphthae particularly, the contents of a tetracycline capsule (250 mg) can be stirred in a little water and held in the mouth for 2–3 minutes, three times daily. Some patients like to use this mouth rinse regularly for 3 days each week if they have frequent ulcers. An antifungal drug may also need to be given to patients who are susceptible to superinfection by *Candida albicans.*

Chlorhexidine.　A 0.2% solution has also been used as a mouth rinse for aphthae. Used three times daily after meals and held in the mouth for at least 1 minute, it has been claimed to reduce the duration and discomfort of aphthous stomatitis. Zinc sulphate or zinc chloride solutions may also have a slight beneficial effect.

Topical salicylate preparations.　Salicylates have an anti-inflammatory action and also have local effects. Preparations of choline salicylate in a gel can be applied to aphthae. These preparations, which are available over the counter, sometimes appear to be helpful.

Treatment of major aphthae.　Major aphthae, whether or not there is underlying disease such as HIV infection, may sometimes be so painful, persistent and resistant to conventional treatment as to be disabling. Reportedly effective treatments include thalidomide, azathioprine, cyclosporin, colchicine and dapsone. All of these are toxic in varying degrees and require specialist supervision. Their use may be justified for major aphthae even in otherwise healthy persons if they are disabled by the pain and difficulty of eating.

BEHÇET'S DISEASE

Behçet's disease comprises oral aphthae, genital ulceration, ocular disease and other lesions. Unlike autoimmune diseases such as the rheumatic diseases, young adult males between 20 and 40 are predominantly affected. Behçet's disease is rare in Britain and most parts of the USA but relatively common in Turkey (Behçet was a Turk), and so common in Japan that its geographical prevalence has been mapped. This racial distribution suggests a strong genetic component. There appears to be an association of HLA-B12 with the mucocutaneous type, HLA-B5 with the ocular, and HLA-B27 with the arthritic type. It is a multisystem disease (Table 13.6) but manifestations appear in various combinations.

Table 13.6 Diagnostic criteria for Behçet's disease

Major criteria	Minor criteria

• Recurrent oral aphthae
• Genital ulceration
• Eye lesions
   (Recurrent hypopyon,
   iritis or iridocyclitis;
   chorioretinitis)
• Skin lesions
   (Erythema nodosum;
   subcutaneous thrombophlebitis;
   hyperirritability of the skin)
	• Arthralgia or arthritis
	• Gastrointestinal lesions
	• Vascular lesions (mainly
	   thrombotic) (Fig. 13.6)
	• Central nervous system
	   involvement

Fig. 13.6 Thrombophlebitis in Behçet's disease. Inflammation and pigmentation highlight the sites of veins and their valves. This is only one of several possible skin manifestations.

The oral aphthae of Behçet's disease are not distinguishable from common aphthae. They are the most consistently found feature and frequently the first manifestation. Behçet's disease should therefore be considered in the differential diagnosis of aphthous stomatitis. The frequency of other manifestations is highly variable. As a result there are no absolute criteria or reliable tests for the diagnosis.

Treatment is difficult and may depend on a multidiscipline approach.

HIV-ASSOCIATED ORAL ULCERATION

Patients with HIV infection (Ch. 24) are susceptible to severe recurrent aphthae which are not otherwise distinguishable from common aphthae. They may also suffer from necrotising mucosal ulceration. Biopsies should be taken to exclude opportunistic infections. Otherwise the aetiology is unknown. Treatment with thalidomide is frequently effective.

LICHEN PLANUS

Lichen planus is a common chronic inflammatory disease of skin and mucous membranes. It mainly affects patients of middle age or over. Oral lesions have characteristic appearances and distribution.

Aetiology

In spite of histological changes, which can be diagnostic, the aetiology of lichen planus remains problematical. The predominantly T lymphocyte infiltrate suggests cell-mediated immunological damage to the epithelium, and a plethora of immunological abnormalities has been reported. Though it has not been possible to demonstrate humoral or lymphocytotoxic mechanisms, the inflammatory infiltrate consists mainly of T lymphocytes. Both CD4 and CD8 cells are present but numbers of CD8 cells may rise with disease progression and they are more numerous in relation to the epithelium. Precise trigger mechanisms remain unclear but lichen planus undoubtedly appears to be a T lymphocyte-mediated disorder.

Disease indistinguishable from lichen planus, induced by drugs (notably gold and antimalarial agents), also suggests involvement of immunological mechanisms. Oral lichen planus is also a virtually invariable feature and an early sign of graft-versus-host disease (Ch. 25), but this does not clarify any immunological mechanisms.

Clinical features

Lichen planus is a chronic disease and typical features are summarised in Table 13.7. The characteristic appearance and distribution of the lesions should be taken into account in making the diagnosis.

Table 13.7 Oral lichen planus — typical features

- Females account for at least 65% of patients
- Patients usually over 40 years old
- Untreated disease can persist for 10 or more years
- Lesions in combination or isolation, comprise:
    Striae
    Atrophic areas
    Erosions
    Plaques
- Common sites are:
    Buccal mucosae
    Dorsum of tongue
    Gingivae (less frequently)
- Lesions usually bilateral and often symmetrical
- Cutaneous lesions only occasionally associated
- Usually good response to corticosteroids

Striae are most common and typically sharply defined, forming lacy, starry or annular patterns (Fig. 13.7). They may occasionally be interspersed with minute, white papules. Striae may not be palpable or may be firmer than the surrounding mucosa.

Atrophic areas are red areas of mucosal thinning (Fig. 13.8) often combined with striae.

Erosions are shallow irregular areas of epithelial destruction. These also can be very persistent and may be covered by a smooth, slightly raised yellowish layer of fibrin (Fig. 13.9). The margins may be slightly depressed due to fibrosis and gradual healing at the periphery. Striae may radiate from the margins of these erosions.

Plaques are occasionally seen in the early stages, particularly on the dorsum of the tongue. Otherwise they may result from persistent disease and mainly affect the buccal mucosa.

Fig. 13.7 Lichen planus, striate pattern. This is the most common site and type of lesion, a lacy network of white striae on the buccal mucosa. The lesions are usually symmetrically distributed.

Fig. 13.8 Lichen planus, atrophic type. There are shallow irregular zones of erythema surrounded by white striae.

Fig. 13.9 Severe lichen planus. Thick plaques of fibrin cover extensive ulcers on the dorsum of the tongue in this severe case.

Distribution

The buccal mucous membranes, particularly posteriorly, are by far the most frequently affected, but lesions may spread forward almost to the commissures. The next most common site is the tongue, either the edges or the lateral margins of the dorsum, or less frequently the centre of the dorsum. The lips and gingivae may also occasionally be affected but the floor of the mouth and palate escape. Lesions are very often symmetrical, often strikingly so (Fig. 13.10).

Symptoms

Striae alone may be asymptomatic and unnoticed by the patient, or cause roughness or slight stiffness of the mucosa. Atrophic lesions are sore, and erosions usually cause more severe symptoms still and may make eating difficult.

Fig. 13.10 Erosive lichen planus of the tongue. Two extensive areas of shallow ulceration have formed symmetrically on the tongue. Lingual involvement is seen, usually in severe cases where the buccal mucosa and other sites are also affected.

Fig. 13.12 Dermal lichen planus. This, the flexor surface of the wrists, is a characteristic site. The lesions consist of confluent papules with a pattern of minute white striae on their surface.

Fig. 13.11 Desquamative gingivitis caused by lichen planus. A well-defined band of patchy erythema extends across the full width of the attached gingiva around several teeth. This change may be localised or widespread. Within the red areas faint white flecks and striae are usually visible.

Gingival lichen planus

The gingivae are occasionally the only site of lichen planus, which needs to be distinguished from other forms of gingivitis. Lesions are usually atrophic so, that the gingivae appear shiny, inflamed and smooth ('desquamative gingivitis') (Fig. 13.11). Striae are uncommon but sometimes present in other parts of the mouth. Gingival lichen planus may involve limited segments.

Soreness caused by atrophic lesions makes toothbrushing difficult. Plaque accumulation and associated inflammatory changes probably aggravate lichen planus. The contribution of local irritation to lichen planus is suggested by disappearance of the lesions when the teeth are extracted. Lichen planus of the denture-bearing area is virtually unknown.

Skin lesions

Lichen planus is a common skin disease but skin lesions are uncommon in those who complain of oral symptoms. Skin lesions typically form purplish papules, 2–3 mm across, with a glistening surface marked by minute fine striae, and are usually itchy. Typical sites are the flexor surface of the forearms and especially the wrists (Fig. 13.12). Skin lesions help, but are not essential, to confirm the diagnosis of oral lichen planus.

Pathology

Corresponding with their clinical features, lesions fall into three distinct histological types (Table 13.8).

Table 13.8 Lichen planus — typical histological features of white lesions (striae) (Figs 13.13–13.15)

- Hyperkeratosis or parakeratosis
- Saw-tooth profile of the rete ridges
- Liquefaction degeneration of the basal cell layer
- Compact, band-like lymphoplasmacytic (predominantly T cell) infiltrate cells hugging the epitheliomesenchymal junction.
- CD8 lymphocytes predominate in relation to the epithelium

Typical histological features of atrophic lesions are summarised in Table 13.9.

Table 13.9 Lichen planus — typical histological features of atrophic lesions (Fig. 13.16)

- Severe thinning and flattening of the epithelium
- Compact band-like, subepithelial inflammatory infiltrate hugging the epitheliomesenchymal junction.

Erosions merely show destruction of the epithelium, leaving only the fibrin-covered, granulating connective tissue floor of the lesion. Diagnosis depends on seeing atrophic lesions or striae nearby.

Fig. 13.13 Lichen planus. The rete ridges have the characteristic pointed (saw-tooth) outline which is frequent in the skin but uncommon in mucosal lichen planus.

Fig. 13.14 Lichen planus. The basement membrane is thickened and lymphocytes from the dense infiltrate below emigrate into the basal cells of the epithelium where they are associated with focal basal cell degeneration.

Diagnosis

The diagnosis of lichen planus can usually be made on the history, the appearance of the lesions and their distribution. However, dysplastic leukoplakias occasionally have a streaky white appearance. A biopsy should be taken, particularly when striae are ill defined, plaques are present or the lesions are in any other ways unusual.

Fig. 13.15 Lichen planus. Lymphocytes infiltrating the basal cells are associated with basal cell apoptosis, loss of a prominent basal cell layer and prickle cells abutting the basement membrane. A cluster of apoptotic bodies is visible centrally, each consisting of a shrunken bright pink cell with a condensed and fragmented nucleus.

Fig. 13.16 Lichen planus. The epithelium is atrophic and greatly thinned. A well-demarcated, dense, broad band of lymphocytes extends along the superficial corium immediately below the epithelium.

Management

Patients are sometimes concerned that lichen planus is infectious and should be reassured that this is not so.

Topical application of potent anti-inflammatory corticosteroids is usually effective but monitoring is required and these preparations are suitable only for hospital use. Possible alternatives are to use similar corticosteroids (such as beclomethasone) from the aerosol inhalers used for asthma. Approximately six puffs from an inhaler daily, can be used to deliver enough of the corticosteroid to an ulcer. Potent corticosteroids used topically may occasionally promote thrush as a side-effect. Triamcinolone dental paste applied to the lesions is an alternative but less effective form of treatment. Gingival lichen planus is the most difficult to treat. The first essential is to maintain rigorous oral hygiene. Corticosteroids should also be used, as already described, and in this situation triamcinolone dental paste may be useful as it can readily be applied to the

Check-list for management of lichen planus

Always check for drugs which might cause a lichenoid reaction. This is indistinguishable clinically but may respond to a change of medication

When inflammation worsens or symptoms become more severe, consider the possibility of superinfection with *Candida*.

Biopsy lesions which appear unusual, form homogeneous plaques or present in unusual sites

Check for skin lesions which may aid diagnosis

Reassure patients that the condition is not usually of great consequence despite the fact that it can produce constant irritating soreness. Tell patients that the severity waxes and wanes unpredictably and the condition may persist for many years

Be aware that squamous carcinoma can develop in lesions, although very rarely. Follow up lesions associated with reddening, and any unusual in site, appearance or severity

Fig. 13.17 Lupus erythematosus. The clinical presentation is often very similar to lichen planus, with ulceration, atrophy and striae. Lesions on the soft palate or with radiating striae, as here, should be investigated for lupus erythematosus.

affected gingivae. In exceptionally severe cases, if topical treatment fails, treatment with systemic corticosteroids is effective. In unresponsive cases, cyclosporin may be effective.

Malignant change in lichen planus

The risk of and possible frequency of malignant change in lichen planus has long been controversial. Probably 1–1.5% of patients suffer this complication after 10 years. Specific risk factors have not been identified with certainty.

LUPUS ERYTHEMATOSUS

Lupus erythematosus is a connective tissue disease which has two main forms: systemic and discoid. Either can give rise to oral lesions which may appear similar to those of oral lichen planus.

Systemic lupus erythematosus has varied effects (Ch. 25). Arthralgias and rashes are most common, but virtually any organ system can be affected. A great variety of autoantibodies, particularly antinuclear, is produced.

Discoid lupus is essentially a skin disease with mucocutaneous lesions indistinguishable clinically from those of systemic lupus. These may be associated with arthralgias but, rarely, significant autoantibody production.

Clinically, oral lesions appear in about 20% of cases of systemic lupus, and can rarely be the presenting sign (Fig. 13.17). Typical lesions are white, often striate, areas with irregular atrophic areas or shallow erosions, but the patterns, particularly those of the striae, are typically far less sharply defined than in lichen planus. They are often patchy and unilateral and may be in the vault of the palate, which lichen planus typically spares.

Lesions can form variable patterns of white and red areas. There may also be small slit-like ulcers just short of the gingival margins. In about 30% of cases, Sjögren's syndrome devel-

Fig. 13.18 Lupus erythematosus stained with PAS to show the thickened basement membrane.

ops and rarely cervical lymphadenopathy (Ch. 26) is the first sign.

Pathology

Lesions show an irregular pattern of epithelial atrophy and acanthosis. Liquefaction degeneration of the basal cell layer is typical and there is PAS-positive thickening of the basement membrane zone and around blood vessels due to deposition of antigen – antibody complexes (Fig. 13.18). In the corium there is oedema and often a hyaline appearance. The inflammatory infiltrate is highly variable in density, typically extends deeply into the connective tissue and may have a perivascular distribution (Fig. 13.19).

Lupus erythematosus shows more irregular patterns of acanthosis and lacks the band-like distribution of lymphocytes in the papillary corium of lichen planus.

Fig. 13.19 Lupus erythematosus. The histological picture is similar to that seen in lichen planus, with a subepithelial band of lymphocytes, basal cell degeneration and epithelial atrophy. The dense perivascular infiltrates of lymphocytes in the deeper tissues are characteristic of lupus erythematosus.

Fig. 13.20 Pemphigus vulgaris. Typical oral presentation with erythema, erosions and persistent ulcers. The surrounding epithelium is friable and disintegrates on gentle stroking.

In frozen sections, a band of immunoglobulins and complement (C3) with a granular texture deposited along the basement membrane may be shown by immunofluorescence. This deposit also underlies normal epithelium in systemic lupus. In paraffin sections, immunoglobulin deposits may be detectable using immunoperoxidase staining. Obvious vasculitis may occasionally be seen in systemic, but not in discoid, lupus erythematosus.

Diagnosis of systemic lupus erythematosus should be confirmed by the pattern of antinuclear autoantibodies. The most specific is that to double-stranded (native) DNA.

Haematological findings in active systemic lupus erythematosus include a raised ESR, anaemia and, often, leukopenia or thrombocytopenia.

Oral lesions of discoid lupus erythematosus may respond in some degree to topical corticosteroids. However, oral lesions in acute systemic lupus erythematosus may not respond to doses of corticosteroids adequate to control systemic effects of the disease. Under such circumstances, palliative treatment is needed until disease activity abates.

Fig. 13.21 Pemphigus vulgaris. The characteristic bullae often appear in the mouth but soon spread over the skin, forming widespread moist or crusted lesions when they rupture.

PEMPHIGUS VULGARIS

Pemphigus is an uncommon autoimmune disease causing vesicles or bullae on skin and mucous membranes. It is usually fatal if untreated. Females, usually aged 40–60 years, are predominantly affected. Lesions often first appear in the mouth but spread widely on the skin. Vesicles are fragile and unlikely to be seen intact in the mouth. Residual erosions often have ragged edges and are superficial, painful and tender (Fig. 13.20). Gently stroking the mucosa can cause a vesicle or bulla to appear (Nikolsky's sign).

Progress of the disease is very variable. It may sometimes be

fulminating with rapid development of widespread oral ulceration, spread to other sites such as the eyes within a few days and very soon afterwards to the skin.

Skin lesions consist of vesicles or bullae varying from a few millimetres to a centimetre or so across (Fig. 13.21). The bullae at first contain clear fluid, which may then become purulent or haemorrhagic. Rupture of vesicles leaves painful ragged erosions. Protein, fluid and electrolytes are lost from the raw areas and they readily become secondarily infected. Without treatment, death usually follows, but immunosuppressive treatment is usually life-saving.

Pathology

An immunopathogenesis can be more convincingly demonstrated in pemphigus vulgaris than in any other oral disease; the histological findings are summarised in Table 13.10. The epithelial cells which lose their attachments become rounded in shape and the cytoplasm contracts around the nucleus. Small groups of these rounded-up acantholytic (*Tzanck*) cells can often be seen histologically in the contents of a vesicle or in a smear from a recently ruptured vesicle.

Table 13.10 Pathology of pemphigus vulgaris

- Loss of intercellular adherence of suprabasal spinous cells (acantholysis)
- Formation of clefts immediately superficial to the basal cells
- Extension of clefts to form intraepithelial vesicles (Fig. 13.22)
- Rupture of vesicles to form ulcers
- High titre of circulating antibodies to epithelial intercellular cement substance
- Binding of antibodies to intercellular substance detectable by fluorescence microscopy

Pemphigus antibodies are tissue-specific and react only to intercellular substance of squamous epithelium (Fig. 13.23). The epithelial cell surface antigen is an intercellular adhesion molecule (ICAM), termed desmoglein 3. The mechanism of breakdown of intercellular attachments appears to result from synthesis of proteases by the epithelial cells.

Management

The diagnosis must be confirmed as early as possible. Biopsy is essential and the changes are sufficiently characteristic to make a diagnosis. Immunofluorescence microscopy should be used to exclude similar but less common diseases. Once the diagnosis has been confirmed, immunosuppressive treatment

Fig. 13.23 Pemphigus vulgaris. Frozen tissue stained with fluorescent antibody to IgG shows fluorescence along the lines of the interepithelial attachments typical of pemphigus. See also Figure 1.6

is required. There is little consensus about dosage but a typical regimen is 80–100 mg/day of prednisolone plus azathioprine (1–1.5 mg/kg daily). Azathioprine is given to allow doses of the corticosteroid to be lowered and reduce their side-effects. Treatment can only be stopped if relapse fails to follow withdrawal, and can itself cause a significant mortality. With combined immunosuppressive treatment, the average mortality is approximately 6%.

Key clinical features are summarised in Table 13.11.

Table 13.11 Pemphigus vulgaris — key clinical features

- Females predominantly affected, usually aged 40–60 years
- Lesions often first in the mouth but spread widely on the skin
- Lesions consist of fragile vesicles and bullae
- Ruptured vesicles form irregular erosions on the mucosa
- Nikolsky's sign may be positive
- Widespread skin involvement is fatal if untreated
- Good response to prolonged immunosuppressive treatment

Fig. 13.22 Pemphigus. The edge of a bulla formed by separation of the epithelium just above the basal cells. There is acantholysis centrally and a layer of basal cells remains covering the dermal papillae.

MUCOUS MEMBRANE PEMPHIGOID

Mucous membrane pemphigoid is an uncommon chronic disease causing bullae, painful erosions and mucosal scarring (Table 13.12). Skin involvement is uncommon and often trivial. Lesions (Fig. 13.24) are rarely widespread and progress is very slow. 'Desquamative gingivitis' can be a manifestation (Fig. 13.25). Nikolsky's sign should be positive and a striking clinical finding is sometimes that the epithelium slides away underneath the edge of the scalpel when a biopsy is attempted. In the mouth, bleeding into bullae can cause them to appear as blood blisters. Rupture of erosions leaves raw areas with well-defined margins. Individual erosions persist for some weeks then slowly heal, usually without scarring. Further erosions may develop nearby and this process may persist for a year or

Fig. 13.24 Pemphigoid. Typical oral presentation with persistent erythema and ulceration of the palate. On close examination tags of epithelium are sometimes seen at the ulcer margins.

Fig. 13.25 Desquamative gingivitis as a result of mucous membrane pemphigoid. There is patchy reddening involving the attached gingivae around several teeth and in places the erythema extends to the alveolar mucosa. Unlike desquamative gingivitis caused by lichen planus, there are no flecks or striae and occasionally tags of separating epithelium may be found.

more. Lesions may remain localised to the mouth for very long periods and may never involve other sites.

Table 13.12 Mucous membrane pemphigoid — typical features
• Females mainly affected and usually elderly
• Oral mucosa often the first site
• Involvement of other mucosae, particularly the eyes, may cause scarring and blindness
• Skin involvement absent or minimal
• Indolent, non-fatal disease
• Oral bullae are subepithelial and frequently seen intact

Pathology

Histologically there is loss of attachment and separation of the full thickness of the epithelium from the connective tissue at the basement membrane. Epithelium, though separated, remains for

Fig. 13.26 Mucous membrane pemphigoid. The full thickness of the epithelium has separated cleanly from the underlying connective tissue to form a fluid-filled bulla. A light inflammatory infiltrate is present in the underlying connective tissue.

Fig. 13.27 Mucous membrane pemphigoid. Frozen tissue stained with fluorescent anti-C3 shows a line of fluorescence along the basement membrane indicating complement activation there. See also Figure 1.6.

a time intact and forms the roof of a bulla (Fig. 13.26). The floor of the bulla is formed by connective tissue alone, infiltrated with inflammatory cells. The disease is immunologically mediated, and binding of immunoglobulin or more frequently of complement components along the basement membrane zone can be demonstrated (Fig. 13.27). Circulating autoantibodies are detectable by sensitive techniques.

Management

The diagnosis is confirmed by biopsy and immunofluorescence microscopy but it is preferable to obtain an intact vesicle or bulla.

Oral mucous membrane pemphigoid can often be effectively controlled with topical corticosteroids. Doses are small and without systemic effects.

Because of the possible risk to sight, ocular examination is necessary if early changes in the eyes are suspected. If the eyes become involved, systemic corticosteroids have to be given and are effective.

Desquamative gingivitis

The term 'desquamative gingivitis' is a clinical description, not a diagnosis. It is used for conditions in which the gingivae appear red or raw. Usually the whole of the attached gingiva of varying numbers of teeth is affected.

Lichen planus is the most common cause. The gingivae then appear smooth, red and translucent due to the thinness of the atrophic epithelium. In older patients mucous membrane pemphigoid may cause gingival erosions. Pemphigus vulgaris is another possible cause. In all cases the appearances are strikingly different from simple marginal gingivitis, and the diagnosis should be confirmed by biopsy.

BULLOUS ERYTHEMA MULTIFORME

This is a mucocutaneous disease but, among dental patients, oral lesions are the most prominent or the only ones present (Table 13.13).

Fig. 13.28   Bullous erythema multiforme. Ulceration of the vermilion border of the lip with bleeding, swelling and crusting is characteristic.

Fig. 13.29   Erythema multiforme. There is ulceration, erythema, sloughing of epithelium and a small vesicle centrally. The anterior part of the mouth and the lips are typically affected.

Table 13.13   Bullous erythema multiforme — typical clinical features

- Occasionally triggered by herpetic infection or drugs
- Adolescents or young adults, particularly males, mainly affected
- Mild fever and systemic upset may be associated
- Lips frequently grossly swollen, split, crusted and bleeding (Fig. 13.28)
- Widespread irregular fibrin-covered erosions and erythema in the mouth (Fig. 13.29)
- Conjunctivitis may be associated
- Cutaneous lesions may consist of widespread erythema alone (Fig. 13.30) or characteristic target lesions
- Attacks may recur at intervals of several months
- Remittant but usually ultimately self-limiting

Target lesions are red macules a centimetre or more in diameter with a bluish cyanotic centre. In severe cases skin lesions are bullous. The attack usually lasts for 3 or 4 weeks, with new crops of lesions developing over a period of about 10 days. Recurrences, usually at intervals of several months, for a year or two are characteristic and are sometimes increasingly severe.

Fig. 13.30   Erythema multiforme. As the name suggests, the rash is variable and ranges from patchy erythema, as here, to the more characteristic target lesions and bullae.

In the most severe cases ocular damage may impair sight and occasionally cause blindness. Very rarely, renal damage can be fatal.

Aetiology and pathology

The aetiology is not clear and, though the disease may be a reaction to a variety of causes, no convincing mechanism has been proposed. Infections, such as herpetic or mycoplasmal, can be triggering factors. Drugs, particularly sulphonamides and barbiturates, have also been implicated, but a positive drug history is also rare. Even when drugs have been taken, coincidence cannot always be excluded and in most patients no precipitating cause can be found.

The histological appearances are variable. Widespread necrosis of keratinocytes with eosinophilic colloid change in the superficial epithelium may be conspicuous. This is not specific but may progress to intraepithelial vesicle or bulla formation (Fig. 13.31). However, subepithelial vesiculation is more frequent (Fig. 13.32). Degenerative changes in the epithelium are associated with infiltration by inflammatory cells which also involve the corium and may have a perivascular distribution. Leakage of immunoglobulins from blood vessels has been reported, but vasculitis is not seen histologically.

Fig. 13.31 Erythema multiforme. At higher power there is necrosis of prickle cells producing intraepithelial vescicles.

Fig. 13.32 Erythema multiforme. There is a dense inflammatory infiltrate immediately below the epithelium and around blood vessels in the deeper corium. The epithelium is separating from the connective tissue, here along the basement membrane, and there is ulceration centrally.

Management

Patients should be warned of the possibility of recurrences but that the disease usually runs a limited course.

There is no specific treatment. Systemic corticosteroids may give symptomatic relief. Antibiotics are usually also given in severe cases, with the idea of preventing secondary infection. Levamisole has also been reported to be effective.

'ALLERGIC' STOMATITIS

Many otherwise harmless substances coming into contact with the skin cause hypersensitisation in susceptible subjects. When this has happened, further contact causes an inflammatory reaction. Examples are eczema or contact dermatitis caused by a wide variety of household and industrial materials. Some mucous membranes, such as those of the eyes, can also become sensitised in this way, but the different parts of the body differ widely in their response. Sulphonamide ointments, for example, are highly sensitising to the skin but cause little trouble in the eyes. The oral mucous membrane appears to show yet other differences and to be unable to mount reactions comparable with contact dermatitis, and there is no such condition as oral eczema. Most so-called allergic reactions of the mouth are due to direct irritation by the substance. Even patients who are sensitised to a material such as nickel can tolerate it in the mouth; it may then cause a characteristic rash but not oral lesions. Amalgam restorations cause no trouble in patients sensitised to mercury, though the material should not be allowed to come into contact with the skin (Ch. 25). Similar considerations apply to methylmethacrylate. Those few people who are sensitised to the monomer can wear acrylic dentures with impunity. Inflammation under acrylic dentures, often in the past described as 'acrylic allergy', is usually candidal infection. Authenticated cases of contact hypersensitisation of the oral mucous membrane are so few as to make it questionable whether the oral mucosa can mount this type of reaction. If it does so it must be phenomenally rare.

MISCELLANEOUS MUCOSAL ULCERS

Eosinophilic ulcer (atypical or traumatic eosinophilic granuloma)

Tumour-like, ulcerated lesions with a microscopic picture resembling that of Langerhans' cell histiocytosis, may occasionally form in the oral soft tissue, particularly the tongue, but also the gingivae and, occasionally, other sites. In some, there is a history of trauma, and, experimentally, crush injury to muscle can induce a proliferative response with tissue eosinophilia.

Clinically, the ulcerated mass may be mistaken for a carcinoma but is typically soft: almost any age can be affected.

Fig. 13.33 Chemical burn. The gingivae are white and necrotic following injudicious use of a caustic agent. On the patient's right side full-thickness ulceration is present.

Pathology

There is typically a dense aggregation of eosinophils and cells which resemble histiocytes beneath the ulcerated surface. The histiocytes lack the ultrastructural features and surface markers of Langerhans' cells but are occasionally pleomorphic.

The differential diagnosis is from Langerhans' cell histiocytosis, which can be excluded by the absence of Langerhans' cells markers (Ch. 9). In practice, lesions usually heal sponta-neously within 3–8 weeks, and management of an isolated soft-tissue mass having these histological characteristics should be expectant.

Ruptured blood bisters (localised oral purpura)

Bullae of mucous membrane pemphigoid sometimes fill with blood but must be distinguished from localised oral purpura (Ch. 23). Rupture of such blisters leaves painful ulcers.

Wegener's granulomatosis

Mucosal ulceration is occasionally a feature of this disease, but mainly in its established form (Ch. 28). Clinically, ulceration may be widespread but is otherwise non-specific.

Oral reactions to drugs

A great variety of drugs can cause mucosal reactions, either as local effects (Fig. 13.33) or through systemic mechanisms which are often obscure.

Systemically-mediated reactions include ulceration, lichenoid reactions and erythema multiforme. These reactions are discussed in more detail in chapter 35.

Table 13.14 Some uncommon mucosal diseases

Disease	Cause	Oral features	Treatment
Epidermolysis bullosa	Autosomal recessive — gravis type due to type VII collagen defect. (junctional type usually lethal at birth)	Subepithelial bullae leading to severe intraoral scarring after minimal trauma, especially in recessive types	None wholly effective. Protect against any mucosal abrasion
Pyostomatitis vegetans	Complication of inflammatory bowel disease, particularly ulcerative colitis	Yellowish miliary pustules in thickened, erythematous mucosa release pus, leaving shallow ulcers. Suprabasal clefting and intraepithelial vesiculation or abscesses containing eosinophils. Sometimes intercellular Ig. Peripheral eosinophilia up to 20% of WBCs	Control of inflammatory bowel disease or systemic prednisolone
Gonorrhoea	*Neisseria gonorrhoeae*, sexually transmitted	Oropharyngeal erythema or ulcers rarely seen	Amoxycillin, spectinomycin or a 4–quinoline
Reiter's disease	Urethritis, conjunctivitis, arthritis. Postinfective reaction	Painless circinate white lesions, histologically psoriasis-like	Oral lesions self-limiting
Leprosy	*Mycobacterium leprae*	Oral ulcers or nodules. Seen mainly in Asia	Dapsone
Paraneoplastic pemphigus	Complication mainly of lymphoreticular tumours and sarcomas	Various vesiculobullous lesions of mucosae. Interepithelial Ig and basement membrane Ig and C3	As for pemphigus vulgaris
IgA pemphigus	Autoimmune	Vesicular bullous lesions resembling pemphigus vulgaris, but with intercellular IgA	Dapsone. Toxic effects often limit duration of treatment
Keratosis follicularis (Darier's disease; warty dyskeratoma)	Genetic. Autosomal dominant	Intraepithelial bullae containing granulocytes and acantholytic cells. Pebbly lesions mainly of palate due to hyperkeratosis, acantholysis with 'corps ronds' and 'grains' (dyskeratosis)	Oral lesions not troublesome but respond to retinoids

SOME UNCOMMON MUCOCUTANEOUS DISEASES

In many of these conditions, the oral lesions are rare or insignificant in comparision with the skin disease (Table 13.14).

SUGGESTED FURTHER READING

Carson P J, Hameed A, Ahmed A R 1996 Influence of treatment on the clinical course of pemphigus vulgaris. J Am Acad Dermatol 34:645–652

Chan L S, Yancey K B, Hammerberg C et al 1993 Immune-mediated subepithelial blistering diseases of mucous membranes. Arch Dermatol 129:448–455

Cribier B, Garnier C, Lausriat D, Heid E 1994 Lichen planus and hepatitis C virus infection: an epidemiologic study. J Am Acad Dermatol 31:1070–1072

Eisen D, Ellis C N, Duell E A, Griffiths C E M, Voorhees J J 1990 Effect of topical cyclosporine rinses on oral lichen planus. A double blind analysis. N Engl J ed 323:290–294

Hietanen J, Pihlman K, Linder E, Reunala T 1987 No evidence of hypersensitivity to dental restorative materials in oral lichen planus. Scand J Dent Res 5:320–327

Ho V C, Gupta A K, Ellis C N, Nickoloff B J, Vorrhees J J 1990 Treatment of severe lichen planus with cyclosporine. J Am Acad Dermatol 22:64–68

Huilgol S C, Bhogal B S, Black M M 1995 Immunofluorescence of the immunobullous disorders. Eur J Dermatol 5:186–195

Karjalainen T K, Tomich C E 1989 A histopathologic study of oral mucosal lupus erythematosus. Oral Surg Oral Med Oral Pathol 67:547–554

Laeijendecker R, van Joost T 1994 Oral manifestations of gold allergy. J Am Acad Dermatol 30:205–209

Laine J, Kalimo K, Forssell H, Happonen R-P 1992 Resolution of oral lichenoid lesions in patients allergic to mercury compounds. Br J Dermatol 26:10–15

Lozada-Nur F, Gorsky M, Silverman S 1989 Oral erythema multiforme: clinical observations and treatment of 95 patients. Oral Surg Oral Med Oral Pathol 67:36–40

MacPhail L A, Greenspan D, Feigal D W, Lennette E T, Greenspan J 1991 Recurrent aphthous ulcers in association with HIV infection. Description of ulcer types and analysis of T-lymphocyte subsets. Oral Surg Oral Med Oral Pathol 1:678–683

Porter S R, Scully C, Flint S 1988 Hematologic status in recurrent aphthous stomatitis compared with other oral disease. Oral Surg Oral Med Oral Pathol 66:41–44

Porter S R, Bain S E, Scully C M 1992 Linear IgA disease manifesting as recalcitrant resquamative gingivitis. Oral Surg Oral Med Oral Pathol 74:179–182

Scully C, Porter S R 1989 Recurrent aphthous stomatitis: current concepts of etiology, pathogenesis and treatment. J Oral Pathol Med 18:21–27

Van Gestel A, Koopman R, Wijnands M, van de Putte L, van Riel P 1994 Mucocutaneous reactions to gold: a prospective study of 74 patients with rheumatoid arthritis. J Rheumatol 21:1814–1819

Vincent S D, Lilly G E, Baker K A 1993 Clinical, historic, and therapeutic features of cicatricial pemphigoid. A literature review and open therapeutic trials with corticosteroids. Oral Surg Oral Med Oral Pathol 76:453–459

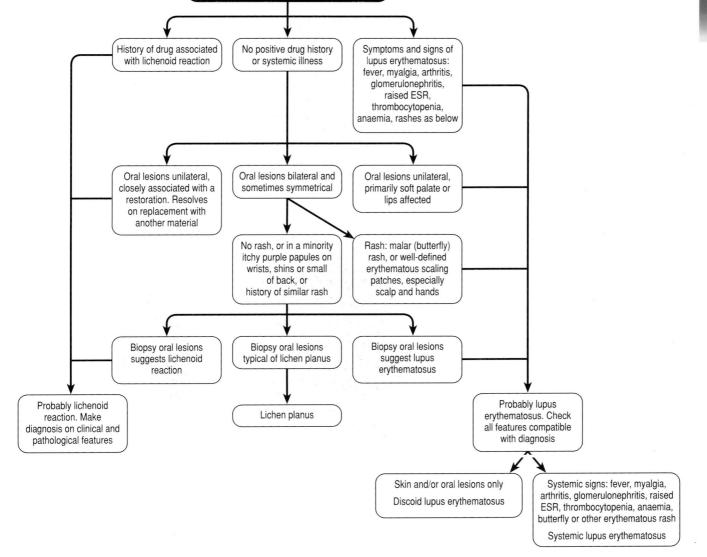

Summary 13.1 Differential diagnosis of oral lichen planus and conditions which mimic it clinically.

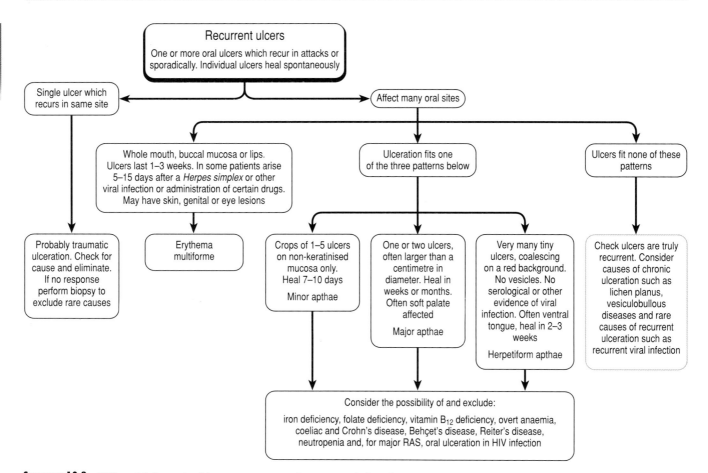

Summary 13.2 Differential diagnosis of the common causes of recurrent oral ulceration.

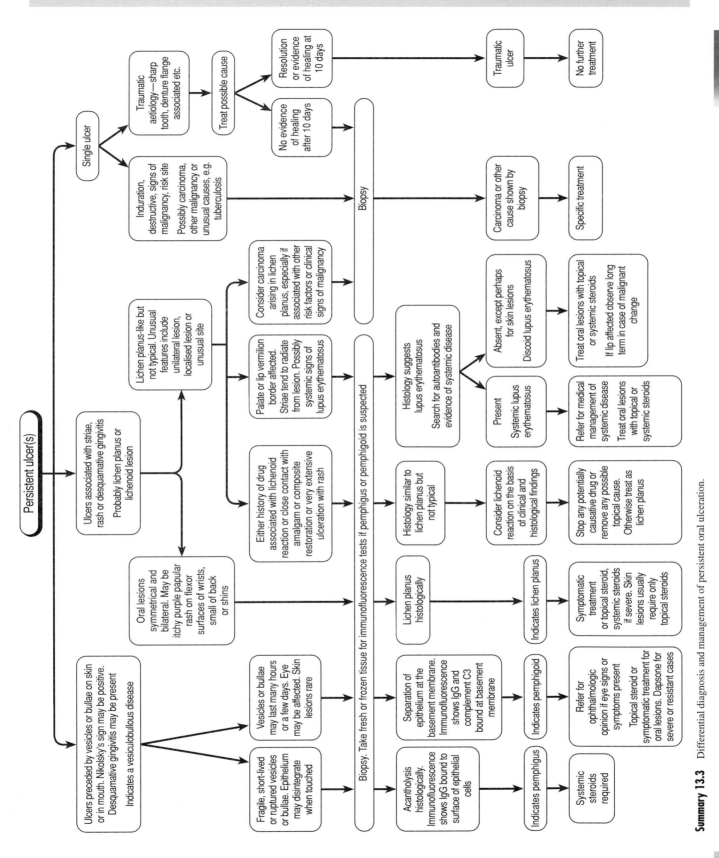

Summary 13.3 Differential diagnosis and management of persistent oral ulceration.

Tongue disorders

The tongue can be involved in generalised stomatitis and show lesions similar to those in other parts of the mouth. The tongue is also the site of lesions or source of symptoms peculiar to itself. For unknown reasons, it can manifest the earliest symptoms of anaemia or latent defects of haemopoiesis.

THE SORE TONGUE

There are several clinical types of sore tongue (Table 14.1).

Table 14.1 Clinical types of sore tongue
• Ulcers (of any type) involving the tongue • Glossitis (red and sore tongue) • The sore, physically normal tongue • Geographical tongue (erythema migrans)

Ulceration of the tongue

The tongue may be involved in, or even be the predominantly affected site of, various types of stomatitis such as herpes simplex or, more frequently, lichen planus (see Fig. 13.10). The tongue may also be the site of solitary ulcers, particularly carcinoma, which when far back may be difficult to see. The lateral borders are affected and carcinoma of the dorsum of the tongue is exceptionally rare.

When there are definable lesions of these kinds, diagnosis is usually straightforward and depends on clinical examination and sometimes biopsy.

Glossitis

Glossitis is the term used for the red, smooth and sore tongue particularly characteristic of anaemia (Ch. 22). These features are a combination of *signs* (redness and smoothness) and a *symptom* (soreness) which are by not always associated. Tongues can be sore in the absence of visible changes or smooth but asymptomatic from a variety of causes (Table 14.2).

Table 14.2 Important causes of glossitis
• Anaemia • Vitamin B group (especially B_{12}) deficiencies • Candidosis

Iron deficiency and pernicious anaemia are the main causes (Fig. 14.1). Women are more frequently affected. Detailed haematological examination is essential. These investigations are important, as a fall in haemoglobin level may lag behind other changes. Thus there may be glossitis, haematological signs of a deficiency state, but a haemoglobin level within normal limits. Abnormalities of the red cells may be seen in a stained film, but the red cell mean corpuscular volume (MCV) is frequently a useful guide. Serum levels of iron and ferritin, vitamin B_{12} or folate (as the case may be) are depressed. When abnormalities such as these are found, specific treatment quickly relieves the symptoms.

Glossitis with angular stomatitis is characteristic of riboflavin deficiency and sometimes of nicotinic acid deficiency, but these are rare. The diagnosis of vitamin deficiency

Fig. 14.1 Glossitis in iron-deficiency anaemia. The tongue is smooth due to atrophy of the papillae, and is red and sore. Anaemia is the commonest diagnosable cause of glossitis and must always be looked for by haematological examination.

Fig. 14.2 Glossitis in antibiotic stomatitis. The tongue is red, smooth and sore as in anaemic glossitis, but the appearance is partly due to inflammatory oedema. Similar changes affect the rest of the mucosa and other features of candidosis, such as thrush, are often present.

Fig. 14.3 Smooth tongue due to lichen planus. This is a late change due to longstanding disease. The tongue is smooth due to atrophy of the papillae, but has a faint silvery sheen. There are usually no symptoms at this stage.

Fig. 14.4 A normal-looking but persistently sore tongue in a doctor's wife who had had repeated but inadequate haematological investigations which failed to detect early pernicious anaemia.

should not be made on oral signs alone in an otherwise healthy patient. These B group vitamins are frequently given in an attempt to relieve sore tongue but are virtually invariably ineffective. Their ineffectiveness makes it clear that deficiency of these vitamins is not the cause.

Candidosis can cause the tongue to be red, sore and oedematous. This is typical of acute antibiotic stomatitis (Fig. 14.2) and often then associated with angular stomatitis and other features of candidosis. This condition is rarely seen now that antibiotics are used less indiscriminately than in the past and topical oral antibiotics have now been discredited for oral infections.

Lichen planus can produce a smooth tongue due to atrophy of the papillae (particularly late in long-standing disease) but there is then no soreness and typically no erythema. There is often a bluish-white sheen to the surface of the tongue, and other signs of lichen planus may be seen in other parts of the mouth (Fig. 14.3).

The sore, physically normal tongue

This type creates the most difficult problems. The symptoms are frequently psychogenic, but it is essential to exclude organic disease, particularly a haematological deficiency.

Haematological deficiencies. Soreness can precede visible, physical changes (Fig. 14.4). The haemoglobin is frequently within normal limits but there are other abnormalities, as described earlier. Treatment of the deficiency quickly relieves the symptoms.

Psychogenic disorders. Soreness of the tongue frequently appears to be psychogenic and is sometimes termed 'burning mouth syndrome'. Some regard it as a variant of atypical facial pain, and clinical features (Table 14.3) may suggest psychogenic factors.

These symptoms are seen in varying combination but psychological disturbance is frequently well disguised or suppressed. In practice, as with atypical facial pain, there are many patients who complain bitterly and persistently of sore tongue, in whom no organic disease can be found and who show no response to psychoactive drugs or any other form of treatment.

Geographical tongue (erythema migrans linguae)

In this condition there is the recurrent appearance and disappearance of red areas on the tongue. The cause is unknown but sometimes there is a clear family history of its presence in sev-

Table 14.3   Features suggestive of 'burning mouth syndrome'

- Middle-aged or older women are mainly affected
- No visible abnormality or evidence of organic disease
- No haematological abnormality
- Pain typically described as 'burning'
- Persistent and unremitting soreness without aggravating or relieving factors. Often of months or years duration. No response to analgesics
- Bizarre patterns of pain radiation inconsistent with neurological or vascular anatomy
- Sometimes, bitter or metallic taste associated
- Associated depression, anxiety or stressful life-situation
- Obsession with symptoms which may rule the patient's life
- Constant search for reasurance and treatment by different practitioners
- Occasionally, dramatic improvement with antidepressive treatment

Fig. 14.5   Erythema migrans. Typical appearance with irregular depapillated patches centred on the lateral border of the tongue. Each patch has a narrow red and white rim.

eral generations. The abnormality can sometimes therefore be seen in infancy, but is probably not often noticed then. Most cases are seen in middle-aged patients. It seems improbable (but not impossible) that the condition has remained unnoticed for so long. In many patients geographical tongue seems to be a developmental anomaly but there also appears to an association with psoriasis.

Clinically, an irregular, smooth, red area appears, usually with a sharply-defined edge, where the filiform papillae stop short (Fig. 14.5). It extends for a few days, then heals, only to appear again in another area (Fig. 14.6). Sometimes the lesion is annular, with a slightly raised pale margin, and several of these areas may coalesce to form a scalloped pattern. Most patients have no symptoms but some adults complain of soreness. One possible reason is that the patient has become anxious that cancer is the cause and needs to be reassured. In others, soreness may be due to an underlying haematological deficiency state and the lesion is coincidental.

However, even children with geographical tongue sometimes complain that it is sufficiently hypersensitive to prevent them eating certain foods. The areas of epithelial thinning and inflammatory changes may therefore cause symptoms in some. Soreness in association with geographical tongue may also be psychogenic, and may then respond to appropriate treatment. Some evidence suggests a significant association between geographical tongue and emotional disturbance. However, there remains a group where no cause for the soreness can be found and no treatment seems to be effective.

Histologically, there is thinning of the epithelium in the centre of the lesion, with mild hyperplasia and hyperkeratosis at the periphery (Fig. 14.7); there are chronic inflammatory cells in the underlying connective tissue. Sometimes the changes are histologically the same as those of psoriasis.

Fig. 14.6   Erythema migrans. Two pictures of an affected tongue taken 6 days apart showing how the outline of patches changes with healing. Lesions heal completely and later new patches of depapillation appear elsewhere on the tongue.

Fig. 14.7 Erythema migrans. The edge of a lesion showing normal mucosa to the right, and to the left the epithelium densely infiltrated by neutrophils. This epithelium at the advancing edge will be shed, leaving the depapillated red patch.

Fig. 14.9 Black hairy tongue. In this patient there is only slight overgrowth of the papillae but dense black staining. In other cases the filiform papillae may be much elongated and hair-like. The posterior part of the tongue is the characteristic site.

Fig. 14.8 Lingual varices. The formation of varicosities in the vessels of the undersurface of tongue and floor of mouth is a common finding with age. Occasionally such varices may be the site of thrombosis.

THE FOLIATE PAPILLAE

The foliate papillae are bilateral, pinkish soft nodules on the lateral borders of the tongue at the junction of the anterior two-thirds and the posterior third (Ch. 2). They enclose lymphoid follicles which sometimes become hyperplastic or inflamed and sore (see Figs 1.1 and 1.2).

The appearance sometimes alarms patients, who need to be reassured that they are normal structures.

LINGUAL VARICOSITIES

Dilated tortuous veins may be seen along the ventral surface of the tongue and tend to become more prominent with age (Fig. 14.8). They may be noticed by patients, who need to be reassured that they are not abnormal.

Fig. 14.10 Hairy tongue. In this patient there are numerous elongated papillae but a brown rather than black pigmentation.

HAIRY TONGUE

The filiform papillae can become elongated and hair-like, forming a thick fur on the dorsum of the tongue. The filaments may be up to half a centimetre long and pale brown to black in colour (Figs 14.9 and 14.10). Adults are affected but the cause is unknown. Heavy smoking, excessive use of antiseptic mouthwashes and defective diet have been blamed, but their effect is questionable. The discolouration is probably caused by pigment-producing bacteria and fungi, but not *Candida albicans*.

Treatment is difficult. The measure most likely to succeed is to persuade the patient to scrape off the hyperplastic papillae and vigorously cleanse the dorsum of the tongue with a firm toothbrush. This removes large numbers of microorganisms mechanically and also, by removing the overgrown papillae, makes conditions less favourable for their proliferation.

Black tongue

The dorsum of the tongue may sometimes become black without overgrowth of the papillae. This may be staining due to drugs, such as iron compounds used for the treatment of anaemia, but is then transient. Occasionally the sucking of antiseptic lozenges causes the tongue to become black, and this may be due to pigment-producing organisms, particularly *Aspergillus* strains.

Furred tongue

The tongue can become coated with desquamating cells and debris in those who smoke heavily, in many systemic upsets, especially of the gastrointestinal tract, and in infections in which the mouth becomes dry and little food is taken. A furred tongue is often seen in the childhood fevers, especially scarlet fever.

MEDIAN RHOMBOID GLOSSITIS

Median rhomboid glossitis is an abnormality in the midline of the dorsum of the tongue at the junction of the anterior two thirds with the posterior third. The site suggests that it is developmental but it is not seen in children and it is no longer accepted that it results from persistence of the tuberculum impar.

Clinically, median rhomboid glossitis is seen in adults and is typically symptomless. It appears as a nodular red or pink area of depapillation (Fig. 14.12). Alternatively it may be white (Fig. 14.11).

Its chief importance is that the histological features have sometimes been mistaken for a carcinoma and it has been treated accordingly. Quite apart from the need for proper histological assessment, carcinoma virtually never develops in this site.

Histologically, the appearances are also variable and include irregular (pseudoepitheliomatous) hyperplasia with an inflammatory infiltrate, a granular cell tumour (Ch. 20) (Fig. 14.13) or candidosis (the white variant).

Management

Reassurance is usually the main requirement. Candidosis can be recognised by finding hyphae in a Gram-stained smear and

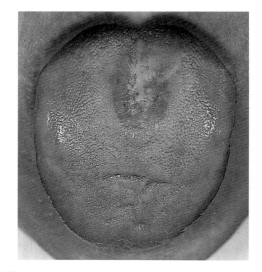

Fig. 14.11   Median rhomboid glossitis. There is a whitish patch of depapillation with sharply demarcated borders in the midline of the tongue.

Fig. 14.12   Median rhomboid glossitis. The typical lozenge-shaped area of depapillation in the midline of the tongue.

Fig. 14.14   Amyloidosis. There is macroglossia and multiple yellowish plaques and nodules along the lateral border of the tongue.

Fig. 14.13   Median rhomboid glossitis. There is hyperplasia with elongated rete processes, hyperparakeratosis and an inflammatory infiltrate of lymphocytes and plasma cells in the connective tissue. There are no signs of a typical candidal infection.

can be treated with an antifungal drug. However, a pink or lobulated abnormality will remain. Observation is required to detect any enlargement of the area but a need for biopsy is unlikely.

MACROGLOSSIA

Important causes are summarised in Table 14.4.

Table 14.4   **Important causes of macroglossia**

- Congenital haemangioma or lymphangioma (Ch. 20)
- Down's syndrome (Ch. 33)
- Cretinism (Ch. 31)
- Acromegaly (Ch. 31)
- Amyloidosis (Fig. 14.14 and Ch. 9)
- Lingual thyroid (Ch. 31)

SUGGESTED FURTHER READING

Dawson T A J, Pielou W D 1967 Geographic tongue in three generations. Br J Dermatol 79:668–671

Field E A, Speechley J A, Rugman F R 1995 Oral signs and symptoms in patients with undiagnosed vitamin B_{12} deficiency. J Oral Pathol Med 24:468–470

Kleinhauz I E M, Baht R, Littner M 1994 Antecedents of burning mouth syndrome (glossodynia) — recent life events vs psychopathologic events. J Dent Res 73:567–572

Morris L F, Phillips C M, Binnie W H et al 1992 Oral lesions in patients with psoriasis. Cutis 49:339–344

O'Connor N, Bunch C 1995 Laboratory diagnosis in haematology. Medicine Int 23:489–494

Pippard M J, Heppleston A D 1996 Microcytic and macrocytic anaemias. Medicine Int 24:4–10

Rojo L, Silvestre F J, Bagan J V, De Vincente T 1994 Prevalence and psychopathology in burning mouth syndrome. Oral Surg Oral Med Oral Pathol 78:312–316

Benign chronic white mucosal lesions

The appearance of mucosal white lesions is usually due to hyperkeratosis; any excess keratin, becoming sodden with saliva, appears white. Apart from the lingual filiform papillae, visible keratinisation of any significant degree is abnormal in the mouth.

Chronic mucosal white plaques have sometimes been termed *leukoplakias*. This term literally means no more than a white plaque but, in the past, was widely but mistakenly regarded as implying premalignancy. However, only a small minority of white patches are premalignant (Ch. 16). The majority without malignant potential are discussed here (Table 15.1).

Table 15.1 Important causes of benign mucosal white lesions

Prevalence	Lesion	Cause
Common	Leukoedema	Normal variation
	Frictional keratosis	Friction
	Cheek-biting	Cheek-biting
	Fordyce's granules	Developmental
	Stomatitis nicotina	Pipe smoking
	Thrush	Candidal infection
Uncommon	Chemical burns	Caustic chemicals
	Hairy leukoplakia	Epstein–Barr virus
	White sponge naevus	Genetic
	Chronic mucocutaneous candidosis	Candidal infection/ immunodeficiency
	Psoriasis	Uncertain
	Oral keratosis of renal failure	Uncertain
	Verruciform xanthoma	Uncertain
	Skin grafts	Iatrogenic

LEUKOEDEMA

Leukoedema is a bilateral, diffuse, translucent, greyish thickening, particularly of the buccal mucosa. It is a variation of normal, present in 90% of black, and variable numbers of white, people.

Histologically, there is thickening of the epithelium with intracellular oedema of the spinous layer.

Treatment is unnecessary but reassurance is sometimes required.

FRICTIONAL KERATOSIS AND CHEEK-BITING

White patches can be caused by prolonged mild abrasion of the mucous membrane by such irritants as a sharp tooth, cheek-biting or dentures.

Clinical features

At first, the patches are pale and translucent (Fig. 15.1), but later become dense and white, sometimes with a rough surface. Habitual cheek-biting causes an area of buccal mucosa to appear patchily red and white with a rough surface (Fig. 15.2).

Pathology

The epithelium is moderately hyperplastic, with a prominent granular cell layer and thick hyperkeratosis but no dysplasia (Fig. 15.3). There are often scattered chronic inflammatory cells in the corium.

Management

Removal of the irritant causes the patch quickly to disappear. Biopsy is necessary only if the patch persists. Frictional kerato-

Fig. 15.1 Frictional keratosis. A poorly-defined patch of keratosis on the buccal mucosa is due to friction from the sharp buccal cusp of a grossly carious upper molar.

Fig. 15.4 Fordyce's spots. Clusters of creamy, slightly elevated papules on the buccal mucosa.

Fig. 15.2 Cheek-biting. There is whitening of the buccal mucosa along a central band and a shredded surface.

Fig. 15.3 Frictional keratosis. There is a slight hyperplasia of the basal cells and a thick layer of orthokeratin at the surface.

Fig. 15.5 Fordyce's spots. Each spot is a histologically normal superficial sebaceous gland without a hair follicle.

sis is completely benign, and there is no evidence that continued minor trauma alone has any carcinogenic potential.

FORDYCE'S GRANULES

Sebaceous glands are present in the oral mucosa in at least 80% of adults. They grow in size with age and appear in the oral mucosa as soft, symmetrically distributed, creamy spots a few millimetres in diameter, particularly in older persons (Fig. 15.4). The buccal mucosa is the main site, but sometimes the lips, and rarely even the tongue, are involved.

These glands are sometimes mistaken for disease but patients

can be reassured that they are of no significance. If a biopsy is carried out it shows a normal sebaceous gland with two or three lobules (Fig. 15.5).

STOMATITIS NICOTINA (SMOKER'S KERATOSIS)

Smoker's keratosis is seen among heavy, long-term pipe smokers and some cigar smokers.

Clinical features

The appearances are distinctive in that the palate is affected, but any part protected by a denture is spared. Changes are then seen only on the soft palate.

The lesion has two components: hyperkeratosis and

Fig. 15.6 Stomatitis nicotina (smoker's palate). There is a generalised whitening with sparing of the gingival margin. The inflamed openings of the minor salivary glands form red spots on the white background.

Fig. 15.7 Stomatitis nicotina (smoker's palate). The epithelium is hyperplastic and hyperkeratotic, especially around the orifice of the duct where there is a concentration of inflammatory cells.

inflammatory swelling of minor mucous glands. Either may predominate but, typically, white thickening of the palatal mucosa is associated with small umbilicated swellings with red centres (Fig. 15.6). The white plaque is sometimes distinctly tessellated (pavement-like).

Microscopy

The white areas show hyperorthokeratosis and acanthosis with a variable inflammatory infiltrate beneath. The diagnostic feature is the swollen, inflamed mucous glands with hyperkeratosis extending up to the margins of the duct orifice (Fig. 15.7).

Management

The clinical appearances, history and ease of management are so distinctive that biopsy should not be necessary. If the patient can be persuaded to stop smoking the lesion resolves within weeks. Key features are summarised in Table 15.2.

Epidemiological evidence suggests that pipe smoking raises the risk of cancer, but when oral cancer develops in association with pipe smoking it typically appears, not in the keratotic area on the palate (one of the least common sites for cancer), but low down in the mouth, often in the lingual retromolar region. This may be the result of carcinogens pooling and having their maximal effect in drainage areas of the mouth. It also suggests that there are different causes for the hyperkeratosis and any carcinomatous change.

Table 15.2 Pipe smokers' keratosis ('stomatitis nicotina') — key features

- Affects mucosa exposed to smoke (mainly the hard palate)
- Areas protected by denture unaffected
- Palate is white (keratotic) with umbilicated swellings with red centres (inflamed mucous glands)
- Responds rapidly to abstinence from pipe smoking
- Statistically, a raised risk of oral cancer but *not* in the hyperkeratinised (palatal) area (Ch. 16)

THRUSH

Thrush (acute candidosis, Ch. 12) is readily distinguishable from other white lesions. The patches can easily be wiped off and Gram-stained smears show a mass of long hyphae.

In a young adult male, thrush in the absence of an obvious predisposing cause strongly suggests HIV infection.

HIV-ASSOCIATED HAIRY LEUKOPLAKIA

Patients with HIV infection may develop a clinically and histologically distinctive white lesion. Hairy leukoplakia is an important manifestation of HIV infection and, though not entirely unique to it, is otherwise exceedingly rare.

Clinical features

Hairy leukoplakia usually has a vertically corrugated or shaggy surface. The plaque is soft, usually painless and most frequently affects the lateral borders of the tongue (Fig. 15.8). Male homosexuals are predominantly affected.

Pathology

Hairy leukoplakia shows hyperkeratosis or parakeratosis or

Fig. 15.8   Hairy leukoplakia in a patient with early symptomatic HIV infection. The surface of the lesion is corrugated, accentuating the normal anatomy of the lateral border of the tongue.

Fig. 15.10   Hairy leukoplakia. Immunocytochemical staining for Epstein–Barr virus shows strong positivity in the prickle cells, indicating viral infection. Details of this technique are included in Chapter 1.

Fig. 15.9   Hairy leukoplakia. There is thickening of the epithelium and a thick superficial layer of parakeratin, below which the pale staining layer of 'koilocyte-like' cells lie. Because this patient is severely immunosuppressed there is no inflammatory reaction to the numerous candidal hyphae which are present in the surface layers of the epithelium.

both, with a ridged or shaggy surface or, rarely, hair-like extensions of keratin. Secondary invasion of the surface by candidal hyphae is relatively common but there is little or no inflammatory infiltration in the submucosa. More important is the presence of *koilocytes*, which are vacuolated and ballooned prickle cells with shrunken, dark (pyknotic) nuclei surrounded by a clear halo (Fig. 15.9).

Epstein–Barr virus (EBV) capsid antigen can be identified by in situ hybridisation in the epithelial cell nuclei (Fig. 15.10). Viral particles resembling EBV can be seen by electron microscopy. This finding appears to be unique to hairy leukoplakia, and the likelihood that EBV is the cause is suggested by reports that hairy leukoplakia responds to treatment with acyclovir or its analogues.

Management

Biopsy confirmation of the diagnosis is essential. In the

absence of symptoms, treatment of hairy leukoplakia is probably not justified, especially as it has a remittant course and can regress spontaneously. Hairy leukoplakia is not premalignant but it indicates advanced immunodeficiency, a more rapid progression to AIDS and a poor prognosis. Key features are summarised in Table 15.3.

Hairy leukoplakia in the absence of HIV infection

Hairy leukoplakia has rarely been seen in other immunodeficient, and even more rarely in immunocompetent, patients. In such patients it appears to resolve spontaneously.

Table 15.3   **Hairy leukoplakia — key features**

- Usually a sign of HIV infection in male homosexuals
- Typically forms soft, corrugated, painless plaques on lateral borders of tongue
- Diagnosis by biopsy
- Histologically, koilocytes in prickle cell layer are typical
- Epstein–Barr virus antigens detectable in epithelial cell nuclei by in situ hybridisation
- Indicates advanced immunodeficiency and poor prognosis but not premalignant
- May regress spontaneously and treatment not usually justified

WHITE SPONGE NAEVUS

White sponge naevus is a developmental anomaly inherited as an autosomal dominant trait.

Clinical features

The appearance is distinctive. The affected mucosa is white, soft and irregularly thickened (Fig. 15.11). The abnormality is usually bilateral and sometimes involves the whole oral

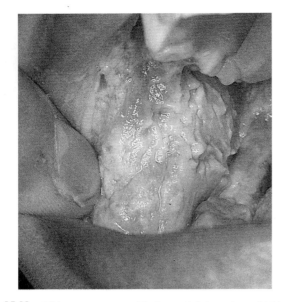

Fig. 15.11   White sponge naevus. The keratosis is irregular and folded and extends into areas which are not subject to friction.

Fig. 15.12   White sponge naevus. The epithelium is acanthotic and the prickle cell layer is composed of large vacuolated cells.

mucosa. There are no defined borders and the edges fade imperceptibly into normal tissue. The anus and vagina can also be affected.

Pathology

The epithelium is hyperplastic, with uniform acanthosis, and the rete ridges have a smooth lower border. Shaggy hyperparakeratosis and intracellular oedema with abnormally prominent cell membranes produce a so-called basket-weave appearance (Fig. 15.12). There is no dysplasia and inflammatory cells in the corium are typically absent.

Management

The appearance is readily recognised, particularly when there is widespread mucosal involvement. A positive family history is virtually confirmatory. If there is any doubt, biopsy confirms the diagnosis. The main requirement is to reassure the patient of the benign nature of the condition.

Key features are summarised in Table 15.4.

Table 15.4   White sponge naevus — key features
● Genetic. Autosomal dominant trait
● Shaggy whitish thickening can involve entire oral mucosa
● White areas lack sharp borders
● Histologically, epithelial hyperplasia with basket-weave appearance
● No dysplasia or inflammation
● No treatment other than reassurance

CHRONIC MUCOCUTANEOUS CANDIDOSIS SYNDROMES

These syndromes are all rare, but difficult to manage. There are four main types (Table 15.5).

Table 15.5   Types of Chronic mucocutaneous candidosis syndrome
● Familial (limited) type
● Diffuse type (*Candida* 'granuloma')
● Endocrine candidosis syndrome
● Late-onset (thymoma syndrome)

Chronic mucocutaneous candidosis (CMCC) is sometimes classed as an immunodeficiency disease but an immune defect cannot always be found. In others cases it is limited to failure to respond to *Candida albicans* or secondary to persistent antigenic stimulation. However, there are more profound defects in the diffuse and late-onset types, while the endocrine candidosis syndrome is part of an autoimmune disease.

Familial (limited) mucocutaneous candidosis

Inheritance is usually as an autosomal recessive trait. The onset is in infancy with persistent thrush in childhood. Later the oral lesions become indistinguishable from those of sporadic cases of chronic hyperplastic candidosis (Figs 15.13 and 15.14).

Fig. 15.13 Chronic mucocutaneous candidosis. There are extensive red and white patches affecting much of the oral mucosa and severe angular cheilitis.

Fig. 15.14 Chronic mucocutaneous candidosis in a child. The tough leukoplakia-like lesions affect the buccal mucosa and the tongue on both sides. This was one of several affected siblings.

There may be mild cutaneous involvement and sideropenia is characteristically associated.

Diffuse type mucocutaneous candidosis

Most cases are sporadic. This is the most severe type and was earlier termed 'monilial granuloma' because of the extensive, warty and often disfiguring overgrowths on the skin. Nevertheless, there is no granuloma formation microscopically. Instead, the lesions are produced by epithelial proliferation and an extreme expression of the same process that produces oral epithelial plaques in response to candidal invasion.

These patients are usually also abnormally susceptible to bacterial diseases, particularly pulmonary and superficial suppurative infections.

Endocrine candidosis syndrome

In this variant, chronic mucocutaneous candidosis is associated with multiple glandular deficiencies and organ-specific autoantibody production. Nevertheless, there is no direct cause-and-effect relationship between the candidosis and the endocrine deficiency. Candidal infection can precede the onset of endocrine deficiency by as long as 15 years but occasionally this sequence is reversed. Treatment of the candidosis does not affect the endocrine deficiency, and vice versa.

Endocrine candidosis syndrome is a manifestation of type I chronic polyendocrinopathy. Addison's disease and hypoparathyroidism are most frequently associated, and other glandular deficiencies can develop, but candidosis is sometimes so mild as to pass unnoticed. Hypoplastic dental defects are frequently also present.

Adrenal failure was the main risk to life in candida-endocrinopathy syndrome but is usually now treated effectively.

Late-onset mucocutaneous candidosis

This syndrome has a clear immunological basis, in that there is a persistent defect of cell-mediated immunity produced by a thymoma. In the full syndrome, myasthenia gravis and pure red cell aplasia are associated. Death from the thymoma or red cell aplasia is the main hazard.

Management of mucocutaneous candidosis syndromes

Microscopic confirmation of chronic candidosis is required (Fig. 15.15 and Ch. 16), but precise categorisation of these

Fig. 15.15 Chronic hyperplastic candidosis. At high power the thick parakeratin layer at the surface of this lesion is seen to be invaded by numerous fungal hyphae.

syndromes may have to await development of other features, such as endocrine deficiency or elucidation of a relevant family history.

Immunological investigation, apart from detection of autoantibodies to glandular tissues in the endocrine candidosis syndrome, is not generally helpful, though detection of impaired or absent cell-mediated immunity to *C. albicans* strongly suggests that the patient has a mucocutaneous candidosis syndrome rather than limited oral hyperplastic candidosis.

The principles of management are therefore to treat the candidal infection with antifungal drugs such as itraconazole and to deal with associated disorders as appropriate. Antibacterial chemotherapy is necessary in diffuse-type chronic mucocutaneous candidosis, and endocrine replacement is essential in endocrine candidosis.

Unlike 'idiopathic' chronic hyperplastic candidosis, chronic mucocutaneous candidosis appears to have little potential for malignant change. Key features are summarised in Table 15.6.

Table 15.6 Chronic mucocutaneous candidosis syndromes — key features

- Onset typically in infancy as persistent thrush
- Gradual transformation into leukoplakia-like lesions
- Ungual and/or mild cutaneous candidosis sometimes associated
- Immune deficiency sometimes present
- Pulmonary and superficial suppurative infections associated in *diffuse CMCC* with gross candidal epithelial proliferation
- In *endocrine candidosis syndrome*, early-onset hypoparathyroidism and/or Addison's disease associated but oral candidosis frequently mild
- In *late-onset CMCC*, thymoma causes defective cell-mediated immunity. Myasthenia gravis and pure red cell aplasia may be associated

---

PSORIASIS

Psoriasis is a common skin disease estimated to affect 2% of the population. Oral psoriatic plaques appear to be very rare but there may be an association between erythema migrans of the tongue (geographical tongue) or other mucosae and cutaneous psoriasis.

The diagnosis should only be considered when there is cutaneous psoriasis. The appearance of the oral lesions varies from translucent plaques to that of erythema migrans. Lesions may be asymptomatic.

Diagnosis is confirmed by biopsy but the histological appearances of psoriasis and erythema migrans (Ch. 14) are sometimes very similar.

ORAL KERATOSIS OF RENAL FAILURE

Leukoplakia-like oral lesions are an occasional and unexplained complication of long-standing renal failure.

Clinically, the plaques are soft, have a crenated surface and are typically symmetrically distributed.

Pathology

The features may not be sufficiently distinctive to allow diagnosis without knowledge of the underlying disease. There is irregular acanthosis with mild atypia of the epithelial cells and moderate parakeratosis. The appearances are somewhat similar to those of hairy leukoplakia. Biopsy is useful also to exclude adherent bacterial plaques, which may develop in patients with renal failure.

Fig. 15.16 Verruciform xanthoma. The epithelium is thin and parakeratotic and forms a series of spiky folds.

Fig. 15.17 Verruciform xanthoma. At higher power dermal papillae within the folded epithelium can be seen to contain many large rounded cells with foamy or vacuolated cytoplasm.

Fig. 15.18 Skin graft. A skin graft placed on the right posterior hard palate appears as a scar-like, pale patch. Hair follicles occasionally survive transplantation to the mouth as has happened here.

Fig. 15.19 Skin graft. This graft placed on the anterior dorsum of the tongue has contracted to produce an irregular margin and surface and might be mistaken for leukoplakia.

Effective dialysis or renal transplantation cause resolution of the lesion. No local treatment is necessary or likely to be effective.

VERRUCIFORM XANTHOMA

Verruciform xanthoma is a rare proliferative lesion which can have a white, hyperkeratotic surface.

Clinically, verruciform xanthoma is most common in the fifth to seventh decades. It is usually found on the gingiva but can form in almost any site in the mouth. It can be white or red in colour, be sessile or pedunculated, have a warty surface, and range in size from one to several centimetres across. It may be mistaken for a papilloma, leukoplakia or carcinoma clinically, but is readily recognisable histologically. Verruciform xanthoma is benign and has no known associations with diseases such as hyperlipidaemia or diabetes mellitus associated with cutaneous xanthoma formation.

Pathology

The warty surface is due to the much infolded epithelium which, in white variants, is hyperkeratinised, but may be parakeratinised. In H & E stained sections, the parakeratin layer stains a distinctive orange colour. The elongated rete ridges are uniformly elongated and extend to a straight, well-defined lower border (Fig. 15.16).

The diagnostic feature is the large, foamy xanthoma cells which fill the connective tissue papillae but extend only to the

lower border of the lesion (Fig. 15.17). These cells contain lipid and PAS-positive granules.

Simple surgical excision is curative.

SKIN GRAFTS

A skin graft may be placed in the mouth to cover a raw area left after excision of (for example) a chronic white lesion.

Skin grafts typically appear sharply demarcated, smooth and paler than the surrounding mucosa (Fig. 15.18). However, grafts on the dorsum of the tongue may become corrugated and less easy to differentiate from a recurrence of leukoplakia (Fig. 15.19).

SUGGESTED FURTHER READING

Cawson R A, Binnie W H, Eveson J W 1995 Color atlas of oral disease, 2nd edn. Mosby-Wolfe, London

Cawson R A, Langdon J D, Eveson J W 1996 Surgical pathology of the mouth and jaws. Wright, Oxford

Eisenberg E, Krutchkoff D, Yamase H 1992 Incidental oral hairy leukoplakia in immunocompetent persons. A report of two cases. Oral Surg Oral Med Oral Pathol 74:332–333

Epstein J B, Fatahzadeh M, Matisic J, Anderson G 1995 Exfoliative cytology and electron microscopy in the diagnosis of hairy leukoplakia. Oral Surg Oral Med Oral Pathol 79:564–569

Higgs J M, Wells R S 1974 Classification of chronic muco-cutaneous candidosis. Clinical data and therapy. Hautartz 25:159–165

Ravina A, Ficarra C, Chiodo M et al 1996 Relationship of circulating CD4[+] T-lymphocytes and p24 antigenemia to the risk of developing AIDS in HIV-infected subjects with hairy leukoplakia. J Oral Pathol Med 25:108–111

Oral premalignancy

Various oral mucosal lesions, particularly red lesions ('erythroplasias') and white lesions ('leukoplakias') have a potential for malignant change (Table 16.1). In some of them, such as chronic hyperplastic candidosis, the risk may be very low. By contrast, the risk with erythroplasia is exceedingly high.

In general, the most common white lesions have the lowest risk of malignant transformation. Practitioners will see many oral white lesions, but few carcinomas. However, they must be able to recognise lesions at particular risk and several features help to assess the likelihood of malignant transformation. The accuracy of such predictions is low, but the process of identifying 'at risk' lesions is fundamental to diagnosis and treatment planning. Important factors are listed in Table 16.2 and information on each of these should be sought.

The best predictor of the potential for malignant transformation is the degree of dysplasia seen histologically. For this reason, and because some lesions will already be malignant, biopsy of red and white patches is mandatory. The term *dysplasia* (literally, *abnormal growth*) is given to the cytological abnormalities seen in both malignant and premalignant cells (Table 16.3). Premalignancy is distinguished from malignancy only by the latter's invasiveness and production of metastases.

It must be emphasised that the implications of *epithelial* dysplasia are quite different from *fibrous* dysplasia, in which there is no risk of carcinomatous change.

Nuclei stain more densely due to heavier nucleic acid content. They are variable in size, out of proportion to that of the cell, so that there may be little surrounding cytoplasm. Mitoses may be frequent and at superficial levels. Loss of polarity refers to the fact that basal cells in particular may lie higgledy-piggledy at angles to one another. Deep cell keratinisation (*dyskeratosis*) refers to individual cells which start to keratinise before the surface is reached and show eosinophilic change deeply within the epithelium. As differentiation is lost, organisation of the individual cell layers deteriorates and clearly defined basal and spinous cell layers cannot be identified. Drop-shaped rete ridges are regarded as a particularly adverse feature. With loss of intercellular adherence, the cells become separated.

Table 16.1 Lesions with potential for malignant change

Lesion/condition	Aetiology	Risk of malignant change*	Prevalence in the UK
Dysplastic leukoplakia	Unknown	High, but can regress	Uncommon
Erythroplasia	Idiopathic/smoking	Very high	Rare
Speckled leukoplakia	Idiopathic/smoking	High	Rare
Tertiary syphilis	*Treponema pallidum*	Very high	No longer seen
Oral submucous fibrosis	'Betel' chewing	High	Uncommon
Dyskeratosis congenita	Genetic	High	Rare
Pipe smokers' keratoses	Pipe smoking	Low and not in the keratotic area	Becoming uncommon
Snuff-dippers' keratoses	Smokeless tobacco	Low	Uncommon
Chronic candidosis	*Candida albicans*	Low	Uncommon
Lichen planus	Idiopathic	Low	Common
Discoid lupus erythematosus	Autoimmune	Unclear (mainly lip)	Uncommon

*Risks of malignant change are difficult to determine accurately and vary with many factors. If more than 25% of lesions become malignant in 5 years this is considered an exceptionally high risk. Malignant change in 2–3% of lesions in 10 years is considered a relatively low risk. Note that the highest risk lesions are uncommon. Common lesions appear in between 1% and 5% of the population.

Table 16.2 Risk factors for malignant change in white lesions

● History	Betel quid usage
	Tobacco smoking or snuff dipping*
	High alcohol intake
	Family history of oral carcinoma
● Clinical features	Advanced age
	Female gender†
	Areas of reddening in the lesion
	Areas of speckling in the lesion
	Nodular areas or ulceration
	High-risk site — posterolateral tongue
	— floor of mouth
	— retromolar region
	— anterior pillar of fauces
	Large lesions
	Lesions present for long periods
	Enlargement or change in character of pre-existing lesion
● Special investigations	Degree of dysplasia on biopsy

*Nevertheless surveys indicate that the risk of malignant change in white lesions is higher in *non-smokers*.
†Surveys indicate that malignant change in white lesions is more frequent in women.

Table 16.3 Epithelial dysplasia — histological features

- Drop-shaped rete ridges
- Nuclear hyperchromatism
- Nuclear pleomorphism and altered nuclear:cytoplasmic ratio
- Excess mitotic activity
- Loss of polarity of cells
- Deep cell keratinisation
- Disordered or loss of differentiation
- Loss of intercellular adherence

A lymphoplasmacytic infiltrate of highly variable intensity is usually present in the corium.

Dysplasia is usually graded as mild, moderate and severe as a guide to patient management (Figs 16.1–16.4). *Carcinoma in situ* is a controversial term sometimes used for the most severe dysplasia where the abnormalities extend throughout the thickness of the epithelium; a state sometimes graphically called 'top-to-bottom change'. In such a lesion all the cellular abnormalities characteristic of malignancy may be present; only invasion is absent. The significance of this grading is discussed below, but the histological assessment of oral epithelial dysplasia is notoriously unreliable because it is subjective and changes are not reliably correlated with behaviour.

PREMALIGNANT LESIONS AND CONDITIONS

Premalignant lesions are those lesions in which carcinoma may

Fig. 16.1 Mild dysplasia. In this lesion there is a thin layer of parakeratin and the structure, maturation and orderly differentiation of the epithelial cells is largely unaffected. However, there is a degree of irregularity of basal cells with variation in size and hyperchromatism. A mitosis is present in the prickle cell layer.

Fig. 16.2 Mild dysplasia. In this lesion there is prominent orthokeratosis and a keratohyaline layer immediately below it. Dysplasia is more prominent than in the previous figure, with enlarged hyperchromatic and bizarre cells in the basal and lower prickle cell layers.

develop. Premalignant conditions are associated with a risk of carcinoma at some site within the mouth, not necessarily marked by a pre-existing lesion.

Fig. 16.3 Moderate dysplasia. The dermal papillae extend close to the surface and there are elongated rete processes, some of which are broader deeply. Enlarged and hyperchromatic cells are visible at this low power in rete processes and in most of the prickle cell layer.

Fig. 16.4 Severe dysplasia. This rete process is composed almost entirely of cells with dark and irregularly shaped nuclei. Only the most superficial layers of cells show maturation to squamous cells and the orderly maturation and differentiation of epithelial cells has been lost.

ERYTHROPLASIA ('ERYTHROPLAKIA')

Erythroplasias are red patches. The surface is frequently velvety in texture and the margin may be sharply defined. Lesions of this type typically do not form plaques (hence the term 'erythroplakia' is inappropriate) but, instead, they are flat or depressed below the level of the surrounding mucosa (Fig. 16.5). Erythroplasia is uncommon in the mouth but carries the highest risk of malignant transformation and lesions are often already malignant on first biopsy.

Fig. 16.5 Erythroplasia. This slightly depressed, well-defined red patch on the dorsolateral tongue showed squamous carcinoma on biopsy.

Fig. 16.6 Speckled leukoplakia. A poorly-defined speckled leukoplakia on the cheek of an elderly female. Carcinoma was present at the first biopsy.

Pathology

Erythroplastic lesions usually show epithelial dysplasia, which may be severe. In other cases, there may be micro- or frankly invasive carcinoma. The epithelium is atrophic and this, together with inflammation, accounts for the red colour seen clinically.

SPECKLED LEUKOPLAKIA

This term applies to lesions consisting of white flecks or fine nodules on an atrophic erythematous base (Figs 16.6 and 16.7). They can be regarded as a combination of or transition between leukoplakia and erythroplasia. Speckled leukoplakia also more

Fig. 16.7 Premalignant lesion in a betel quid chewer. The classical appearance of a speckled leukoplakia such as this is almost always associated with either severe dysplasia or invasive carcinoma. Note also the brown betel quid staining on the teeth.

Fig. 16.8 Homogeneous leukoplakia. There is a bright, white, sharply-defined patch extending from the gingiva on to the labial mucosa. The surface has a slightly rippled appearance and no red areas are associated.

frequently shows dysplasia than lesions with a homogeneous surface. The histological characteristics are usually, therefore, intermediate between leukoplakia and erythroplasia.

Many cases of chronic candidosis have this appearance.

HOMOGENEOUS LEUKOPLAKIA

A leukoplakia is defined as a white patch which cannot be wiped off the mucosa or ascribed to any specific disease process. Although the term is often used loosely for any white patch, it should be reserved for idiopathic lesions. If investigations fail to reveal any cause, the term may be appropriate.

The most extensive follow-up studies on white patches suggest that idiopathic leukoplakia now has the highest risk of developing cancer, especially now that late stage syphilis forms a negligibly small group. Nevertheless, the malignant transformation rate of leukoplakia is relatively low, around 1–2% in 5 years, and even in smokers the vast majority of leukoplakias show no dysplasia histologically and carry no risk of malignant transformation.

Clinical features

Idiopathic leukoplakias and dysplastic lesions do not have any specific clinical appearance, but are tough and adherent and typically form plaques whose surface is slightly raised above the surrounding mucosa. The surface is usually irregular. Small and innocent-looking white patches are as likely to show epithelial dysplasia as large and irregular ones (Figs 16.8 and 16.9). However, lesions with red, nodular or verrucous areas (Fig. 16.10) should be regarded with particular suspicion. The most common sites are the posterior buccal mucosa, retromolar region, floor of mouth and the tongue.

Fig. 16.9 An innocent-looking, poorly-defined inconspicuous white patch which showed dysplasia on biopsy. Despite excision, malignant transformation followed several months later.

Pathology

The histopathology is highly variable but there is always parakeratosis or orthokeratosis, or both in different areas, and the two may alternate along the length of the specimen. The keratin gives the lesion its white appearance. The epithelium ranges from thinner than normal (atrophic) to much thicker (acanthotic) (see Figs 16.1 and 16.2).

Most leukoplakias show no dysplasia histologically. A minority display a range of dysplasia from mild to severe and treatment is planned partly on this basis. An inflammatory reaction of lymphocytes and plasma cells induced by the abnormal dysplastic cells is often present in the underlying connective tissue.

Fig. 16.10 White patch with dysplasia. This postcommissural lesion is poorly defined and comprises both red and white areas. Lesions at this site are frequently due to candidosis.

Fig. 16.11 Sublingual keratosis. This white patch involving the entire ventral tongue and floor of mouth has a uniformly wrinkled appearance. No red areas are associated but the site alone indicates a high risk of malignant transformation.

SUBLINGUAL KERATOSIS

The term sublingual keratosis is applied to white lesions on the floor of the mouth and ventral tongue. Whether this lesion is a different entity from other leukoplakias is unclear. Malignant change was reported in an unusually high proportion of cases (30%) in one series but this has not been widely confirmed. Probably the risk of malignant transformation is less than 10%, and possibly much lower.

Clinical features

Sublingual keratosis is a white, soft plaque, usually with a finely wrinkled surface, an irregular but well-defined outline, and sometimes bilateral with a butterfly shape. The plaque typically extends from the anterior floor of the mouth to the undersurface of the tongue (Figs 16.11 and 16.12). There is usually no associated inflammation.

Pathology

Sublingual keratosis is not distinctive histologically and the appearances are those described above for leukoplakia.

PIPE SMOKERS' KERATOSIS

As noted earlier (Ch. 15), palatal keratosis due to pipe smoking

Fig. 16.12 Sublingual keratosis. This more irregular white patch is associated with some reddening in the floor of the mouth.

is benign. Any carcinomas related to pipe smoking appear in another site in the mouth and may not be preceded by keratosis.

SMOKELESS TOBACCO-RELATED KERATOSES

Hyperkeratotic mucosal lesions can result from smoking or use of smokeless tobacco ('topical tobacco' — snuff dipping and tobacco chewing). By contrast, there is no characteristic hyperkeratotic lesion associated with the far more common habit of cigarette smoking.

Tobacco chewing and snuff dipping (holding flavoured

tobacco powder in an oral sulcus) are popular habits in the USA and some parts of Europe. Loose oral snuff appears to cause more severe changes than tobacco chewing but not all topical tobacco habits are associated with a risk of malignant change. The use of Scandinavian-type snuff sachets appears to carry no risk and it is important to ascertain exactly what type of tobacco is used and how it is prepared. Many smokeless tobacco users also smoke and, regardless of this, all lesions in the mouths of tobacco users should be regarded with suspicion.

Clinical features

The habit of snuff dipping or tobacco chewing may be maintained for decades and gives rise to keratoses in the buccal or labial sulcus, where the tobacco is held. Early changes are erythema and mild, whitish thickening. Long-term use gives rise to extensive white thickening and wrinkling of the buccal mucosa. Malignant change can follow, but only after several decades of use. A high proportion of carcinomas in snuff users are verrucous in type (Ch. 17), but if they remain untreated invasive squamous carcinoma may develop.

Pathology

The main changes are thickening of the epithelium with plump or squared-off rete ridges. There are varying degrees of hyperorthokeratosis or parakeratosis and there may be subepithelial fibrosis in the area where the tobacco is held. Dysplasia may eventually be seen.

Management

Diagnosis is based on the history of snuff use and the white lesion in the area where the tobacco is held. Biopsy is required to exclude dysplasia or early malignant change.

Snuff-dippers' lesions will resolve on stopping the habit, even after 25 years of use. This therefore is the main measure. If this fails, regular follow-up and biopsies are required.

CHRONIC HYPERPLASTIC CANDIDOSIS (CANDIDAL LEUKOPLAKIA)

Chronic oral candidosis produces a tough adherent plaque, distinguishable only by biopsy from other leukoplakias.

Clinical features

Adults, typically males of middle age or over, are affected. The usual sites are the dorsum of the tongue and the postcommissural buccal mucosa. The plaque is variable in thickness and often rough or irregular in texture, or nodular with an erythematous background (speckled). Angular stomatitis may be associated, is sometimes continuous with intraoral plaques and

Fig. 16.13 Chronic hyperplastic candidosis. This white localised patch and its associated erythema are the result of candidal infection alone and no dysplasia was present despite the sinister clinical appearance.

Fig. 16.14 Chronic hyperplastic candidosis. The typical site is the postcommissural buccal mucosa. This florid example is white and slightly nodular.

suggests the candidal nature of the lesion (Figs 16.13 and 16.14).

Pathology

Unlike thrush, the plaque cannot be wiped off, but fragments can be detached by firm scraping. Gram- or PAS-staining then shows candidal hyphae embedded in clumps of detached epithelial cells.

Like thrush, the plaque of chronic candidosis is parakeratotic, but more coherent because it is not widely infiltrated by inflammatory exudate. In H & E stained sections, hyphae are difficult to see as faint tracks through the epithelium. PAS stain clearly shows the hyphae growing (as in thrush) through the full thickness of the keratin to the prickle cell layer, where the inflammatory cells tend to be more concentrated.

Electron microscopy shows *Candida albicans* to be an intracellular parasite growing within the epithelial cytoplasm (Fig. 16.15). The hyphae, therefore, grow in relatively straight lines and do not follow a tortuous path along the intercellular spaces.

Fig. 16.15 Two candidal hyphae growing through superficial keratinocytes of the oral mucosa.

Induction of epithelial proliferation by *C. albicans* infection has been demonstrated experimentally, and in candidal plaques there is often rete hyperplasia with rounded downgrowths and acanthosis. Dysplasia may be present, especially in speckled lesions.

The chronic inflammatory infiltrate in the corium is variable and a fibrinous inflammatory exudate may be seen at the basement membrane.

Management

After confirmation of the diagnosis by histology, treatment should be with a systemic antifungal drug such as fluconazole, but this may have to be continued for several months. Other factors likely to perpetuate candidal infection should be controlled. Stopping the patient from smoking and elimination of candidal infection from under an upper denture are important. Any iron deficiency should also be treated.

Excision of candidal plaque alone is of little value, as the infection can recur in the same site even after skin grafting. Vigorous antifungal therapy is therefore essential, but sometimes some residual (uninfected) plaque may persist after treatment and lesions often recur and require long-term intermittent antifungal therapy.

The potential for malignant change exists. The level of risk is controversial but low.

ORAL SUBMUCOUS FIBROSIS

In oral submucous fibrosis (Ch. 11) affected areas of the oral mucosa such as the palate or buccal mucosa appear almost white. The pallor is due to the underlying fibrosis and ischaemia rather than a superficial plaque, and the mucosa is typically smooth, thin and atrophic (see Figs 11.1 and 11.2).

However, erythroplasia and leukoplakia may be associated (see Fig. 16.7) and the epithelium may show dysplasia on biopsy.

Surveys suggest that oral submucous fibrosis undergoes malignant transformation in 4.5–7.6% of cases and may contribute to the high incidence of oral cancer in the Indian subcontinent and in Asian immigrant populations in other countries. Submucous fibrosis is probably premalignant because of its association with betel quid chewing.

LICHEN PLANUS

As noted in Chapter 13, it is estimated that 1–4% of patients develop carcinomas after 10 years. Specific types of lesion and other risk factors have not been firmly identified but plaque-type and erosive lichen planus in unusual sites, such as the fauces and tongue, should be regarded with particular suspicion.

In view of the great frequency of lichen planus, its importance as a precursor of malignant change may be considerable. Lichen planus of the skin appears to carry no risk of malignant change.

LUPUS ERYTHEMATOSUS

Lupus erythematosus is an uncommon connective tissue disease (Chs 12 and 25). There is a small risk of malignant change in cutaneous lupus, especially in lesions of the lower lip.

DYSKERATOSIS CONGENITA

Dyskeratosis congenita is a rare heritable recessive or dominant trait. The main features are dysplastic white or red lesions of the oral mucosa, cutaneous pigmentation, dystrophies of the nails and haematological abnormalities. Many patients may also be immunodeficient or have other abnormalities.

Causes of death include cancers of the mouth or other sites, and bleeding (gastrointestinal or cerebral), but in 50% of cases from infections, which are frequently opportunistic.

SYPHILITIC LEUKOPLAKIA

Leukoplakia of the dorsum of the tongue is a characteristic complication of tertiary syphilis but is of little more than historical interest.

Clinical features

Syphilitic leukoplakia has no distinctive features, but typically affects the dorsum of the tongue and spares the margins. The

Fig. 16.16 Syphilitic leukoplakia. Carcinoma has developed in a patch of leukoplakia on the tongue of a patient who had had tertiary syphilis for many years.

lesion has an irregular outline and surface. Cracks, small erosions or nodules may prove on histology to be foci of invasive carcinoma (Fig. 16.16). Carcinoma developing near the centre of the dorsum of the tongue is typically a sequel to syphilitic leukoplakia and, as a consequence of the great decline in late-stage syphilis, is exceedingly rare in this site now.

Pathology

In addition to hyperkeratosis and acanthosis, often with dysplasia, the characteristic late syphilitic chronic inflammatory changes, with plasma cells predominating, may be seen. Giant cells and, rarely, granulomas may be present. Endarteritis of small arteries is particularly characteristic. However, distinctive features of a syphilitic tissue reaction may be lacking.

Behaviour and management

The diagnosis is confirmed mainly by the serological findings. However, even if positive, biopsy is still essential, as minute areas of malignant change may be found and the management is affected accordingly. In particular, the presence of syphilitic endarteritis may be a contraindication to radiotherapy.

Antibiotic treatment of syphilis does not cure the leukoplakia, which persists and can undergo malignant change even after serology has become negative.

EARLY CARCINOMA

Occasionally an early carcinoma produces surface keratin and appears as a white patch. It should not be interpreted as malignant change in a leukoplakia.

MANAGEMENT OF DYSPLASTIC LESIONS

As noted in Chapter 17, the prognosis in oral carcinoma is good only when the diagnosis is made early and the tumour is small. Accurate assessment of the risk of malignant change in red and white patches is therefore very important, but is an ideal, not an objective reality. The level of risk cannot be reliably assessed from the histopathology alone and the clinical features listed in Table 16.2 should be used to help gauge the risk for an individual lesion.

The best predictor of malignant potential is the presence of dysplasia on biopsy. However, even this is rather poorly correlated with behaviour, for reasons such as inadequate sampling at biopsy and variability of assessment.

In the most extensive study based on no fewer than 782 cases of histologically unspecified oral white lesions followed for an average of 12 years, 2.4% underwent malignant change in 10 years and fewer than 5% after 20 years. However, even this low rate represents a risk of malignant change 50–100 times that in the normal mouth. It was also conspicuous that, in this and in other studies, the rate of malignant change in oral leukoplakias has been up to *10 times higher in non-smokers than in smokers* and more frequent in women. Other, smaller, series have suggested rates of malignant change of 30% or more in unspecified types of white lesions, though in many cases no time-scale has been indicated, and the wide variation in the rate of malignant change in these different series suggests that the findings have been significantly affected by selection of cases.

It must be emphasised that these large follow-up studies have been on oral keratoses which had not been histologically assessed. Because of the rarity of dysplastic oral lesions, there are very few studies, and none on a large scale, that have followed their progress for adequate periods. In a study of 45 patients with oral dysplastic lesions, followed for up to 8 years, 11% underwent malignant change in this period and up to 30% of them regressed or even ultimately disappeared spontaneously.

The principles of the management of dysplastic lesions are summarised in Table 16.4. The management of dysplastic oral lesions remains controversial, as their relative rarity has made it impossible as yet to accumulate enough data to make reliable predictions or evaluate treatment. It has to be assumed that dysplasia represents an early stage in the development of

Table 16.4 **Principles of management of dysplastic lesions**

- Stop any associated habits, e.g. betel quid or smoking
- Treat candidal infection and/or iron deficiency if present
- Biopsy to assess dysplasia
- Assess risk of premalignant change on clinical and histological findings
- Consider ablation of individual lesions (Table 16.5)
- Maintain observation for signs of malignant change

carcinoma and provides an opportunity to treat carcinoma at an exceptionally early, and potentially curative, preinvasive stage.

Unfortunately, these assumptions are not well supported by clinical evidence. Lesions which are excised appear more likely to become frankly malignant, though this may reflect selection of the highest risk cases for surgery. If lesions are of manageable size, it is tempting to excise them — this can presumably do no harm, but it is essentially a treatment of hope rather than certainty. An alternative approach is to observe the lesions for signs of deterioration, in the hope of detecting carcinoma as early as possible. Once carcinoma develops, the treatment options are much more clear-cut.

A dysplastic lesion is associated with a higher risk of developing lesions elsewhere in the mouth and of developing more than one oral carcinoma. This process is sometimes described as 'field change', to convey the idea that large areas of the oral epithelium may be premalignant. Regular examination of the whole mouth is therefore essential.

Some dysplastic lesions regress spontaneously, and published surveys suggest that dysplastic lesions may regress as frequently as they undergo malignant change. However, disappearance of a white lesion does not necessarily indicate resolution of dysplasia, and continued observation may still be indicated. Photographs or video records of lesions are an invaluable aid to long-term observation of lesions and should be used for high-risk lesions.

In practice, an attempt is usually made to remove lesions with moderate or severe dysplasia or high-risk clinical features (Table 16.5). Surgical excision is the most common approach. It provides an excision biopsy specimen which can be examined for the extent of the dysplasia and for possible carcinoma. Unfortunately, lesions in the highest risk areas in the posterior floor of mouth are technically difficult to excise and large lesions may require grafting.

Table 16.5 **Options for management of premalignant lesions**

- Observation for early detection of carcinoma
- Surgical excision with grafting, if required
- Cryotherapy
- Laser excision or vaporisation
- Topical chemotherapy
- Retinoids

The effectiveness of other treatments has not yet been assessed on any adequate scale.

After cryotherapy ablation the area heals rapidly to leave an apparently normal mucosa. However, there is some uncertainty about the risk of invasive carcinomas subsequently arising in these sites. Carbon dioxide laser ablation has also been advocated, but the same objections may apply. Topical chemotherapeutic agents, such as bleomycin, have also been used experimentally. Treatment with systemic or topical retinoids has also been tried. Topical retinoids are largely ineffective and, though a proportion of white lesions resolve with systemic treatment, toxic effects are usually unacceptable. Further, lesions which resolve with treatment recur on withdrawal of the drugs.

With all such treatments the lesion is not available for histoloical examination and multiple biopsy before treatment is required to ensure that malignant change is not already present. This option may be of value in those for whom surgery is not practical because of, for instance, unfitness for anaesthesia.

In summary, frequent clinical observation, preferably with photographic records, and immediate biopsy of any areas that are suspicious or change in appearance is generally the best option. Selected lesions with clinical features of high risk or severe dysplasia on biopsy are probably best excised.

SUGGESTED FURTHER READING

Abbey L M, Kaugars G E, Gunsolley J C et al 1995 Interexaminer and intraexaminer reliability in the diagnosis of oral epithelial dysplasia. Oral Surg Oral Med Oral Pathol Oral Radiol Endod 80:188–191

Barnard N A, Scully C, Eveson J W et al 1993 Oral cancer development in patients with oral lichen planus. Oral Pathol Med 22:421–424

Borle R M, Borle S R 1991 Management of oral submucous fibrosis: a conservative approach. J Oral Maxillofac Surg 49:788–791

Cawson R A 1966 Chronic oral candidiasis and leukoplakia. Oral Surg Oral Med Oral Pathol 22:582–591

Cawson R A 1973 Induction of epithelial hyperplasia by *Candida albicans*. Br J Dermatol 89:497–503

Cawson R A, Binnie W H 1980 Candida leukoplakia and carcinoma: a possible relationship. In: Mackenzie I C, Dabelsteen E, Squier C A (eds) Oral premalignancy. Proceedings of the first Dow symposium. University of Iowa, pp 59–66

Cawson R A, Rajasingham K C 1972 Ultrastructural features of the invasive phase of *Candida albicans*. Br J Dermatol 87:435–443

Cawson R A, Binnie W H, Eveson J W 1994 Color atlas of oral disease, 2nd edn. Mosby-Wolfe, London

Cawson R A, Langdon J D, Eveson J W 1996 Surgical pathology of the mouth and jaws. Wright, Oxford

Daniels T E, Hansen L S, Greenspan J S et al 1992 Histopathology of smokeless tobacco lesions in professional baseball players. Associations with different types of tobacco. Oral Surg Oral Med Oral Pathol 73:720–725

Davidson H R, Connor J M 1988 Dykeratosis congenita. J Med Genet 25:843–846

Einhorn J, Wersall J 1967 Incidence of oral carcinoma in patients with leukoplakia of the oral mucosa. Cancer 20:2184–2193

Eveson J W 1983 Oral premalignancy. Cancer Surv 2:403–424

Higgs J M, Wells R S 1974 Classification of chronic muco-cutaneous candidosis. Clinical data and therapy. Hautartz 25:159–165

Kaugars G E, Silverman S, Lovas J G L et al 1996 Use of antioxidant supplements in the treatment of human oral leukoplakia. Review of the literature and current studies. Oral Surg Oral Med Oral Pathol Oral Radiol Endod 81:5–14

Kramer I R H, El-Labban N, Lee K W 1978 The clinical features and risk of malignant transformation in sublingual keratosis. Br Dent J 144:171–176

Larrson A, Axéll T, Andersson G 1991 Reversibility of snuff dippers' lesion in Swedish moist snuff users: a clinical and histologic study. J Oral Pathol Med 20:258–264

Mincer H H, Coleman S A, Hopkins K P 1972 Observations on the clinical characteristics of oral lesions showing histologic epithelial dysplasia. Oral Surg 33:389–399

Murti P R, Bhonsle R B, Pindborg J J, Daftary D K, Gupta P C, Mehta F S 1985 Malignant transformation rate in oral submucous fibrosis over a 17-year period. Community Dent Oral Epidemiol 13:340–341

Murti P R, Daftary D K, Bhonsle R B, Gupta P C, Meahta F S, Pindborg J J 1986 Malignant potential of oral lichen planus: observations in 722 patients from India. J Oral Pathol 15:71–77

Pillai R, Balaram P, Reddiar K S 1992 Pathogenesis of oral submucous fibrosis. Relationship to risk factors associated with oral cancer. Cancer 69:2011–2020

Pindborg J J, Roed-Petersen B, Renstrup G 1972 Role of smoking in floor of the mouth leukoplakias. J Oral Pathol 1:22–27

Silverman S, Bhargava R, Mani N J, Smith L W, Malaowalla A M 1976 Malignant transformation and natural history of oral leukoplakia in 57 518 industrial workers in Gujerat, India. Cancer 38:1790–1795

Silverman S, Gorsky M, Lozada F 1984 Oral leukoplakia and malignant transformation. A follow-up study of 257 patients. Cancer 53:563–568

Voute A B E, de Jong W F B, Schulten E A J M, Snow G B, van der Waal I 1992 Possible premalignant character of oral lichen planus; the Amsterdam experience. J Oral Pathol Med 21:326–329

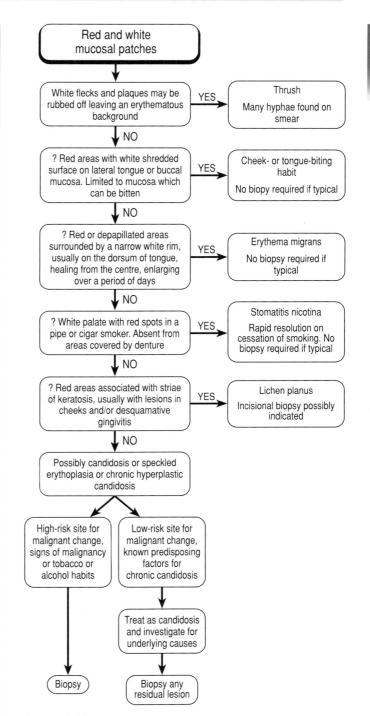

Summary 16.1 Differential diagnosis and management of the common causes of red and white patches of the oral mucosa.

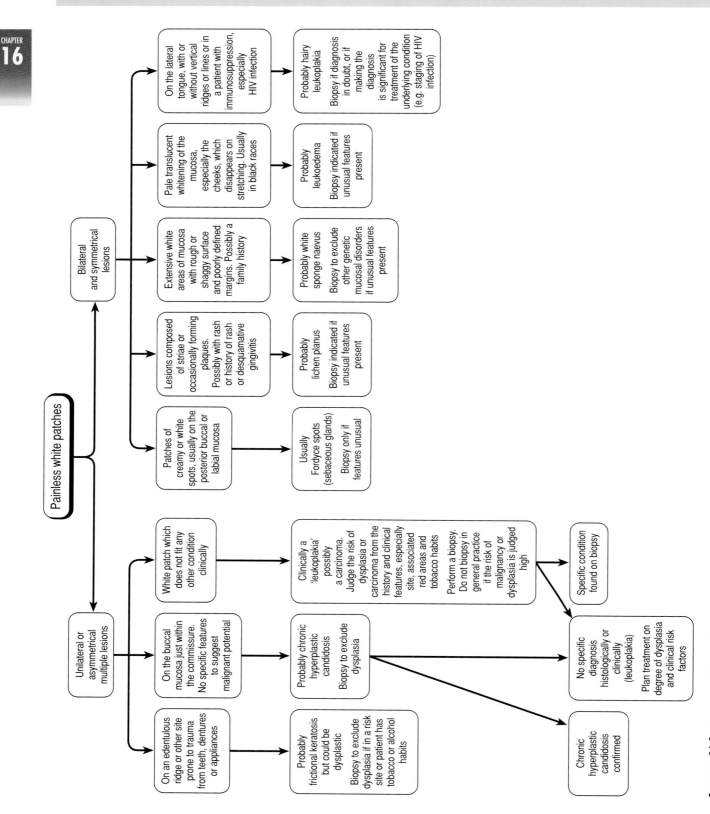

Summary 16.2 Summary of the key features of the common and important oral white patches.

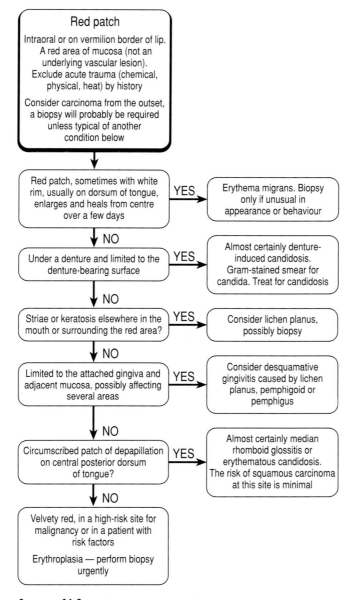

Summary 16.3 Differential diagnosis of common and important red patches affecting the oral mucosa.

Oral cancer

Over 90% of malignant neoplasms (cancers) of the mouth are squamous cell carcinomas arising from mucosal surface epithelium. Most of the remainder are adenocarcinomas of minor salivary glands; only a few are undifferentiated or metastases.

Epidemiology

Oral carcinoma accounts for only about 2% of all malignant tumours in such countries as the UK and the USA. In most countries where data are available, the incidence of cancer of the mouth, though variable, is low. India and Sri Lanka are, however, exceptional, and cancer of the mouth accounts for approximately 40% or more of all cancer there, though the incidence varies widely in different parts of this subcontinent.

Approximately 2000 cases of intraoral and lip carcinoma are registered each year in the UK. For most of this century the incidence of oral cancer has declined, but it appears to be rising again and, though it is rare, cases are now more frequently seen in those aged 30–50.

Age and sex incidence

Oral cancer is an age-related disease, and 98% of patients are over the age of 40. While the overall incidence in the population is only about 1 in 20 000, this rises to 1 in 1100 in males of 75 and over. There is a sharp and virtually linear increase in incidence of mouth cancer with age, as with carcinoma in many other sites.

Cancer of the mouth is considerably more common in men than women in most countries, and carcinoma of the lip is at least eight times as common in men as in women in Britain. Intraoral cancer used to be several times more frequent in men than women, but the male to female ratio is overall about 3:2, and in south-east England recent figures show little difference in incidence between the sexes. The change is the result of the progressive decline in oral cancer in men in former years, but a low, static rate in women.

The incidence of oral cancer rises steeply with age and, with an ageing population, oral cancer will become more common.

Aetiology

It has not been possible to prove conclusively a causative association between specific aetiological factors and oral cancer. This is partly because the quality of cancer statistics is very variable and partly because the aetiology of malignancy is complex and multifactorial. Causative factors operate over a long period and the process of malignant change is so slow that there is a prolonged lag period before disease appears. This has been shown strikingly in Japan, where cancers were still developing half a century after the radiation exposure from atomic bombs.

Significant or speculative risk factors for oral squamous cell carcinoma are summarised in Table 17.1.

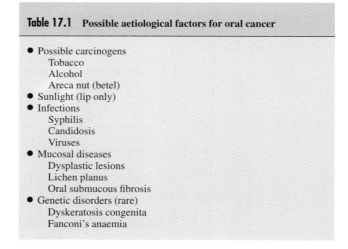

Table 17.1 **Possible aetiological factors for oral cancer**

- Possible carcinogens
    Tobacco
    Alcohol
    Areca nut (betel)
- Sunlight (lip only)
- Infections
    Syphilis
    Candidosis
    Viruses
- Mucosal diseases
    Dysplastic lesions
    Lichen planus
    Oral submucous fibrosis
- Genetic disorders (rare)
    Dyskeratosis congenita
    Fanconi's anaemia

Tobacco use

The effects of tobacco on the mouth depend on the way it is used, and this varies in different countries. In Westernised countries, cigarette smoking predominates and pipe smoking has declined. In some countries, notably in India, the southern states of the USA, and Sweden, tobacco chewing or snuff dipping (unsmoked tobacco held in the mouth for prolonged periods) is a habit. Methods of processing tobacco before use also vary widely, so that its products, released into the mouth, differ considerably in their effect. This is particularly noticeable in India where, in some areas, the use of a particular type of tobacco appears to be associated with a very high incidence of cancer.

Cigarette smoking

Smoking is considered to be a major aetiological factor, particularly in association with alcohol, and its importance is that it is preventable. However, it is difficult to demonstrate a direct causal link between cigarette smoking and oral cancer. Epidemiological studies have shown that oral cancer in males steadily *declined* over a period of more than three-quarters of a century while cigarette consumption grew steadily. However, the incidence of oral cancer in males appears to be rising again, despite the fact that males are now smoking less.

Equally difficult to explain is the fact that mouth cancer in women has remained at a steady low level despite their widespread adoption of cigarette smoking. The escalation of their cigarette consumption is shown by the fact that the lung cancer rate in women has risen to nearly equal that of men in the USA.

Also puzzling is that, unlike pipe smoking or smokeless tobacco use, there is no specific oral lesion related to cigarette smoking.

Nevertheless, many studies have closely linked smoking, particularly in association with alcohol, to oral carcinoma. In case–control studies which take account of the amount and duration of tobacco consumption, the specific site, and other factors such as alcohol, cigarette smoking has been shown to be closely associated and carry a significant relative risk. The risk of developing a second primary carcinoma is also closely linked to smoking and alcohol. Smoking cigarettes occasionally appears to carry a very low risk, whereas the risk rises dramatically in heavy smokers.

Pipe smoking

Epidemiological evidence has associated oral cancer with pipe smoking but the habit has steadily declined in most Westernised countries and has never become popular with women. Pipe smokers are also likely to develop stomatitis nicotina of the palate (Ch. 15), a white patch with no premalignant potential.

Smokeless tobacco

In the southern USA, snuff dipping and tobacco chewing, in which either dry snuff or a plug of chewing tobacco (often with various other ingredients) is held in the lower buccal sulcus for prolonged periods, is well established. These habits cause extensive hyperkeratotic plaques and, after decades of continuous use, may lead to verrucous carcinoma (see below) as well as squamous carcinoma.

Tobacco is frequently included in betel quid (see below) and it is significant that in these habits carcinomas tend to arise at the site in the mouth where the tobacco is habitually held.

Nevertheless, the greatest consumption of smokeless tobacco is in Sweden, where there is no evidence of related oral cancer development.

Alcohol

Alcohol consumption has steadily risen in Britain, particularly in the past half-century when oral cancer was declining. However, as noted earlier, the incidence may now be rising. In some countries, such as Denmark, there is good epidemiological evidence to link alcohol intake with oral carcinoma and in the Bas Rhin of France, alcohol is held to be responsible for the highest oropharyngeal cancer incidence in Europe.

It is generally considered that the combination of smoking and drinking is the most important aetiological factor for mouth cancer and, as noted above, many oral cancer patients smoke and drink heavily. The low incidence of mouth cancer among Mormons and Seventh Day Adventists, who neither drink nor smoke, supports this idea. The relative risks for alcohol and tobacco consumption are shown in Figure 17.1

Alcoholic drinks are not usually allowed to reside in the mouth for long periods, and there is no specific alcohol-related oral lesion. The mechanism by which alcoholic drinks might

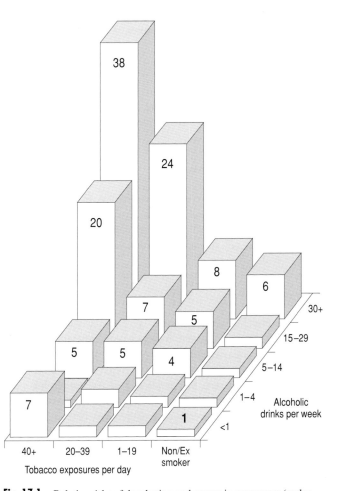

Fig. 17.1 Relative risks of developing oral cancer in consumers (males in a western population) of tobacco and alcohol. The relative risk for a non-smoker and non-alcohol consumer is taken as 1. A smoker consuming 30 cigarettes a day and 20 alcoholic drinks a week is seven times more likely to develop carcinoma.

cause carcinomas is unclear and may not be their ethanol content. Drinks with the highest content of congeners, such as raw home-brewed spirits, appear to have the closest association with carcinoma. By contrast, evidence from the USA suggests that beer drinking is associated with a greater risk. It is also possible that alcohol might predispose to carcinoma through its action on the liver, and some studies have found a correlation between mouth cancer and cirrhosis. As with smoking, the total consumption is probably a critical factor.

Concern over the possible carcinogenic effects of alcohol has led to a proposal that it should be banned from mouthwashes, some of which contain more than 25% alcohol. There is as yet no strong link between mouthwash use and oral carcinoma.

Viruses

Human papilloma virus DNA, particularly type 16, has been found in oral cancers. Papilloma viruses are closely associated with cervical cancer but the association with oral carcinoma remains speculative and the virus may also be found in apparently normal epithelium and papillomas. Human papilloma viruses may induce p53 gene mutation, of which there is a high frequency in oral cancer.

Syphilis

Syphilitic leukoplakia, developing in late-stage disease, has a high malignant potential but is no longer a significant risk factor (Ch. 16).

Chronic candidosis

Chronic candidosis can lead to formation of hyperkeratotic plaques or speckled leukoplakias with epithelial dysplasia. There have been isolated reports of malignant change in such lesions, but, overall, this accounts for a very small proportion of cases (Ch. 16).

Malnutrition

There is a high incidence of mouth as well as oesophageal cancer in Paterson–Kelly syndrome, in which iron deficiency is a feature. However, this disease is no longer a significant risk factor.

Epidemiologically, a low vitamin A intake has been associated with oral carcinoma but deficiency of β-carotene has now been dismissed as a contributing factor. In India, malnutrition is widespread and may contribute, together with betel quid chewing, to the high incidence. However, there appears to be no comparably high frequency of mouth cancer in other areas, such as many parts of Africa, where malnutrition is at least as severe.

Oral sepsis

Oral sepsis has traditionally been regarded as contributing to

mouth cancer. The latter is most common in low socioeconomic groups, which tend to have the most neglected mouths. Oral cancer also progressively declined in frequency in Britain, where a slow but steady improvement in oral health is well documented.

Despite such considerations the aetiological role of oral sepsis in mouth cancer remains unproven.

Betel (pan) chewing

Use of a quid of areca nut, lime, tobacco and spices wrapped in betel leaf is a widespread habit in the Indian subcontinent and among immigrant Asian populations in the UK. The quid is held in the sulcus. Areca nut releases arecolin which, experimentally, is carcinogenic, while the tobacco contains numerous carcinogens. In South-east Asia, the quid frequently consists of areca nut with flavouring agents, but no betel leaf, and is also associated with a high cancer incidence. White patches may develop where the quid is held and these have a high risk of malignant change. Betel or areca nut chewing may also cause oral submucous fibrosis (Ch. 11), which also appears to be premalignant. The trismus resulting from submucous fibrosis also makes diagnosis and treatment of oral carcinoma very difficult. Betel quid chewing should be vigorously discouraged by dentists.

Sunlight

Exposure to the ultraviolet component of sunlight is a risk factor, with the result that lip cancer is predominantly a disease of outdoor workers, particularly farmers and fishermen. As with other skin cancers, fair-skinned persons are at most risk. There may be multiple lesions in the most severely affected.

The relationship between exposure to sunlight and lip cancer has been clearly shown in hot countries, such as Australia and the USA, with large immigrant, fair-skinned populations of European origin. In the USA, for example, the risk of lip cancer approximately doubles for every 250 miles nearer the equator the site of residence is.

Dysplastic lesions caused by sunlight may precede the carcinoma, and the sun-damaged lip may be identified clinically by its loss of elasticity and atrophic epithelium. Damage due to sunlight is preventable and dentists should encourage the wearing of a high factor sun-block during exposure to strong sunlight.

Genetic factors

There are a few genetic disorders, notably dyskeratosis congenita (Ch. 16), of which oral cancer is a frequent feature, but such disorders are rare. Mice with a high susceptibility to oral cancer have also been bred. However, there is no other convincing evidence of any genetic trait predisposing to oral cancer in humans.

Precancerous lesions

Several premalignant lesions are recognised (Ch. 16). In general, the risk of malignant transformation in the more common white lesions is very low, but it is not known what proportion of carcinomas arise in recognisable premalignant lesions.

Key features of oral cancer are summarised in Table 17.2.

Table 17.2   Cancer of the mouth — key features
• Account for approximately 2% of all cancers in the UK but one of the most common cancers in the Indian subcontinent • Males more frequently affected • Most patients are over 40 and incidence rises rapidly with age • Lower lip is the most common site and related to actinic damage • Tongue, posterolaterally, is the most common site within the mouth • Some arise in pre-existing white or red lesions • Heavy tobacco smoking and alcohol consumption tend to be associated • In India and South-east Asia, betel or areca nut chewing may be more important

Sites of oral cancer

The lower lip is the most frequent site of oral cancer overall, while the tongue is the most frequently affected site *within* the mouth. In the oral cavity, the majority of cancers are concentrated in the lower part of the mouth, particularly the lateral borders of the tongue, the adjacent floor of the mouth and lingual aspect of the alveolar margin, forming a U-shaped area extending back towards the oropharynx (Fig. 17.2). This accounts for only about 20% of the whole area of the interior of the oral cavity, but 70% of oral cancers are concentrated there.

This distribution may possibly be due to carcinogens pooling and concentrating in the lower mouth before swallowing. For the same reason, the hard palate and central dorsum of tongue are very rarely affected.

Early squamous cell carcinoma

In their earliest stages carcinomas appear as painless red, speckled (Fig. 17.3) or white patches (Fig. 17.4), and only a minority are ulcerated. As noted in Chapter 16, a high proportion of erythroplasias and speckled leukoplakias are already malignant on first biopsy. The similar appearances of early carcinoma and premalignant lesions result from the processes of keratinisation and epithelial atrophy and do not necessarily indicate that the carcinoma has arisen in a pre-existing lesion.

As a carcinoma enlarges it may develop into a raised nodule or become ulcerated. Induration results from inflammation and

Fig. 17.3   Squamous carcinoma of the soft palate and mucosa posterior to the tuberosity appearing as a speckled leukoplakia.

Fig. 17.2   High-risk sites for development of oral carcinoma. The shaded U-shaped area accounts for only about 20% of the whole area of the interior of the mouth but is the site of over 70% of oral cancers.

Fig. 17.4   Early squamous carcinoma. Despite its inconspicuous appearance this small white patch on the lateral border of the tongue was found to be a squamous carcinoma on biopsy.

Fig. 17.5 Advanced squamous carcinoma. The classical ulcer with a rolled border and central necrosis is a late presentation. Note the surrounding areas of keratosis and erythema which had been present for many years before the carcinoma developed.

Fig. 17.6 Squamous carcinoma of lip. There is an indurated, crusted ulcer with keratosis at one margin in the centre of the lower lip.

fibrosis and infiltration of the tissues. By the time a carcinoma has formed an indurated ulcer with the typical rolled border, it will have been present for some time (Fig. 17.5). As noted below, diagnosis at this late stage is associated with a very poor prognosis and every attempt must be made to identify carcinomas as early as possible.

Ulceration may cause soreness, or stinging pain when sharply flavoured food is eaten. Pain is of no value in the diagnosis of carcinoma, but is typically severe in the late stages. Bleeding, either spontaneously or from mild trauma, is also a late feature.

Carcinoma of the lip

The lip is the most common single site for oral cancer but this is infrequently seen in dental practice. Being visible, it is often recognised at a very early stage and so has a better prognosis than intraoral cancer. The usual site is the vermilion border of the lower lip to one side of the midline. Men of middle age or over are predominantly affected.

An area of thickening, induration, crusting or shallow ulceration of the lip, less than a quarter of an inch (6 mm) in diameter, is a common early presentation (Fig. 17.6). Advanced, neglected tumours (Fig. 17.7) are unlikely to be seen now. Spread to lymph nodes tends to be slow. The submental nodes are usually the first to be affected.

Carcinoma of the tongue and floor of mouth

The anterior part of the tongue, particularly the lateral border, and the adjacent ventral tongue and floor of mouth are frequently involved, and presentation is often late, with an ulcer 2 cm or more in diameter. Approximately 60% or more patients with localised lesions less than 2 cm in diameter survive for 5 or

Fig. 17.7 Advanced carcinoma of lip. There is extensive ulceration and necrosis and distortion as a result of scarring. Nowadays such extensive lesions are unusual.

more years after treatment. In more advanced disease the usual picture is of a typical malignant ulcer several centimetres in diameter, hard in consistency, with rolled or irregular, raised edges and a rough infected floor which bleeds readily. As growth proceeds the carcinoma becomes fixed to surrounding tissues and infiltrates the tongue, which becomes progressively stiffer and more painful. Eating, swallowing and talking become difficult. By this time pain is usually the main symptom and may radiate widely. The lymph nodes also become involved.

Affected lymph nodes are enlarged and hard, the surface becomes irregular and they become fixed to deeper tissues and skin. The growth has spread beyond the tongue when the majority of patients are first seen. In these circumstances the prognosis is poor. Only one patient in six survives for 5 years or longer. In the late stages, local spread of the growth causes gross destruction of adjacent parts with widespread sloughing. The tongue becomes fixed; pain is severe and persistent; swallowing and speech are difficult. Affected lymph nodes may ulcerate through the skin. The combination of pain, infection and difficulty in eating causes loss of weight, anaemia and deterioration of general health. This state (malignant cachexia) is ultimately fatal. In other patients aspiration of septic material from the mouth causes bronchopneumonia, and, in a few, haemorrhage from the growth is the cause of death.

A small, but possibly growing, proportion of patients survive treatment of the primary growth but die later from distant metastases.

Carcinoma of the alveolar ridge, cheek and palate

These show essentially the same features as carcinoma elsewhere. Carcinoma of the buccal mucosa is particularly associated with betel quid chewing. Carcinoma of the alveolar ridge and palate are more likely to erode bone at an earlier stage, making treatment more complex.

Pathology

The essential feature of carcinoma is the invasion of surrounding tissues by the malignant epithelial cells. The invading cells grow into the tissues, forming irregular branching processes, the tips of which are often cut off in a section to give the appearance of separate islands of tumour (Fig. 17.8). In the more infiltrative, higher grade carcinomas, single cells and small clusters of cells detach along the invasive front of the lesion. Tumour cells invade deeper tissues, regardless of their nature. Muscle, fat, nerves and eventually bone are infiltrated and destroyed (Fig. 17.9). Invading cancer cells excite an inflammatory reaction and become surrounded by lymphocytes and plasma cells.

The individual cells show the features of malignancy. Large and irregularly-shaped nuclei, darkly-stained nuclei (hyperchromatism), frequent and sometimes abnormal mitoses and loss of the well-ordered architecture of epithelium are seen (Fig. 17.10). These are essentially the same changes as are seen in dysplastic epithelium (Ch. 16).

Squamous carcinoma is graded according to its degree of differentiation, that is the degree to which the malignant cells differentiate to form prickle cells and keratin. In well-differentiated tumours, the cells have cytoplasm which stains palely with eosin or may form concentric layers of keratin (cell nests) or keratin pearls (fig. 17.11). In poorly-differentiated tumours the

Fig. 17.8 A small squamous carcinoma. At low power the epithelium is seen to invade deeply into the connective tissue and underlying muscle. At this early stage there is no ulceration.

Fig. 17.9 Squamous carcinoma. Higher power showing strands of malignant epithelium invading the connective tissue.

cells tend to be more plemorphic and darkly staining, and show less evidence of a squamous pattern. In the most poorly-differentiated carcinomas, the cells have little cytoplasm and may not be recognisable as epithelial cells by routine microscopy (Fig. 17.12). Poorly-differentiated carcinomas tend to infiltrate more widely at an early stage, are more likely to metastasise and carry a poorer prognosis.

Spread of oral carcinoma

Carcinoma invades adjacent tissue by direct extension. Bone initially forms a barrier but is eventually destroyed, usually by superficial erosion, but once the cortex is breached carcinoma may invade laterally along the medullary cavity.

Fig. 17.10 Squamous carcinoma. At high power a group of tumour cells shows typical cytologic irregularity. Surrounding and beneath the tumour, muscle fibres are being destroyed.

Fig. 17.11 Squamous carcinoma. In this moderately well-differentiated tumour many of the neoplastic epithelial cells are forming keratin pearls.

Fig. 17.12 Squamous carcinoma. In this poorly-differentiated carcinoma there is little or no keratin formation and the malignant cells show great pleomorphism with variably-sized nuclei, many of which are hyperchromatic, and frequent mitotic figures.

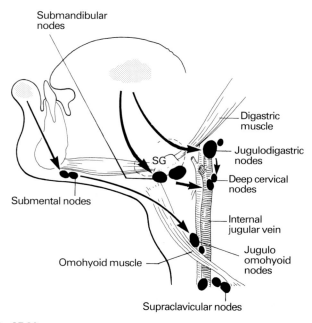

Fig. 17.13 Typical routes of lymphatic spread from lip and intra-oral squamous carcinomas.

Metastatic spread is primarily via the lymphatics to the regional lymph nodes. The specific sites of metastasis depend on the drainage of the tumour site but, because most carcinomas arise posteriorly in the lower mouth, the submandibular and jugulodigastric nodes are most frequently involved. Lymphatic drainage from the tip of the tongue is to the submental nodes and then to the jugulo-omohyoid group, low down in the neck. From the dorsum and sides of the tongue, drainage is to the submandibular nodes and then to the jugulodigastric group (Fig. 17.13). Lip and floor of mouth carcinomas may spread bilaterally. Spread of cancer may be by an abnormal route, and all the lymph nodes of both sides of the neck must be examined.

Oral cancer spreads progressively down the jugular lymphatic chain and it is unusual for it to involve supraclavicular lymph nodes until a late stage. Perineural infiltration and vascular invasion are less common (Fig. 17.14 and 17.15).

Metastatic carcinoma is initially limited to the affected node but, in time, spreads through the capsule into the tissues of the neck. Excision is then difficult and the chances of survival are diminished. This extracapsular spread is evident clinically as fixation of the node. Metastatic carcinoma forms a solid mass when small, but in larger masses the central areas become necrotic and may break down so that the metastasis becomes cystic and fluctuant clinically.

Fig. 17.14 Squamous carcinoma. In this carcinoma malignant epithelium is invading around nerve sheaths. Although this is infrequent, occasionally carcinoma may spread some distance from the main tumour mass along nerve trunks.

Fig. 17.15 Squamous carcinoma. Less frequent than perineural invasion is vascular invasion. Here a cluster of poorly-differentiated malignant epithelial cells have eroded the wall of the vessel and entered the circulation.

Bloodstream spread is an uncommon, late feature of the disease. Key features are summarised in Table 17.3.

Management of oral carcinoma is complex and depends on the age and medical condition of the usually elderly patient, as well as its exact site, degree of spread (stage) and histological type. An appropriate treatment protocol must be selected for each individual case, taking these features into account.

Treatment may be by surgery or radiotherapy and either may be used for cure or palliation. In practice, most intraoral carcinomas are treated by surgery combined with radiotherapy ('multimodality therapy'). Surgery alone is preferred for small carcinomas of the tongue which may be easily excised, for those involving bone because of the risk of later radionecrosis, and for verrucous carcinoma.

Actual and potential dental infection in the mouth must be dealt with before starting treatment, particularly if this is to be by irradiation. Dental infection or extractions may lead to extensive osteomyelitis in irradiated bone because of its poor

Table 17.3 Oral cancer — clinicopathological features and behaviour

- Early cancers appear as white or red patches or shallow ulcers and are painless
- Later carcinomas appear as ulcers with prominent rolled edges and induration and become painful
- Over 70% or oral cancers form on the lateral borders of the tongue and adjacent alveolar ridge and floor of mouth
- Over 95% are well- or moderately well-differentiated squamous cell carcinomas
- Spread is by direct invasion of surrounding tissues and by lymphatic metastasis
- The submandibular and jugulodigastric nodes are most frequently involved
- The prognosis deteriorates sharply with local spread and nodal involvement

vascularity: it is very resistant to treatment. The sockets should be healed, as nearly as possible, before radiotherapy is begun. In practice, teeth with extensive caries, or periapical lesions for which rapid succesful treatment cannot be guaranteed, are usually extracted because of the need to start treatment quickly.

Treatment by irradiation provides a more acceptable cosmetic and functional result than major surgery but involves considerable discomfort during a long course of treatment and has unwanted effects in the long term (Table 17.4).

Radiotherapy is carried out by implantation of radioactive material into and around the neoplasm (brachytherapy), or by exposure to beams of X-rays or γ-rays from X-ray generators or radioactive isotopes such as cobalt (teletherapy). Ionising radiation damages normal as well as neoplastic tissue, so that treatment planning is critical. The lesion is accurately localised by imaging techniques and a dose, usually in the region of 60 Gy for oral lesions, is given. Damage to surrounding tissues is limited by fractionating the dose over many visits (perhaps 30 daily fractions) and by applying external beams from many angles, but avoiding radiosensitive tissues such as the eye and bone. For teletherapy, a mask is made to fit the patient's head to allow reproducible beam angulation between visits. Radiotherapy planning and mask construction are complex and involve a short delay before treatment can start.

Table 17.4 Unwanted effects of radiotherapy to the oral region

● During treatment	Severe xerostomia
	Mucositis and ulceration
	Acute candidosis
	Skin erythema
● Long term	Xerostomia
	Mucosal and skin atrophy
	Risk of osteomyelitis (osteoradionecrosis)
	Scarring and fibrosis of tissues
	Cataract if eye irradiated (e.g. in antral carcinoma)
	Risk of late radiation-induced malignancy

Surgery is mainly indicated when cancer has invaded bone or when there has been a poor response to, or recurrence after, irradiation. The aim is to excise the carcinoma with as wide a margin as possible, ideally 1 cm or more. Modern surgical methods allow excision, reconstruction, grafting or bypassing of almost any structure in the oral regions. However, a margin of more than a few millimetres is rarely achieved in practice, because the carcinoma may be too extensive and its margin may be difficult to identify at operation. Also, wider excision may make reconstruction difficult. Such a small margin is insufficient to guarantee removal of the carcinoma, which may recur at the original site.

Reconstructive surgery is normally performed at the same operation as excision, to provide a better cosmetic and functional result.

Recurrence after treatment may be at the primary site or in lymph nodes. Primary site recurrence usually signifies a poor prognosis because either a full course of radiotherapy or as large an excision as practical will already have been performed. Recurrence in lymph nodes usually appears within 2 years after treatment. The metastases probably arise from microscopic deposits of carcinoma already in the lymph nodes at the time of initial therapy (occult metastases). They may be treated surgically by block dissection or by radiotherapy and do not necessarily indicate failure of treatment. Block dissection of clinically normal cervical lymph nodes is sometimes performed to remove occult metastases, but is a controversial procedure.

A recent approach to treatment is photodynamic therapy. In principle, a light-sensitising drug is administered and localises to the tumour site. Exposure of the tumour to light of an appropriate wavelength triggers a photochemical reaction which should kill the cancer cells. One problem is to find a drug which has a sufficiently selective effect and the method overall requires long-term assessment of its value.

Palliative treatment is given to patients who have advanced tumours or for treatment failures. Radiotherapy is the most practical method for palliative care but surgery is occasionally used when a large tumour compromises the airway or becomes grossly necrotic. Chemotherapy is little used in the UK, being reserved for widespread metastases or salvage therapy. It causes serious complications and may not improve survival.

Survival from oral cancer

Duration of survival after treatment depends on many factors (Table 17.5). In comparison with malignant neoplasms at other body sites, oral carcinoma has a poor prognosis. The quality of life in the terminal stages is also poor. The poorer survival of older people is probably because they are less able to withstand radiotherapy or surgery. The reason for the poorer survival rates for males is uncertain, although later presentation seems likely. Tumour stage at the start of treatment depends both on its growth rate and on delay in diagnosis. Some small (early) carcinomas are fast-growing and aggressive, but large tumours, even if slow-growing, are more difficult to manage. In either case

Table 17.5 Some factors adversely affecting survival from oral cancer

- Delay in treatment
- Advanced age
- Male gender
- Tumour size
- Posterior location
- Lack of histological differentiation
- Lymph node spread

delay in treatment allows further tumour spread and lessens chances of long survival.

The highest mortality from oral cancer is in the first 2 years; the disease then continues to claim victims but at a slower rate, and those few that survive for 10 years have a reasonable chance of having been cured. As a guide as to survival rates, nearly 90% of males with early-stage disease survive the first years, about 65% survive for up to 5 years, while just under 55% survive for 10 years. Of males with late-stage disease, well under 45% survive the first year, about 16% survive for 5 years, and 12% survive for 10 years.

As to the site of the growth, the extremes are seen in cancer of the lip, where the 5-year survival rate for males is over 77%. For cancer of the tongue it is 26%, and in the mesopharynx it is only 17.6%. Tumours, particularly of the posterior third of the tongue, are not readily detectable and more difficult to excise. In general therefore the more posterior the tumour is, the poorer the survival.

Role of the dentist

Early diagnosis is critical if patients are to be cured. Small carcinomas are more easily excised, less likely to have metastasised and have the best prognosis. Unfortunately, most carcinomas present at a relatively late, incurable stage and health care workers, including dentists, have frequently either failed to make the diagnosis or have actively delayed referral.

Dentists must be alert to the possibility of carcinoma, even though they may encounter it only once or twice in a practising lifetime. The nature of a chronic ulcer, white or red lesion, or swelling of the mucous membrane *must* be confirmed by biopsy. Indecision about taking a biopsy or trying the effect of local measures or antibiotics can prove fatal.

The dental practitioner is likely to see more patients with white mucosal patches. As noted in Chapter 15, the vast majority of such lesions are benign and may be biopsied in a practice setting. However, it is inadvisable to perform a biopsy of a high-risk lesion (for instance, an erythroplasia or speckled leukoplakia) because the practitioner may be forced into the unenviable position of having to tell the patient that they have cancer, a task for which most dentists are not trained.

Any high-risk premalignant lesion or suspected carcinoma should be referred the same day to a specialist treatment centre.

An appropriately worded referral letter should state the urgent nature of the referral and the suspected malignant nature of the lesion.

Although much of a patient's treatment has to be performed in hospital, patients may continue to see their practitioner after treatment. The dental practitioner is also ideally placed for the prevention of oral cancer and can contribute in other ways (Table 17.6).

Table 17.6   Role of the dental practitioner in cancer prevention and diagnosis

Prevention
- Actively discourage smoking and betel quid use
- Encourage moderation of alcohol intake
- Health promotion and education on oral carcinoma
- Provide check-ups for the edentulous and/or institutionalised elderly and other high-risk non-attenders

Early diagnosis
- Be vigilant and suspicious
- Always examine mucosa as well as the teeth
- Monitor low-risk premalignant lesions
- Refer all high-risk lesions on discovery
- Perform biopsy appropriately

After treatment
- Manage simple denture problems after surgery
- Alleviate the effects of postirradiation dry mouth, e.g. preventing caries (Ch. 3)
- Monitor for recurrence, new premalignant lesions and second primary tumours
- Monitor for cervical metastasis
- Maintain morale of and provide additional support to patients and their relatives

---

Oral cancer screening

Screening is the process of applying a rapid test to, or examining, a population to identify a group at risk from a disease. This group can then be referred for accurate and earlier diagnosis. An example is the national cervical carcinoma screening scheme using the cervical smear test. Oral carcinoma screening should be possible because the tumour is so accessible and because those at most risk (elderly persons who smoke and drink alcohol) are readily identified. A simple effective screening test is an examination of the mouth for red and white lesions. Because screening is not designed to be accurately diagnostic it may be performed by appropriately trained health care workers in the community. Such oral cancer screening schemes have proved successful in several countries with a high incidence. In the UK such a scheme would have the advantage that it might reach the most at risk individuals, who tend to be irregular dental attenders. It would also provide an opportunity for preventive advice to the same group.

Although a national screening scheme for the UK has been widely discussed, it has only been applied on a limited scale. In the meantime, oral cancer screening continues to fall within the remit of the general dental and medical practitioner.

Toluidine blue rinsing

Toluidine blue is a dye which binds to nucleic acids and can be used as an oral rinse to stain carcinoma and premalignant lesions blue. The technique was extensively evaluated many years ago and is now the subject of a resurgence of interest. It may be of value when deciding which part of an extensive lesion should be biopsied or when the clinician does not feel confident about a clinical diagnosis. However, the technique is not an accurate test for either carcinoma or premalignancy and is no more than an adjunct to diagnosis. Toluidine blue is itself mutagenic and it seems inadvisable to use it as a general screening test. The general rule should be that any suspicious lesion must be subjected to biopsy as soon as possible, regardless of the pattern of staining with toluidine blue.

VERRUCOUS CARCINOMA

This variant of squamous cell carcinoma is a low-grade neoplasm. In the UK it is more frequent in the elderly, particularly males, and has a characteristic white, warty appearance, forming a well-circumscribed mass raised above the level of the surrounding mucosa (Fig. 17.16). If small, it may easily be mistaken for a papilloma. Verrucous carcinoma is particularly associated with the habit of snuff dipping (see above).

Pathology

Verrucous carcinoma consists of close-packed papillary masses of well-differentiated squamous epithelium which is heavily keratinised. The lower border of the lesion is well defined and formed by blunt rete processes which indent but do not invade the underlying tissues. There is typically chronic inflammation in the stroma (Fig. 17.17).

Fig. 17.16   Verrucous carcinoma. An extensive lesion covering most of the buccal mucosa and starting to involve the skin at the commissure. Such longstanding lesions are likely to develop invasive squamous carcinoma and may then metastasise. (By kind permission of Professor S J Challacombe.)

Fig. 17.17 Verrucous carcinoma. The epithelium is thickened and thrown into a series of folds with a spiky parakeratotic surface. Deeply the carcinoma retains a broad pushing invasive front.

Verrucous carcinoma is slow-growing and spreads laterally rather than deeply. It can be excised relatively easily unless it is extensive. If left untreated for a period of years, a focus within verrucous carcinoma may progress to invasive squamous carcinoma and release metastases. The neoplasm must then be treated as a conventional squamous carcinoma.

SUGGESTED FURTHER READING

Anderson D L 1971 Cause and prevention of lip cancer. J Can Dent Assoc 37:138–143

Caniff J P, Harvey W, Harris M 1986 Oral submucous fibrosis: its pathogenesis and management. Br Dent J 160:429–434

Cawson R A, Binnie W H, Eveson J W 1994 Color atlas of oral disease, 2nd edn. Mosby-Wolfe, London

Cawson R A, Langdon J D, Eveson J W 1996 Surgical pathology of the mouth and jaws. Wright, Oxford

Girod S C, Pfahl M 1996 Retinoid actions and implications for prevention and therapy of cancer. Int J Oral Maxillofac Surg 25:69–73

Goldberg H I, Lockwood S A, Wyatt S W, Crossett L S 1994 Trends and differentials from cancers of the oral cavity and pharynx in the United States, 1973–1987. Cancer 74:565–572

Hogewind W F C, van der Waal I, van der Kwast, Snow G B 1989 The association of white lesions with oral squamous cell carcinoma. A retrospective study of 212 patients. Int J Oral Maxillofac Surg 18:163–164

Hopper C 1996 The role of photodynamic therapy in the management of oral cancer and precancer. Oral Oncol Eur J Cancer 32B:71–72

Kusama K, Okutso S, Takeda A et al 1996 p53 gene alterations and p53 protein in oral epithelial dysplasia and squamous cell carcinoma. J Pathol 178:415–421

Link J O, Kaugars G E, Burns J C 1992 Comparison of oral carcinomas in smokeless tobacco users and nonusers. J Oral Maxillofac Surg 50:452–455

Lukinmaa P-L, Hietanen J, Söderholm A-L, Lindquist C 1992 The histologic pattern of bone invasion by squamous cell carcinoma of the mandibular region. Br J Oral Maxillofac Surg 30:2–7

Murti P R, Bhonsle R B, Pindborg J J, Daftary D K, Gupta P C, Mehta F S 1985 Malignant transformation rate in oral submucous fibrosis over a 17-year period. Community Dent Oral Epidemiol 13:340–341

Ogden G R, Kiddie R A, Lunny D P, Lane D P 1992 Assessment of p53 protein expression in normal, benign and malignant oral mucosa. J Pathol 166:389–394

Neoplastic and non-neoplastic diseases of salivary glands

Normal function and health of the mouth depend on normal secretion of saliva by the major and minor glands. Failure of salivary secretion causes a dry mouth, which is both distressing and promotes oral infections.

OBSTRUCTION

Salivary calculi

A stone can form in a salivary gland or duct. At least 80% of calculi form in the submandibular gland, about 6% in the parotid and about 2% in the sublingual and minor salivary glands.

Clinical features

Adults are mainly affected — males twice as often as females. Calculi are usually unilateral. The classical symptom is pain when the smell or taste of food stimulates salivary secretion. Alternatively duct obstruction leads to infection, pain and swelling of the gland.

Occasionally there are no symptoms until the stone passes forward and can be palpated in the duct or seen at the duct orifice (Fig. 18.1). Alternatively the stone may be seen in a radiograph. However, about 40% of parotid and 20% of submandibular stones are not radiopaque, and sialography may be needed to locate them.

Calculi are *not* a cause of dry mouth.

Pathology

Salivary calculi are usually caused by deposition of calcium salts around a nidus of organic material, and have a layered structure. The roughness of their surface may cause the duct lining to undergo squamous metaplasia (Fig. 18.2).

Management

If sufficiently far forward in the duct, a stone may sometimes be milked forward and manipulated out of the orifice. Otherwise the duct has to be opened. An incision, usually under local

Fig. 18.1   Salivary calculus. This stone has impacted just behind the orifice of the submandibular duct forming a hard nodule. The yellow colour of the stone is visible through the thin mucosa.

Fig. 18.2   Salivary calculus in a duct. To the left is the salivary calculus which has a lamellar structure and an irregular surface. On the surface is a thick layer of microbial flora filling the space between the stone and the epithelial lining. In the surrounding wall there is an infiltrate of lymphocytes and plasma cells and neutrophils are migrating through the duct epithelium into the lumen.

anaesthesia, is made along the line of the duct just long enough to release the mass. A temporary suture should be put through the duct behind the calculus to prevent it from slipping backwards. The papilla should be left unsutured or the margins of the opening sutured to the mucosa on either side to prevent subsequent scarring and fibrous obstruction. If the gland has become damaged by recurrent infection and fibrosis, or calculi have formed within the gland itself, it may have to be excised.

Key features of salivary calculi are summarised in Table 18.1.

Table 18.1 Salivary calculi — key features

- Adult males mainly affected
- Usually (80%) in submandibular gland
- Usually form by accretion of calcium salts round organic nidus
- Typically cause pain by obstructing food-related surge of salivary secretion
- Occasionally asymptomatic until palpable in the mouth or seen in routine radiograph
- Do *not* cause dry mouth
- Should be removed by manipulation or incision of duct

Parotid papilla and duct strictures

The usual cause is chronic trauma (from such causes as projecting clasps, faulty restorations or sharp edges of broken teeth) leading to fibrosis. Fibrosis makes the duct papilla difficult to find and may prevent insertion of a probe.

Fibrosis and stenosis of a duct may be caused by ulceration round a calculus or result from incompetent surgery.

Sialography should show the degree of narrowing of the duct or papilla and dilatation behind. Once the cause has been removed, treatment depends on the site of the obstruction. The papilla may have to be excised and the duct lining sutured to the oral mucosa on either side. Alternatively the duct may be dilated with bougies.

Salivary fistula

Salivary fistula, a communication between the duct system or gland with the skin or mucous membrane, is uncommon. Internal fistulae drain into the oral cavity and cause no symptoms. By contrast, a parotid fistula on the skin is troublesome and often persistent. It may be the result of an injury to the cheek or a complication of surgery. Infection often becomes superimposed and persistent leakage of saliva prevents healing. The treatment is primarily by surgical repair but is difficult, especially because of the risk of damage to branches of the facial nerve.

Mucoceles — cysts

The most common type of salivary and soft-tissue cyst is the mucous extravasation cyst (mucocele) of minor glands, but retention cysts occasionally form. Mucoceles mainly affect the minor salivary glands, particularly of the lip. The cause is usually damage to the duct of a mucous gland. This may be caused

by a blow on the lip, as might happen to a football referee holding a whistle in the mouth.

Clinical features

Mucoceles most often form in the lower lip but occasionally on the buccal mucosa or floor of the mouth (ranula). They are usually superficial and rarely larger than 1 cm in diameter. In the early stages they appear as rounded fleshy swellings. Later, they are obviously cystic, hemispherical, fluctuant and bluish due to the thin wall (Fig. 18.3). A mucous extravasation cyst cannot be distinguished from a retention cyst clinically, but this is of little practical importance.

Pathology

Saliva leaking from a damaged duct into the superficial surrounding tissues excites an inflammatory reaction (Figs 18.4 and 18.5). The pools of saliva gradually coalesce to form a rounded cyst, usually surrounded by compressed connective tissue, without an epithelial lining. Occasionally the duct may become obstructed but less severely damaged so that saliva does not escape into the surrounding tissues. A retention cyst thus forms, with a lining of compressed duct epithelium (Fig. 18.6).

Treatment

A small superficial mucocele should be excised with the underlying gland. The latter is usually found to have been removed with the cyst but, if not, recurrence is likely. Key features are summarised in Table 18.2.

Fig. 18.3 Mucous extravasation cyst. The typical presentation at the commonest site: a rounded bluish, translucent cyst in the lower lip.

Fig. 18.4 Mucous extravasation cyst. To the left is a cavity of spilt mucin with the remnants of the ruptured duct lining-epithelium at its edge. To the right is the associated minor mucous salivary gland.

Fig. 18.5 Mucous extravasation cyst. Higher power showing the lining of the mucin-filled space. Macrophages are migrating into the mucin and in phagocytosing it develop a foamy or vacuolated cytoplasm.

Table 18.2 Mucoceles — key features

- Most common soft tissue cyst
- Most frequently on lower lip
- Usually caused by damage to duct and extravasation of saliva
- Saliva leaking into surrounding tissues causes mild inflammation
- Saliva eventually pools up to form cyst with connective tissue lining
- Rarely due to duct obstruction and dilatation forming a retention cyst with epithelial lining

Ranula

A ranula is an uncommon type of mucocele arising from the sublingual or submandibular salivary glands.

The structure is essentially the same as other mucoceles, though there is usually an epithelial lining. Ranulae are usually unilateral and 2 or 3 cm in diameter (Fig. 18.7). Occasionally they extend across the whole of the floor of the mouth. They are soft, fluctuant and bluish. They are typically painless but may interfere with speech or mastication. Treatment is preferably by marsupialisation with removal of the related gland. A simple incision leads to recurrence, and enucleation is difficult because of the very thin wall.

SIALADENITIS

Mumps

Mumps is due a paramyxovirus (the mumps virus) and causes painful swelling of the parotids and sometimes other glands. It is highly infectious and is the most common cause of acute parotid swelling.

Clinical features

Children are mainly affected. An incubation period of about 21

Fig. 18.7 Ranula. A large bluish, translucent swelling in the floor of the mouth caused by a mucous extravasation or retention cyst.

Fig. 18.6 Mucous retention cyst. Remnants of the minor mucous salivary glands are visible, together with their dilated duct, the epithelium of which is continuous with the epithelial lining of the cyst (above).

days is followed by headache, malaise, fever and tense, painful and tender swelling of the parotids. Permanent nerve deafness or, rarely, meningitis are possible complications. Adults who contract mumps may develop orchitis or oophoritis and may have severe and prolonged malaise. After an attack immunity is long lasting.

The diagnosis is usually obvious from the history and clinical findings, especially in a child. However, mumps may be mistaken for a dental infection or bacterial sialadenitis, if unilateral. Rarely, when the submaxillary or sublingual glands are affected, mumps may have to be differentiated from lymphadenitis. In cases of doubt a history of mumps earlier in life usually excludes this diagnosis. If necessary, the diagnosis can be confirmed by a rise in titre of complement-fixing antibodies. Afterwards, antibodies to the S antigen disappear relatively quickly, and their presence indicates recent mumps. The V antibody is persistent and only indicates an infection at some time previously.

With wide use of immunisation, childhood mumps is becoming infrequent and mumps in adults may take atypical forms.

Suppurative parotitis

Suppurative parotitis traditionally affected debilitated patients, particularly postoperatively, as a result of xerostomia secondary to dehydration. Currently, suppurative parotitis is more commonly seen in ambulant patients with severe xerostomia, particularly Sjögren's syndrome, and as an uncommon complication of tricyclic antidepressant treatment. Important bacterial causes include *Staphylococcus aureus*, streptococci and anaerobes. Typical clinical features are pain in one or both parotids with swelling, redness and tenderness and often increasing malaise. The regional lymph nodes are enlarged and tender, and pus exudes or can be expressed from the parotid duct. The progress of the infection depends largely on the patient's underlying physical state.

Pathology

An intense acute inflammatory infiltrate extends along and dilates the ducts. Inflammation also extends into the periductal tissues and to a varying degree into acini. If neglected, abscesses form and there are varying degrees of acinar destruction.

Management

Treatment can be started with flucloxacillin, but only after pus has been obtained for culture and sensitivity testing. The antibiotic can be changed if the bacteriological findings dictate, and drainage is rarely necessary.

Chronic sialadenitis

Chronic sialadenitis is usually a complication of duct obstruction. It is usually unilateral and asymptomatic or with intermit-

Fig. 18.8 Chronic sialadenitis resulting from obstruction. The ducts contain casts of mucin and neutrophils and are surrounded by a layer of fibrosis. There is marked acinar atrophy and the space previously occupied by acinar cells now contains infiltrates of lymphocytes and plasma cells.

tent painful swelling of the gland. Sialography may show dilatation of ducts behind the obstruction.

Pathology

There are varying degrees of destruction of acini, duct dilatation and a scattered chronic inflammatory cellular infiltrate, predominantly lymphoplasmacytic. (Fig. 18.8). Extensive interstitial fibrosis, and sometimes squamous metaplasia in the duct epithelium, follow. Calculus formation may be seen in the dilated ducts.

If possible, the obstruction should be removed, but more often the gland has to be excised and the mass examined histologically to exclude a neoplasm.

DRY MOUTH (XEROSTOMIA)

Many patients with severe xerostomia make no complaint of dry mouth, though they may, for instance, admit that they have difficulty in eating dry food. Some complain of an unpleasant taste in the mouth. Conversely, some who complain of dry mouth have normal salivary flow rates on objective testing and the problem is neurotic in nature. Salivary flow studies are valuable when patients complain of dry mouth. Important causes are summarised in Table 18.3.

SJÖGREN'S SYNDROME

In 1933, Sjögren noticed the association of dryness of the mouth and dryness of the eyes. Later he found that there was a significant association with rheumatoid arthritis. These combinations of complaints are caused by two closely related but distinct diseases:

Table 18.3   Causes of Xerostomia

Organic Causes
Sjögren's syndrome
Irradiation
Mumps (transient)
HIV infection
Sarcoidosis
Amyloid
Iron deposition (haemochromatosis, thalassaemia)

Functional causes
Dehydration
Fluid deprivation
Haemorrhage
Persistent diarrhoea
Psychogenic
   Anxiety states
   Depression
Drugs
   Diuretic overdosage
   Drugs with antimuscarinic effects
      Atropine, ipratropium, hyoscine and other analogues
      Tricyclic and some other antidepressants
      Antihistamines
      Antiemetics (including antihistamines and phenothiazines)
      Neuroleptics, particularly phenothiazines
      Some older antihypertensives (ganglion blockers and clonidine)
   Drugs with sympathomimetic actions
      'Cold cures' containing ephedrine, etc.
      Decongestants
      Bronchodilators
      Appetite supresants, particularly amphetamines

Table 18.4   Oral effects of Sjögren's syndrome

- Discomfort
- Difficulties with eating or swallowing
- Disturbed taste sensation
- Disturbed quality of speech
- Predisposition to infection

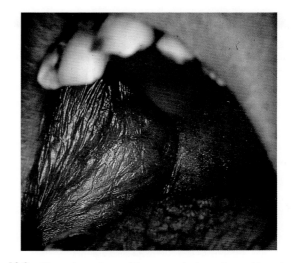

Fig. 18.9   Sjögren's syndrome. The mucosa is dry, red, atrophic and wrinkled and sticks to the fingers or mirror during examination. These changes are common to all causes of xerostomia.

Fig. 18.10   Tongue in Sjögren's syndrome. Longstanding dry mouth and repeated candidal infection produce this depapillated but lobulated tongue.

- *Primary Sjögren's syndrome*, which comprises dry mouth and dry eyes unassociated with any connective tissue disease.
- *Secondary Sjögren's syndrome*, which comprises dry mouth and dry eyes associated with rheumatoid arthritis or other connective tissue disease.

Clinical features

Females are affected nearly 10 times as frequently as males. Sjögren's syndrome affects 10–15% of patients with rheumatoid arthritis, possibly 30% of patients with lupus erythematosus and a variable proportion of patients with or without other connective tissue diseases. Sjögren's syndromes are therefore relatively common. In the absence of drug treatment or radiotherapy, they are the main cause of dry mouth but their most serious consequence is damage to the eyes and the risk of lymphoma. Primary Sjögren's syndrome tends to cause more severe oral and ocular changes and has a higher risk of lymphomatous change than secondary.

Major oral effects of Sjögren's syndrome are summarised in Table 18.4.

In the early stages, the mucosa may appear moist but salivary flow measurement shows diminished secretion. In established cases the oral mucosa is obviously dry, often red, shiny and parchment-like (Fig. 18.9). The tongue is typically red, the papillae characteristically atrophy and the dorsum becomes lobulated with a cobble-stone appearance (Fig. 18.10). With diminished salivary secretion the oral flora changes and candidal infections are common. The latter are the main cause of soreness of the mouth in Sjögren's syndrome and cause generalised erythema of the mucosa, often with angular stomatitis. Plaque accumulates (Fig. 18.11) and there may be rapidly progressive dental caries. The most severe infective complication is suppurative parotitis.

Swelling of the parotids is not common, but a history of

Fig. 18.11 Sjögren's syndrome. Extensive cervical caries is a frequent complication of dry mouth. In addition to the lack of saliva, patients may attempt to stimulate salivary flow with sweets or chewing gums.

Fig. 18.12 Salivary gland swelling in primary Sjögren's syndrome. The outline of the parotid gland is clearly demarcated.

swelling at some stage may be obtained in about 30% of patients. Swelling due to the syndrome itself shows no inflammation and is rarely painful (Fig. 18.12). A hot, tender parotid swelling with red, shiny overlying skin indicates suppurative parotitis. Parotid swelling appearing years after the onset strongly suggests lymphoma.

Sjögren's syndrome can have serious ocular effects (Table 18.5).

Table 18.5 Ocular effects of Sjögren's syndrome

- Failure of tear secretion
- Failure of clearance of foreign particles from the cornea and conjunctiva
- Gritty sensation in the eyes and inflammation (*keratoconjunctivitis sicca*)
- Risk of impairment or loss of sight

Aetiology and pathology

Sjögren's syndrome is an autoimmune (connective tissue) disease which shows a corresponding variety of immunological abnormalities (Table 18.6).

Table 18.6 Typical patterns of autoantibodies in primary and secondary Sjögren's syndrome (SS)

Autoantibodies	Primary SS %	Secondary SS %
Salivary duct antibody	10–36	67–70
Rheumatoid factor	50±	90±
SS-A antibodies	5–10	50–80
SS-B antibodies	50–75	2–5
Rheumatoid arthritis precipitin	5±	75±

A retrovirus or other virus is as yet unconfirmed as a cause. Histological changes are shown in Table 18.7 and Figs 18.13 and 18.14. The final result is replacement of the whole gland by a dense lymphocytic infiltrate. However, the infiltrate remains confined within the gland capsule and does not cross the intraglandular septa.

Table 18.7 Histological changes in salivary glands in Sjögren's syndrome

- Polyclonal infiltration by CD4 lymphocytes and plasma cells
- Infiltrate initially periductal
- Progressive spread of infiltrate through the glandular tissue
- Progressive destruction of secretory acini
- Proliferation of some duct tissue as epimyoepithelial islands

Fig. 18.13 Sjögren's syndrome. The histological appearance is typical. Dense, well-defined foci of lymphocytes surround the larger ducts in the centre of the lobules. In the area occupied by the lymphocytes there is complete acinar atrophy and a rim of residual salivary parenchyma remains around the periphery of the lobule.

Fig. 18.14 Sjögren's syndrome. In late disease no salivary acini remain and the gland is replaced by a confluent infiltrate of lymphocytes. A few ducts remain and proliferate to form the epimyoepithelial islands. Such extensive changes sometimes suggest that there has been progression to a low-grade lymphoma.

Table 18.9 Principles of management of Sjögren's syndrome

- Salivary gland damage is irreversible
- Give reassurance and help with dry mouth
- Opthalmological investigation for *keratoconjunctivitis sicca*
- Refer to specialist if connective tissue disease is untreated
- Check for any associated drug treatment contributing to dry mouth
- Alleviate dry mouth
    Frequent small sips of water
    Prescribe saliva substitutes
- Control caries in dentate patients
    Avoid sweets (e.g. lemon drops)
    Suggest sugar-free gum
    Check diet for excess sugary foods
    Maintain good oral hygiene
    Fluoride applications
    Chlorhexidine (0.2%) rinses
- Monitor for mucosal candidosis
    Give antifungal mixtures (not tablets) as necessary
- Treat difficulties with dentures symptomatically
- Observe regularly for possible development of ascending parotitis and lymphoma

---

Diagnosis

Other causes of xerostomia must be excluded (see Table 18.3).

Diagnostic tests in Sjögren's syndrome are summarised in Table 18.8. Normal salivary flow is between 1 and 2 ml/min but may be reduced to 0.5 ml/min or less. Pathological changes in labial salivary glands correlate closely with those in the parotids and biopsy of them avoids the risks of damage to the facial nerve or a parotid fistula inherent in parotid gland biopsy. A snowstorm appearance on sialography (so-called sialectasis) is due to leakage of contrast material through the duct walls (Fig. 18.15).

Table 18.8 Diagnostic tests in Sjögren's syndrome

- Diminished mixed salivary flow rate
- Labial salivary gland biopsy showing periductal lymphocytic infiltrate
- Antibody screen, especially rheumatoid factor and SS-A and SS-B
- Sialectasis on sialography
- Diminished tear secretion

Management

Many aspects need to be taken into account (Table 18.9), but the combination of painful arthritis and dryness of the mouth in secondary Sjögren's syndrome can reduce life to prolonged misery.

Ophthalmological examination is particularly important to exclude keratoconjunctivitis sicca which, in its early stages, is symptomless. Anaemia should be excluded, particularly when there is rheumatoid arthritis.

Dryness of the mouth can be relieved to some degree by providing artificial saliva (Table 18.10). Cholinesterase inhibitors

Fig. 18.15 Sjögren's syndrome. The sialogram shows the typical snowstorm appearance of blobs of contrast medium that have leaked from the duct system. Emptying and clearance of the contrast medium are also much delayed because of the reduced salivary flow.

such as pilocarpine are sometimes recommended to stimulate salivary secretion but any benefits may be conterbalanced by side-effects such as nausea, diarrhoea and bradycardia.

Table 18.10 Types of artificial saliva currently available

- Glandosane spray. Carmellose (carboxymethyl cellulose) solution with sorbitol and electrolytes: neutral, lemon or peppermint flavoured
- Luborant spray. Carmellose solution with electrolytes and preservatives
- Saliva Orthana spray. Gastric mucin, xylitol, sodium fluoride with preservatives and flavouring
- Saliva Orthana lozenges. Mucin with xylitol in sorbitol base
- Salivace spray. Carmellose with xylitol, electrolytes and preservative
- Salivix pastilles. Sugar-free. Contain gum acacia and malic acid

Dryness of the eyes is treated with artificial tears such as methyl cellulose solution. In dentate patients, sweet-eating should be prohibited, a high standard of oral hygiene maintained and frequent dental checks are necessary. Topical fluorides should be applied regularly and 0.2% chlorhexidine mouth rinses may help to reduce plaque formation. Soreness of the mouth due to infection by *Candida albicans* can be treated with nystatin or amphotericin mixture, *not* tablets. Ascending parotitis should be treated as described earlier.

In view of the risk of malignant lymphoma, immunosuppressive treatment or irradiation to reduce the size of swollen glands is contraindicated. In any case, such measures have no lasting benefit in Sjögren's syndrome. Key features are summarised in Table 18.11.

Table 18.11 Sjögren's syndromes — key features

- Middle-aged or elderly women mainly affected
- Rheumatoid arthritis or other connective tissue disease associated in secondary Sjögren's syndrome
- Dry mouth
- Dry eyes
- Polyclonal infiltration of salivary glands by CD4 lymphocytes with acinar destruction
- Multiple autoantibodies particularly SS-A and SS-B
- Significant risk of salivary gland and extrasalivary lymphomas

Benign lymphoepithelial lesion (myoepithelial sialadenitis, autoimmune sialadenitis)

Benign lymphoepithelial lesion is a term that has been used to describe salivary gland swelling with the histological features of Sjögren's syndrome. Other features of Sjögren's syndrome were thought to be absent but this was probably due to inadequate investigation. Benign lymphoepithelial lesion is a misleading term which should be avoided, as there is a high risk of lymphomatous change and it is probably not a separate entity from Sjögren's syndrome.

IRRADIATION DAMAGE

Salivary tissue is highly sensitive to ionising radiation. Irreversible destruction of acini and fibrous replacement can result from therapeutic radiation of the head and neck. Troublesome xerostomia with its attendant complications, such as rampant dental caries, is the typical result.

The management of dry mouth is as described earlier. However, it is especially important to control dental caries and its sequelae because of the danger of irradiation-associated osteomyelitis (Ch. 6) secondary to periapical infection or extractions.

HIV-ASSOCIATED SIALADENITIS

Chronic parotitis in children is said to be almost pathognomonic of HIV infection. In adults, xerostomia, sometimes with cystic parotid gland swellings, may develop and be associated with generalised lymphadenopathy (Ch. 24). Young males are predominantly affected.

Pathology

The histological features are essentially similar to those of Sjögren's syndrome, apart from gross cyst formation. Also, the infiltrate is by CD8 lymphocytes, and autoantibodies typical of Sjögren's syndrome are lacking.

As in Sjögren's syndrome, lymphomatous change is a hazard.

SJÖGREN-LIKE SYNDROME IN GRAFT-VERSUS-HOST DISEASE

A disease similar to primary Sjögren's syndrome develops in about a third of all cases of graft-versus-host disease, particularly when severe. The histological changes in lip biopsies are the same as in Sjögren's syndrome and serve to distinguish graft-versus-host disease from salivary gland damage secondary to irradiation used for immunosuppression before marrow transplantation.

HYPERSALIVATION (PTYALISM)

True ptyalism is not a significant complaint as any excess of saliva can readily be swallowed. 'False ptyalism' is more common and is either delusional (a disturbed patient may suddenly become alarmed at 'water' continually appearing in the mouth) or due to faulty neuromuscular control that leads to drooling, despite normal salivary flow (Table 18.12).

Table 18.12 Causes of ptyalism

- Local reflexes
    Oral infections (e.g. acute ulcerative gingivitis)
    Oral wounds
    Dental procedures
    New dentures
- Systemic
    Nausea
    Acid regurgitation (reflux oesophagitis)
- Toxic
    Iodine. Heavy metal poisoning
- 'False ptyalism'
    Psychogenic
    Bell's palsy
    Parkinson's disease
    Stroke

SALIVARY GLAND NEOPLASMS

Salivary gland tumours comprise a significant proportion of oral tumours and are the next most common neoplasms of the mouth after squamous cell carcinoma. However, tumours of the minor intraoral salivary glands are less common than in the parotids. The incidence of salivary gland cancers in Europe is estimated to be about 1.2 per 100 000, and in England and Wales about 600 salivary gland cancers are registered each year. However, over 75% of salivary gland tumours are benign, so that the total number (benign and malignant) seen annually in Britain may be approximately 2400. Women are slightly more frequently affected. About 70% of salivary gland tumours develop in the parotid and a few affect the submandibular glands. Tumours in the sublingual glands are a rarity but usually malignant (Fig. 18.16).

Little is known of the aetiology of salivary gland tumours except that they can result from irradiation to the head area. In survivors of the atomic blasts at Hiroshima and Nagasaki there has been an excess of salivary gland tumours. Similarly, these tumours can follow therapeutic irradiation of, for example, the thyroid and, it is suggested, multiple dental diagnostic radiographs.

Classification

The World Health Organization 1972 classification of salivary gland tumours is still widely used and a modified version is summarised in Table 18.13.

The 1990 WHO typing of salivary gland tumours includes no fewer than 32 types of epithelial tumours, but only polymorphous low-grade adenocarcinoma and epithelial–myoepithelial carcinoma are included in the following descriptions.

General clinical features of salivary gland tumours

Adults are predominantly affected. The usual intraoral site is the palate, often at the junction of the hard and soft palate

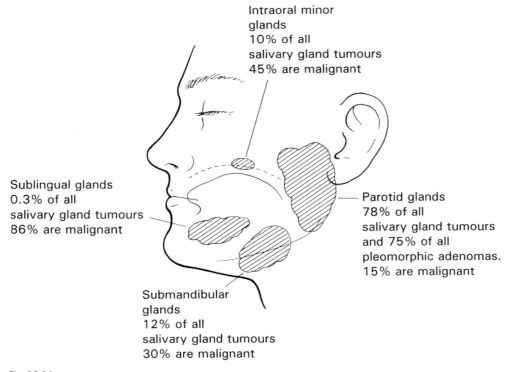

Intraoral minor glands
10% of all salivary gland tumours
45% are malignant

Sublingual glands
0.3% of all salivary gland tumours
86% are malignant

Parotid glands
78% of all salivary gland tumours
and 75% of all pleomorphic adenomas.
15% are malignant

Submandibular glands
12% of all salivary gland tumours
30% are malignant

Fig. 18.16 The distribution of salivary gland neoplasms showing the approximate overall frequency of tumours in different sites and the relevant frequency of benign and malignant tumours by site.

Table 18.13 Salivary gland neoplasms (modified 1972 classification)

Epithelial tumours
Adenomas
    Pleomorphic adenoma ('mixed tumour')
    Monomorphic adenomas — adenolymphoma — oxyphilic adenoma
Carcinomas
    Mucoepidermoid carcinoma
    Acinic cell carcinoma
    Adenoid cystic carcinoma
    Adenocarcinoma
    Epidermoid carcinoma
    Undifferentiated carcinoma
    Carcinoma in pleomorphic adenoma (malignant mixed tumour)

Non-epithelial tumours
Lymphomas
Sarcomas

Table 18.14 Salivary gland tumours — typical clinical features

Benign salivary gland tumours	*Malignant salivary gland tumours*
Slow-growing	Sometimes fast-growing
Soft or rubbery consistency	Sometimes hard consistency
85% of parotid tumours are benign	45% of minor gland tumours are malignant
Do not ulcerate	May ulcerate and invade bone
No associated nerve signs	May cause cranial nerve palsies*

*Malignant parotid tumours can cause facial palsy in particular. Adenoid cystic carcinoma can cause multiple cranial nerve lesions especially of lingual, facial or hypoglossal nerves.

Fig. 18.17 Pleomorphic adenoma. The junction of hard and soft palates is a common intraoral site; the tumour usually feels rubbery and lobulated on palpation.

Fig. 18.18 Pleomorphic adenoma. This slowly enlarging lump in the lower pole of the parotid gland is caused by a pleomorphic adenoma but the appearance is not specific and any benign and some low-grade malignant neoplams could appear the same.

(Fig. 18.17) or occasionally the cheek or lip. Typical clinical features of benign and malignant salivary gland tumours are shown in Table 18.14. However, in their early stages, benign and malignant salivary gland tumours cannot be distinguished clinically.

Pleomorphic adenoma

Pleomorphic adenomas ('mixed tumours') account for about 75% of parotid tumours but a lower proportion of intraoral salivary gland tumours (Fig. 18.18). They arise mainly from duct

epithelium or myoepithelial cells. A wide variety of structures may be seen (Table 18.15).

Table 18.15 Pleomorphic adenomas — important histological features

- Capsule — never complete
- Ducts
- Sheets or strands of dark-staining epithelial cells
- Squamous metaplasia and foci of keratin
- Fibrous and elastic tissue
- Myxoid tissue
- Cartilage, sometimes calcified. Rarely true bone formation

These varied tissues are completely disordered in arrangement and the proportions of the different components also vary

Fig. 18.19 Pleomorphic adenoma. The histological appearances are very varied. In this typical area there are clusters of ducts containing eosinophilic material surrounded by stellate cells lying in a mucinous stroma.

Fig. 18.22 Pleomorphic adenoma. At the margins of pleomorphic adenomas there are often extensions of the tumour into and beyond the capsule, rendering enucleation an ineffective treatment.

Fig. 18.20 Pleomorphic adenoma. In this area there has been maturation of the mucinous stroma to form a cartilage-like material within which there are more cellular islands with ducts.

Fig. 18.23 This excised pleomorphic adenoma is 3 cm across and the lobular shape is clearly seen.

Fig. 18.21 Plemorphic adenoma. In this lesion there is formation of true cartilage which is undergoing ossification.

widely (Figs 18.19–18.22). The fibrous, myxoid or cartilaginous mesenchymal elements are due to the pluripotential properties of myoepithelial cells. Some tumours are predominantly myxoid and can burst at operation if not gently handled, and then recur. Myoepithelial cells cannot be identified by light microscopy and can appear dark and angular, spindle-shaped or resemble plasma cells. However, immunohistochemistry shows their typical double staining with epithelial (cytokeratin) markers and mesenchymal markers, particularly S-100 protein, vimentin and actin. Myoepithelial cells may occasionally predominate or are the only cells present. Such a tumour is termed a *myoepithelioma*.

Growth of pleomorphic adenomas is slow and may take several years to reach an inch (2.5 cm) in diameter. They form rubbery, often lobulated swellings (Fig. 18.23). When close under the mucosa the tumour may appear bluish. The swelling is typically attached to the overlying mucosa but mobile on the deeper tissues. If neglected, pleomorphic adenomas can grow to a great size and occasionally undergo malignant change.

Treatment is by wide excision: recurrence is otherwise inevitable. The reputation of the pleomorphic adenoma for recurrence is due to the great surgical difficulties of complete removal of tumours from the parotid (the common site), where the facial nerve, in particular, makes dissection hazardous. Pleomorphic adenomas have an unusually strong tendency to seed and recur in the incision scar if opened at operation or if incompletely excised. In the case of parotid tumours, therefore, recurrences are prevented only by removing the gland with the tumour intact. The recurrence rate is low in skilled hands, but recurrences are typically multifocal and difficult to eradicate.

Warthin's tumour (adenolymphoma)

Warthin's tumour arises in the parotid glands and accounts for about 9% of tumours there. It has a highly characteristic histological appearance consisting of tall, eosinophilic columnar cells which form a much-folded layer covering dense lymphoid tissue, including many germinal centres (Fig. 18.24). These structures line and form papillary projections into cystic spaces (Fig. 18.25).

Fig. 18.24   Warthin's tumour. Tall columnar cells surround lymphoid tissue and line a convoluted cystic space.

Fig. 18.25   Warthin's tumour. At higher power the tall columnar epithelial cells are readily identified and beneath them the lymphoid tissue.

Warthin's tumour is benign and responds to enucleation but is sometimes multiple.

Oncocytoma

Oncocytoma is a rare benign tumour that virtually only affects the parotids, particularly in the elderly. It consists of large, eosinophilic cells with small compact nuclei ('oncocytes'), which are typically arranged in solid cords.

Oncocytosis is the term given to replacement or transformation of acinar cells of the parotid (or rarely other glands) by cells having the same appearance as those of an oncocytoma but without loss of the normal lobular architecture. Oncocytosis is usually an age-related change and, when widespread, the gland becomes swollen and soft.

Other adenomas

Other adenomas lack the connective tissue components of the pleomorphic adenoma and may have a uniform cellular structure, often with a tubular or trabecular pattern. Canalicular adenomas particularly affect the upper lip and consist of small darkly-staining cells in a tubular or trabecular pattern but sometimes resembling an adenoid cystic carcinoma.

Adenomas other than pleomorphic adenoma respond to enucleation or simple excision.

Mucoepidermoid carcinoma

Mucoepidermoid carcinomas account for between 3% and 9% of salivary gland neoplasms.

Histologically, they consist of two cell types: large, pale mucus-secreting cells which are surrounded by epidermoid (squamous) cells. Either may be predominant. If mainly mucoid, the tumour tends to be cystic; if mainly epidermoid, the tumour is solid and often then more aggressive (Figs 18.26 and 18.27). There is no well-defined capsule but the tumour usually grows slowly.

Despite benign cytological appearances, mucoepidermoid carcinomas can be invasive and occasionally metastasise. Those which are obviously malignant microscopically are uncommon but are more likely to metastasise.

Treatment is by wide excision but the tumour may recur.

Acinic cell carcinoma

Acinic cell carcinomas are rare and account for about 1% of salivary gland tumours. Their behaviour is also unpredictable.

Histologically, they show an almost uniform pattern of large cells, similar to serous cells, with granular basophilic cytoplasm, often in an acinar arrangement (Fig. 18.28). A characteristic feature is scattered round 'holes', thought to be entrapped secretion. Sometimes these are so numerous as to give the tumour a lace-like appearance.

Despite apparently benign histological appearances, acinic

Fig. 18.26 Mucoepidermoid carcinoma. The mucous cells surround microcysts. Underlying the mucous cells are the epidermoid (squamous) cells.

Fig. 18.27 Mucoepidermoid carcinoma. At higher power the finely granular mucous cells are seen to the right with the underlying epidermoid cells to the left.

Fig. 18.28 Acinic cell carcinoma. The tumour is composed of granular acinar-type cells, sometimes arranged in acinus-like clusters and sometimes forming irregular sheets. Cytological atypia is uncommon.

Fig. 18.29 Adenoid cystic carcinoma. There is an ulcerated mass arising from a minor gland in the palate. The clinical appearance would be the same with other malignant salivary neoplasms.

Adenoid cystic carcinoma

Adenoid cystic carcinoma usually has a highly characteristic histological pattern consisting of rounded groups of small, darkly-staining cells of almost uniform size, surrounding multiple small clear spaces (cribriform or 'Swiss cheese' pattern) (Figs 18.29 and 18.30). Adenoid cystic carcinomas usually grow relatively slowly but tend to infiltrate along nerve sheaths. When they reach and spread along bony canals their extent is considerably greater than radiographs show. Metastases usually appear late. The prognosis is poor unless the tumour is vigorously treated by early wide excision at the earliest possible stage, often combined with radiotherapy.

Adenocarcinoma

Adenocarcinomas of the salivary glands show a variety of appearances. Some show attempts at duct formation typical of adenocarcinomas, while others have a papillary cystic pattern. Some are so poorly differentiated that their glandular origin is difficult to discern.

cell carcinomas can be invasive and occasionally metastasise. More obviously malignant variants with nuclear pleomorphism and hyperchromatism are also occasionally seen microscopically.

Fig. 18.30 Adenoid cystic carcinoma. The small darkly staining cells of the adenoid cystic carcinoma form cribriform islands with large holes which have been likened, rather inappropriately, to Swiss cheese.

Fig. 18.31 Polymorphous low-grade adenocarcinoma. At the margin of the carcinoma islands of epithelium form ducts and sheets and invade the surrounding tissue.

Fig. 18.32 Carcinoma arising in a pleomorphic adenoma. In longstanding pleomorphic adenomas the stroma may become hyalinised, dense and acellular. In such tumours there is a risk of transformation to carcinoma, as shown here by clusters of cells showing cytological atypia.

Polymorphous low-grade adenocarcinoma

Polymorphous low-grade adenocarcinoma arises in minor glands, particularly of the palate. It consists of cytologically benign-looking pale-staining cells in lobular, papillary or papil-

Fig. 18.33 Necrotising sialometaplasia. The clinical appearances are similar to those of a malignant salivary neoplasm.

Fig. 18.34 Necrotising sialometaplasia. The histological features may also be mistaken for malignancy. There is necrosis of all the acinar cells, and only hyperplastic ducts showing squamous metaplasia remain.

Fig. 18.35 Sialadenosis. In this case of idiopathic sialadenosis there is conspicuous swelling of the parotid glands producing a characteristic appearance.

lary cystic, cribriform or trabecular configurations (Fig. 18.31). It is invasive and can spread along nerve sheaths but rarely metastasises.

Epithelial–myoepithelial carcinoma

Epithelial–myoepithelial carcinoma is a tumour of major glands. It consists of ducts or trabeculae of benign-looking, dark-staining cells with an outer layer of clear cells. The latter sometimes predominate and the tumour has to be distinguished from other clear cell tumours, most of which are malignant.

Squamous cell carcinoma

This can also affect salivary glands by metaplasia of glandular cells, as seen in pleomorphic adenoma, but is rare. It does not differ from a mucosal carcinoma histologically.

Undifferentiated carcinomas

These usually consist of closely set, small, darkly-staining cells with little cytoplasm. Rapid spread and metastasis are typical.

Malignant change in pleomorphic adenoma

Pleomorphic adenoma is one of the few benign tumours that can undergo malignant change. Clinically, this is sometimes suggested by a sudden spurt in growth or development of pain or facial palsy.

Histologically, malignant change in pleomorphic adenoma is shown by obviously carcinomatous features adjacent to the benign cellular picture of the remainder of the tumour (Fig. 18.32). This is typically a late phenomenon, usually only after the tumour has been present for many years or in recurrences after inadequate excision.

Secondary tumours

Carcinomas, and occasionally other tumours, can metastasise to the salivary glands, particularly the parotid. Such secondaries can sometimes resemble primary salivary gland carcinomas: renal cell carcinoma metastases in particular can closely resemble epithelial–myoepithelial carcinoma. Diagnosis may depend on finding a primary elsewhere but usually the prognosis is almost hopeless in view of the dissemination of the tumour.

Non-epithelial tumours

The most common non-epithelial tumours of salivary glands are lymphomas. Some of these arise as a complication of Sjögren's syndrome of 'benign lymphoepithelial lesion'. In other cases salivary gland lymphoma is the first sign of wide-spread disease. Such a possibility must always be investigated because the prognosis is heavily dependent on the tumour's stage.

Juvenile haemangioma of the parotids

Juvenile haemangioma is a rare tumour which may be present at birth or first seen in childhood. Girls are more frequently affected. It forms a soft, sometimes bluish, swelling.

Histologically, the parotid structure is largely replaced by angiomatous tissue, among which glandular elements can be found. This angiomatous proliferation may occasionally be so vast as to form an arteriovenous fistula.

Sometimes these tumours regress spontaneously but if this has not happened by the age of 10 years, excision is required. Corticosteroids may delay tumour growth and facilitate later surgery.

Intraosseous salivary gland tumours

Ectopic salivary gland tissue is occasionally present in the mandible, either in a cavity in the bone near the angle (Stafne bone cavity) or occasionally in other sites. Rarely, salivary gland tumours of any type can develop within the jaw (presumably from this ectopic salivary tissue) and may be mistaken for odontogenic tumours by an unsuspecting pathologist. However, they are most frequently mucoepidermoid carcinomas.

Radiographically, intraosseous salivary tumours produce cyst-like or poorly circumscribed areas of radiolucency. The diagnosis can only be made histologically. Wide excision is required

TUMOUR-LIKE SALIVARY SWELLINGS

Necrotising sialometaplasia

This tumour-like lesion mainly affects the minor glands of the palate. It is of unknown cause. Middle-aged males are predominantly affected and are often cigarette smokers.

Typically, a relatively painless, ulcerated swelling, 15–20 mm in diameter, forms on the hard palate, often in the first molar region (Fig. 18.33). The margins are irregular and heaped-up or everted. Clinically, it resembles a carcinoma, for which it has sometimes also been mistaken histologically.

Pathology

There is chronic inflammation of minor salivary glands and necrosis of acini. The duct tissue undergoes squamous metaplasia and proliferates to produce a pseudoepitheliomatous appearance (Fig. 18.34).

Necrotising sialometaplasia is often excised for diagnosis, but usually heals spontaneously after 8–10 weeks.

Sialadenosis

Sialadenosis is a non-neoplastic, non-inflammatory enlargement of salivary glands, most noticeably of the parotids, due to a variety of causes (Fig. 18.35 and Table 18.16). Histologically, there is hypertrophy of serous acini and oedema of interstitial connective tissue.

Table 18.16   Important causes of sialadenosis

- Alcoholism
- Diabetes mellitus
- Other endocrine diseases
- Pregnancy
- Drugs (e.g. sympathomimetics)
- Bulimia
- Idiopathic

SUGGESTED FURTHER READING

Barnes L, Rao U, Krause J, Contis L, Schwartz A, Scalamonga P 1994 Salivary duct carcinoma. Part I. A clinicopathologic evaluation and DNA analysis of 13 cases with review of the literature. Oral Surg Oral Med Oral Pathol 78:64–73

Brook I 1992 Diagnosis and management of parotitis. Arch Otolaryngol Head Neck Surg 118:469–471

Brookstone M S, Huvos A G 1992 Central salivary gland tumors of the maxilla and mandible: a clinicopathologic study of 11 cases with an analysis of the literature. J Oral Maxillofac Surg 50:229–236

Callender D L, Frankenthaler R A, Luna M A, Lee S S, Goepfert H 1992 Salivary gland neoplasms in children. Arch Otolaryngol Head Neck Surg 118:472–476

Cawson R A, Langdon J D, Eveson J W 1996 Surgical pathology of the mouth and jaws. Wright, Oxford

Delgado R, Vuitch F, Albores-Saavedra J 1993 Salivary duct carcinoma. Cancer 72:1503–1512

Ellis G L, Corio R L 1983 Acinic cell adenocarcinoma. A clinicopathologic analysis of 294 cases. Cancer 52:542–549

Epstein J B, Scully C 1992 The role of saliva in oral health and the causes and effects of xerostomia. Can Dent Assoc J 58:217–221

Epstein J B, Stevenson-Moore P, Scully C 1992 Management of xerostomia. Can Dent Assoc J 58:140–143

Eveson J W, Cawson R A 1986 Warthin's tumor (cystadenolymphoma) of salivary glands. A clinicopathologic investigation of 278 cases. Oral Surg Oral Med Oral Pathol 61:256–262

Falzon M, Isaacson P G 1991 The natural history of benign lymphoepithelial lesion of the salivary gland in which there is a monoclonal population of B cells. A report of two cases. Am J Surg Pathol 15:59–65

Gleeson M J, Cawson R A, Bennett M H 1986 Benign lymphoepithelial lesion: a less than benign disease. Clin Otolaryngol 11:47–51

Gleeson M J, Bennett M H, Cawson R A 1986 Lymphomas of salivary glands. Cancer 58:699–704

Hamper K, Brugmann M, Koppermann R et al 1989 Epithelial-myoepithelial duct carcinoma of salivary glands: a follow-up and cytophotometric study of 21 cases. J Oral Pathol Med 18:299–304

Hamper K, Lazar F, Dietel M et al 1990 Prognostic factors for adenoid cystic carcinoma of the head and neck: a retrospective evaluation of 96 cases. J Oral Pathol Med 19:101–107

Hickman R E, Cawson R A, Duffy S W 1984 The prognosis of specific types of salivary gland tumors. Cancer 54:1620–1624

Holliday R A, Cohen W A, Schinella R A et al 1988 Benign lymphoepithelial parotid cysts and hyperplastic cervical lymphadenopathy in AIDS-risk patients: a new CT appearance. Radiology 168:439–441

Labrouyie E, Merlio J P H, Beylot-Barry M et al 1993 Human immunodeficiency virus type I replication within cystic lymphoepithelial lesion of salivary glands. Am J Clin Pathol 100:41–46

Lewis J E, Olsen K D, Weiland L H 1991 Acinic cell carcinoma. Clinicopathologic review. Cancer 68:172–179

McCluggage G, Sloan J, Cameron S, Hamilton P, Toner P 1995 Basal cell adenocarcinoma of the submandibular gland. Oral Surg Oral Med Oral Pathol 79:342–350

O'Connell J E, George M K, Speculand G B, Pahor A L 1993 Mycobacterial infection of the parotid gland: an unusual cause of parotid swelling. J Laryngol Otol 107:560–564

Qureshi A A, Gitelis A, Templeton A A, Piasecki P A 1994 'Benign' metastasizing pleomorphic adenoma. A case report and review of the literature. Clin Orthop Rel Res 308:192–198

Raad I I, Sabbagh M F, Caranasos G J 1990 Acute bacterial sialadenitis: a study of 29 cases and review. Rev Infect Dis 12:591–601

Seifert G, Miehlke A, Haubrich J, Chilla R 1986 Diseases of the salivary glands. Thieme, Stuttgart

Seifert G, Brocheriou C, Cardesa A, Eveson J W 1990 WHO International Histological Classification of Tumours. Pathol Res Pract 186:555–581

Takeichi N, Hirose F, Yamamoto H, Ezaki H, Fujikura T 1983 Salivary gland tumors in atomic bomb survivors, Hiroshima, Japan. II Pathologic study and supplementary epidemiologic observations. Cancer 52:377–385

Thackray A C, Lucas R B 1974 Tumors of the major salivary glands. Atlas of tumor pathology, second series, fascicle 10. Armed Forces Institute of Pathology, Washington DC

Toynton S C, Wilkins M J, Cook H T, Stafford N D S 1994 True malignant mixed tumour of a minor salivary gland. J Laryngol Otol 108:76–79

Van der Wal J E, Snow G B, van der Waal I 1990 Intraoral adenoid cystic carcinoma. The presence of perineural spread in relation to site, size, local extension and metastatic spread in 22 cases. Cancer 66:2031–2033

Vincent S D, Hammond H L, Finkelstein M W 1994 Clinical and therapeutic features of polymorphous low-grade adenocarcinoma. Oral Surg Oral Med Oral Pathol 77:41–47

Waldron C A, Koh M L 1990 Central mucoepidermoid carcinoma of the jaws: report of four cases with analysis of the literature and discussion of the relationship to mucoepidermoid, sialodontogenic and glandular odontogenic cysts. J Oral Maxillofac Surg 48:871–877

Wolvius E B, van der Valk P, van der Wal J E et al 1996 Primary non-Hodgkin lymphoma of the salivary glands. An analysis of 22 cases. J Oral Pathol Med 25:177–181

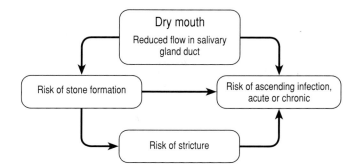

Summary 18.1   Inter-relationships between dry mouth, calculi and their complications (see p. 242).

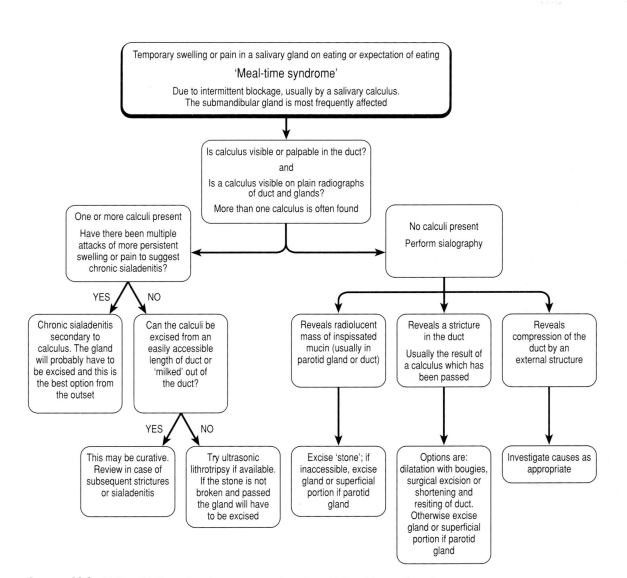

Summary 18.2   Differential diagnosis and management of a patient with 'mealtime syndrome'.

CHAPTER
18

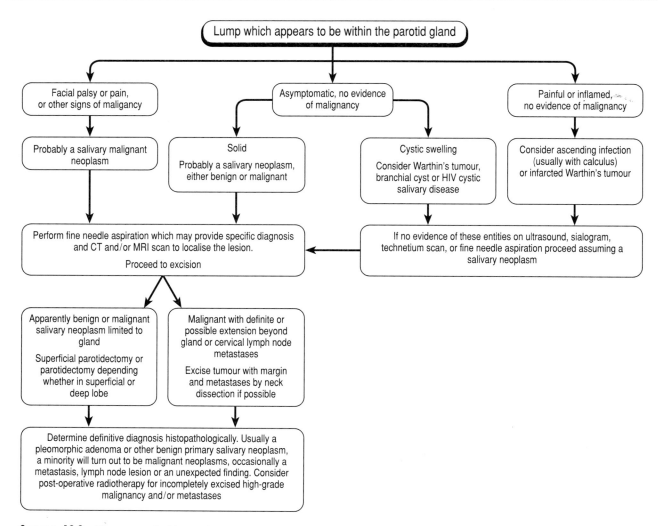

Lump which appears to be within the parotid gland

Facial palsy or pain,
or other signs of malignancy

Asymptomatic, no evidence
of malignancy

Painful or inflamed,
no evidence of malignancy

Probably a salivary malignant
neoplasm

Solid

Probably a salivary neoplasm,
either benign or malignant

Cystic swelling

Consider Warthin's tumour,
branchial cyst or HIV cystic
salivary disease

Consider ascending infection
(usually with calculus)
or infarcted Warthin's tumour

Perform fine needle aspiration which may provide specific diagnosis
and CT and/or MRI scan to localise the lesion.

Proceed to excision

If no evidence of these entities on ultrasound, sialogram,
technetium scan, or fine needle aspiration proceed assuming a
salivary neoplasm

Apparently benign or malignant
salivary neoplasm limited to
gland

Superficial parotidectomy or
parotidectomy depending
whether in superficial or
deep lobe

Malignant with definite or
possible extension beyond
gland or cervical lymph node
metastases

Excise tumour with margin
and metastases by neck
dissection if possible

Determine definitive diagnosis histopathologically. Usually a
pleomorphic adenoma or other benign primary salivary neoplasm,
a minority will turn out to be malignant neoplasms, occasionally a
metastasis, lymph node lesion or an unexpected finding. Consider
post-operative radiotherapy for incompletely excised high-grade
malignancy and/or metastases

Summary 18.3   Management decisions and treatment for a lump in the parotid gland.

Summary 18.4   Summary of the diagnosis of persistent bilateral swelling of the parotid glands.

Common benign mucosal swellings

FIBROUS POLYPS, EPULIDES AND DENTURE-INDUCED GRANULOMAS

Fibrous nodules are the most common soft-tissue swellings of the mouth. They are not neoplasms but hyperplastic swellings that develop in sites subject to chronic minor injury and/or low-grade infection (Table 19.1). Fibromas are not recognised as an entity and in any case cannot be distinguished from fibrous hyperplasia. The term *epulis* (literally 'on the gingiva') refers only to the site. It has no implications for the histology, but in practice most epulides are fibrous.

Irritation of the gingival margin by the sharp edge of a carious cavity or by calculus may lead to the formation of a fibrous epulis; irritation of alveolar or palatal mucosa by a rough area on a denture may provoke development of a denture granuloma. Though different names are given to these lesions they are similar in origin and structure.

Clinical features

A fibrous epulis is most common near the front of the mouth between two teeth on the gingiva (Fig. 19.1). Fibrous polyps can also form on the buccal mucosa (Fig. 19.2). Denture-induced hyperplasias ('denture granulomas') often form at the edge of dentures (Fig. 19.3). These swellings are pale and firm but may be abraded and ulcerated, and then inflamed.

Leaf fibroma is another fibrous overgrowth which forms

Fig. 19.2 Fibrous polyp. This lesion on the buccal mucosa has arisen as a result of cheek biting and is a firm, painless polyp covered by mucosa of normal appearance.

Fig. 19.1 Fibrous epulis. This lesion arising from the gingival margin between the lower central incisors is firm, pink and not ulcerated.

Fig. 19.3 Denture-induced granuloma. Fibrous hyperplasia at the posterior border of this upper partial denture has resulted in a firm mucosal swelling moulded to fit the denture.

Fig. 19.4 'Leaf fibroma'. Flat lesions formed between the denture and mucosa are often termed leaf fibromas because of their shape. Raising this example with a probe reveals its pedunculated shape.

Fig. 19.6 Fibrous epulis with ossification. Much of the surface of this pedunculated nodule is ulcerated and hyperplastic epithelium covers the margins. Centrally the lesion is very cellular, partly as a result of inflammatory infiltrate, and trabeculae of woven bone are being deposited and maturing into lamellar bone. The presence of bone in a fibrous epulis appears to be of no clinical significance.

Fig. 19.7 Papillary hyperplasia of the palate. A small leaf fibroma is also present in the anterior palate.

Fig. 19.5 Fibrous polyp. The lesion is composed of mature fibrous tissue covered by hyperplastic epithelium with spiky rete processes. A few inflammatory cells are present near the base.

under a denture but is flattened against the palate (Fig. 19.4). It may be difficult to see until lifted away from its bed.

Pathology

These nodules consist of irregular interlacing connective tissue fibres without encapsulation but covered by epithelium, which is usually hyperplastic (Fig. 19.5).

Bone formation is sometimes seen in a fibrous epulis (Fig. 19.6). In American texts a fibrous epulis is termed (in an

Fig. 19.8 Papillary hyperplasia. The mucosa is thrown into a series of convoluted folds covered by hyperplastic epithelium. Inflammatory change is greater when candidal infection is present.

Fig. 19.9 Pyogenic granuloma. A bright red polypoid swelling. The gingiva is a common site.

Fig. 19.10 Giant cell epulis. Typical lesion in a child showing the bluish or maroon colour of the gingival nodule. (By kind permission of Mrs H Pitt-Ford.)

Fig. 19.11 Giant cell epulis. At high magnification clusters of giant cells in vascular fibrous tissue may be seen lying immediately below the covering epithelium.

apparent desire to cause confusion) a 'peripheral ossifying fibroma', even though it has no relation to the ossifying fibroma of bone and is not a fibroma.

Fibrous nodules should be excised, together with the small base of normal tissue from which they arise. In the case of a fibrous epulis the underlying bone should be curetted. There should be no recurrence if this is done thoroughly and the source of irritation is removed.

Histological examination is needed to confirm that an epulis is fibrous and not a giant cell lesion, pyogenic granuloma or a malignant tumour, which can very rarely form on the gingival margin and simulate a simple epulis.

Fig. 19.12 Papilloma arising at the commissure.

Fig. 19.13 Papilloma. The lesion consists of thickened fingers of epithelium. Slender vascular cores of connective tissue support each frond.

Table 19.1 Fibrous nodules — practical points

- The most common oral tumour-like swellings
- Most frequently form at gingival margins (fibrous epulis) or in relation to a denture
- They are hyperplastic responses to chronic irritation
- Should be excised complete and sent for histological examination

Giant cell fibroma

This variant is relatively common. It is distinguished microscopically by large, mononucleate, stellate, darkly-staining cells (quite unlike the multinucleate cells of a giant cell granuloma), scattered between short, coarse fibrous tissue bundles. Clinically, giant cell fibromas are typically pedunculated and usually arise from the gingivae. The surface is frequently verrucous.

The treatment is the same as for a fibrous epulis.

PAPILLARY HYPERPLASIA OF THE PALATE

Nodular overgrowth of the palatal mucosa is occasionally seen, particularly under dentures in older persons in whom low-grade trauma or infection exacerbates the proliferation (Fig. 19.7). Candidosis is sometimes superimposed but is not the cause. Mild palatal papillary hyperplasia is also occasionally seen in non-denture wearers.

Histologically, palatal papillary hyperplasia shows close-set nodules of vascular fibrous tissue with a variable chronic inflammatory infiltrate and a covering of hyperplastic epithelium (Fig. 19.8).

There is no justification for stripping palatal papillary hyperplasia. Dentures should be kept clean and not worn overnight. Any superimposed candidal infection should be treated with an antifungal drug.

PYOGENIC GRANULOMA AND PREGNANCY EPULIS

Pyogenic granuloma is relatively uncommon. Clinically it is usually red and relatively soft (Fig. 19.9). Microsopically it consists of many dilated blood vessels in a loose oedematous connective tissue stroma. There is typically a dense acute inflammatory infiltrate but this is sometimes scanty or absent. A pregnancy epulis has the same histological appearances and can only be distinguished by the nature of the patient and, usually, an associated pregnancy gingivitis (Ch. 5).

GIANT CELL EPULIS

The giant cell epulis, like the fibrous epulis, is probably hyperplastic, but less common.

Clinically, a giant cell epulis is usually found on the gingival margin between teeth anterior to the permanent molars. Its development may therefore be related to the resorption of deciduous teeth. The swelling is rounded, soft and typically maroon or purplish (Fig. 19.10).

Histologically, numerous multinucleate cells lie in a vascular stroma of plump, spindle-shaped cells. The appearance is similar to that of a giant cell granuloma of the jaw, but for the fact that the epulis is extraosseus and has a covering of stratified squamous epithelium (Fig. 19.11). Very rarely a giant cell epulis is a manifestation of hyperparathyroidism, in which case changes in blood chemistry confirm the diagnosis (Ch. 10).

A giant cell epulis should be excised, together with its gingival base and the underlying bone curetted. Adjacent teeth need not be extracted if they are healthy, and if treatment is thorough there should be no recurrence.

BENIGN EPITHELIAL TUMOURS AND TUMOUR-LIKE LESIONS

Squamous cell papilloma

Papillomas mainly affect adults and have a distinctive, clinically recognisable, cauliflower-like or branched structure of finger-like processes (Fig. 19.12).

Histologically, the papillae consist of stratified squamous epithelium supported by a vascular connective tissue core (Fig. 19.13). When keratinised, they appear white.

Human papilloma virus (HPV) of various subtypes is associated but no inclusion bodies or other signs of viral infection are histologically evident. Oral papillomas appear to have no potential for malignant change and respond to local excision.

Infective warts (verruca vulgaris)

Oral warts are uncommon but seen particularly in children and frequently result from autoinoculation from warts on the hands.

Histologically, the structure is generally similar to that of papillomas but there are typically large clear cells (koilocytes) with pyknotic nuclei and prominent keratohyaline granules in the superficial layers of the prickle cells. There is also positive staining of the nuclei with peroxidase-labelled antiserum to HPV.

Oral warts are occasionally multiple but, if numerous or confluent, HIV infection or other cause of immunodeficiency should be suspected.

Adenoma

Intraoral adenomas arise from minor salivary glands. They typically form smooth, round or lobulated, painless firm swellings and are most frequently found on the palate (Ch. 18).

Other benign neoplasms

Benign neoplasms such as neurofibroma and lipoma which are occasionally found in the mouth are discussed in the following chapter.

SUGGESTED FURTHER READING

Abbey L M, Page D G, Sawyer D R 1980 The clinical and histopathologic features of a series of 464 oral squamous cell papillomas. Oral Surg 49:419–427

Anneroth G, Sigurdson A 1983 Hyperplastic lesions of the gingiva and alveolar mucosa. A study of 175 cases. Acta Odontol Scand 41:75–86

Cawson R A, Binnie W H, Eveson J W 1994 Color atlas of oral disease, 2nd edn. Mosby-Wolfe, London

Cawson R A, Langdon J D, Eveson J W 1996 Surgical pathology of the mouth and jaws. Wright, Oxford

Ellis G L, Jensen J L, Reingold I M, Barr R J 1977 Malignant neoplasms metastatic to the gingivae. Oral Surg Oral Med Oral Pathol 44:238–245

Giansanti J S, Waldron C A 1969 Peripheral giant cell granuloma: review of 720 cases. J Oral Surg 27:787–791

Hirshberg A, Leibovich P, Buchner A 1993 Metastases to the oral mucosa: analysis of 157 cases. J Oral Pathol Med 22:385–390

Houston G D 1982 The giant cell fibroma. A review of 464 cases. Oral Surg 53:582–587

Zain R B, Fei Y J 1990 Fibrous lesions of the gingiva: a histopathologic analysis of 204 cases. Oral Surg Oral Med Oral Pathol 70:466–470

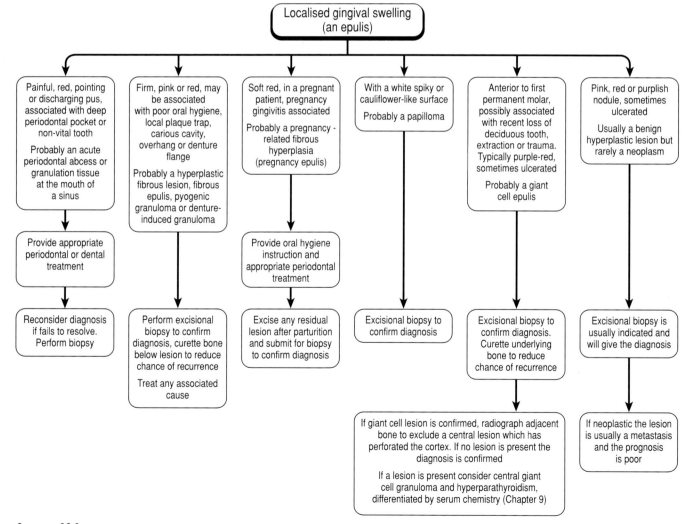

Summary 19.1   Differential diagnosis and management of the common localised gingival swellings.

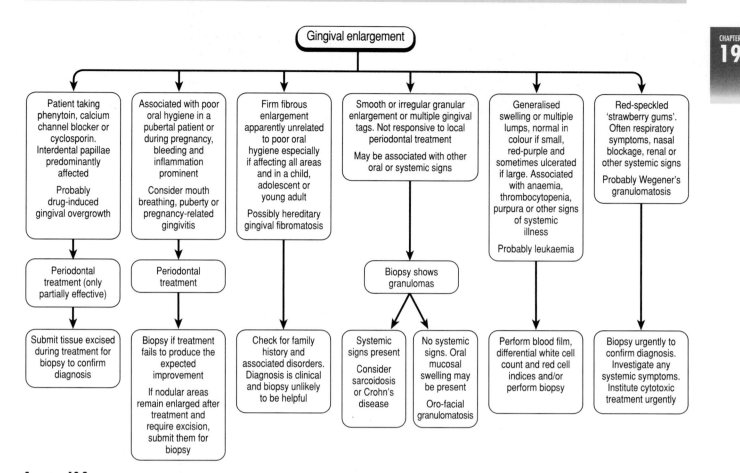

Summary 19.2 Differential diagnosis of the common and important causes of gingival enlargement.

Soft-tissue (mesenchymal) neoplasms and lymphomas

BENIGN TUMOURS

Neurofibromas

These uncommon tumours arise from nerve sheaths. They form smooth, painless lumps in the mouth. When seen in the mouth, neurofibromatosis should be suspected.

Histologically, neurofibromas are cellular, with plump nuclei separated by fine, sinuous collagen fibres, among which mast cells can usually be found (Fig. 20.1). Excision is curative.

Neurilemmomas

Neurilemmomas arise from axon sheaths and are also uncommon. They too form painless smooth swellings.

Histologically, the appearance is distinctive, with multiple rounded masses of elongated spindle cells with palisaded nuclei (Antoni A tissue, Fig. 20.2). There is also a variable amount of unorganised loose connective tissue with scanty pleomorphic nuclei (Antoni B tissue). Excision is curative.

Fig. 20.2 Neurilemmoma. The compact bundles of fibroblast-like cells with grouped (palisaded) nuclei (Antoni A tissue) are characteristic.

Fig. 20.1 Submucosal neurofibroma. The highly cellular structure with collagenous fibrous tissue and sharp demarcation from the surrounding connective tissue are characteristic.

Lipoma and fibrolipoma

Lipomas can occasionally grow, particularly from the buccal fat pad, as soft, sometimes yellowish, swellings, which may be pedunculated (Fig. 20.3). They grow slowly and cause no symptoms unless bitten, or become conspicuous because of their size.

Histologically, lipomas consist of globules of fat supported by areolar tissue (Fig. 20.4). Sometimes, fibrous tissue forms a large part of the tumour (fibrolipoma). They should be excised.

Granular cell tumour

Clinically, granular cell tumours typically form painless smooth swellings. The tongue is the most common site.

Pathology. Large granular cells form the bulk of the lesion but pseudoepitheliomatous hyperplasia of the overlying epithelium may be conspicuous (Fig. 20.5). Electron microscopy sug-

Fig. 20.3   Lipoma of the cheek. The tumour forms a pale, very soft yellowish swelling.

Fig. 20.5   Granular cell tumour. The irregular proliferation of the epithelium (pseudoepitheliomatous hyperplasia) may mimic a squamous carcinoma in superficial biopsy specimens.

Fig. 20.4   Lipoma. The fat cells are closely packed between septa of fibrous tissue and often only partially encapsulated at the margin.

Fig. 20.6   Granular cell tumour. At high power the granular cells apparently merging with muscle fibres are characteristic and indicate the diagnosis.

gests that the granular cells originate from Schwann cells. However, the presence of all stages of apparent transition of striped muscle cells into granular cells is a striking histological feature (Fig. 20.6). Elsewhere, the granular cells are large, with clearly-defined cell membranes and filled with eosinophilic granules.

The pseudoepitheliomatous hyperplasia is such that granular cell tumours have been mistaken histologically for carcinomas, with resulting overtreatment. Simple excision should, however, be curative.

Congenital (granular cell) epulis

The rare congenital epulis is typically present at birth as a smooth but prominent soft nodule, usually on the alveolar ridge (Fig. 20.7). Females are predominantly affected and occasionally the mass is so large as to obstruct respiration.

Histologically, large pale granular cells with sharply-defined cell membranes are covered by epithelium which lacks pseudoepitheliomatous hyperplasia. Immunohistochemistry suggests that the origin is myogenous.

Excision is curative but spontaneous regression is also seen.

Fig. 20.7 Congenital epulis. A firm pink non-ulcerated nodule on the alveolar ridge of a neonate is the typical presentation.

Fig. 20.8 Cavernous haemangioma of the cheek. The colour is deep purple and the structure, a mass of thin-walled blood sinuses is visible through the thin epithelium. A mass engorged with blood and as prominent as this is liable to be bitten and bleed profusely.

Fig. 20.9 Capillary haemangioma. Numerous large and small closely packed capillary vessels extend from the epithelium into the deeper tissues.

Haemangiomas

Haemangiomas are mostly vascular malformations. Vascular neoplasms (apart from Kaposi's sarcoma) are rare.

Haemangiomas may be localised but are occasionally diffuse and associated with similarly affected areas of the face. Rarely, the meninges are also involved, causing epilepsy and mental defect (Sturge–Weber syndrome). Isolated haemangiomas form purple, flat or nodular lesions which blanch on pressure (Fig. 20.8).

Histologically, haemangiomas are either capillary, cavernous or mixed. The capillary type consists of innumerable minute blood vessels and vasoformative tissue — mere rosettes of endothelial cells (Fig. 20.9). The cavernous type consists of large, blood-filled sinusoids.

Excision of mucosal haemangiomas should be avoided unless trauma causes repeated episodes of bleeding. Cryosurgery may allow removal of a haemangioma without excessive bleeding.

Lymphangioma

These uncommon tumours usually form pale, translucent,

smooth or nodular elevations of the mucosa. However, they may be noticed because they suddenly swell and become dark purple due to bleeding into the lymphatic spaces. Rarely lymphangiomas are diffuse and extensive, and cause generalised enlargement of the tongue (macroglossia) or lip (Fig. 20.10).

Histologically, lymphangiomas consist of thin-walled vascular spaces containing pinkish amorphous material as a result of fixation of lymph (Fig. 20.11).

Localised lymphangiomas can be excised but this is more difficult in the diffuse type, where the operation may have to be done in stages.

MALIGNANT CONNECTIVE TISSUE TUMOURS

Sarcomas of virtually any type can affect the oral soft tissues, but most are rare. Kaposi's sarcoma has become the most common type, but among HIV-negative persons rhabdomyosarcoma is the most common. Sarcomas tend to affect a considerably younger age group than carcinomas, and rhabdomyosarcomas in particular may be seen in children. Sarcomas grow rapidly, are invasive, destroy surrounding tissues, and usually spread by the bloodstream. Many sarcomas are clinically indistinguish-

Fig. 20.10 Lymphangioma of the lip. The lip and tongue are common sites for lymphangioma and a characteristic swelling such as this is sometimes produced.

Fig. 20.11 Lymphangioma. There is a localised aggregation of cavernous lymphatics which formed a pale superficial swelling. Bleeding into these lesions causes them suddenly to become purple or almost black.

able from one another, but others such as Kaposi's sarcoma and malignant melanoma are pigmented and must be differentiated from benign pigmented lesions.

Rhabdomyosarcoma

Rhabdomyosarcomas can affect children or young adults and form rapidly growing soft swellings.

Histologically, several types are recognised. The embryonal type, which more frequently affects children, consists of cells of variable shape and size. Some are strap- or tadpole-shaped, while muscle-like cells with cross-striations may be difficult to find. The alveolar type consists of slit-like spaces into which hang tear-shaped, darkly-staining cells attached to the walls. These alveoli are separated by a fibrous stroma.

Treatment is by excision and combination chemotherapy but the prognosis is poor.

Fibrosarcoma

Fibrosarcomas consist of broad interlacing bands of fibroblasts

Fig. 20.12 Fibrosarcoma of the tongue. There are streams of neoplastic fibroblasts, but the striking feature is the dense masses of spindle-shaped, darkly staining nuclei and their variation in size.

with a streaming or herring-bone pattern (Fig. 20.12). Some produce abundant collagen; others are highly cellular with close-packed nuclei, among which there are often mitoses.

Treatment is by radical excision. Local recurrence and spread are common but metastasis is rare.

Kaposi's sarcoma

Since the outbreak of AIDS, Kaposi's sarcoma has become the most common type of intraoral sarcoma. It mainly affects male homosexuals with AIDS, and rarely intravenous drug addicts or haemophiliacs who have acquired HIV infection from blood products.

Within the mouth, the palate is the most frequent site and the tumour appears as a purplish area or nodule which bleeds readily (Fig. 20.13). In any male below the age of about 50 with such a lesion, Kaposi's sarcoma must be excluded, as (in the absence of immunosuppressive treatment) it is pathognomonic of AIDS. Kaposi's sarcoma is occasionally the first manifestation of HIV infection but is usually associated with a low CD4 count and opportunistic infections. Human herpes virus 8 (HHV-8) DNA can be found in Kaposi's sarcoma cells and patients with both HIV and HHV-8 infection appear to have a high risk of developing Kaposi's sarcoma.

Fig. 20.13 Kaposi's sarcoma. Lesions are red, maroon or bluish and highly vascular. They may be flat or form tumour masses and the gingivae or palate are characteristic sites. (By kind permission of Professor W H Binnie.)

Fig. 20.14 Kaposi's sarcoma. The tumour is composed of spindled and plump cells with cytological atypia and frequent mitoses. Many of the small holes visible are the result of formation of capillaries.

Histologically, Kaposi's sarcoma is a vascular tumour in which factor VIII antigen (a marker for endothelial cells) can be identified. The early 'presarcomatous' lesion consists of a mass of capillary-sized blood vessels, sometimes with mononuclear cell cuffing. It resembles granulation tissue, particularly in the mouth where superficial lesions can be traumatised and become secondarily inflamed. Later, there is increasingly widespread angiomatous proliferation, and in some areas the vessels may be slit-shaped when obliquely sectioned. There is also proliferation of angular or spindle-shaped interstitial cells (Fig. 20.14). Ultimately, the latter predominate and show increasing numbers of mitoses. Central necrosis may develop and extravasation of red cells can leave deposits of haemosiderin.

Associated HIV infection is usually suggested by other clinical manifestations (such as opportunistic infections) and lymphopenia in the blood picture.

Kaposi's sarcoma must be distinguished from AIDS-associated thrombocytopenic purpura, which may appear similar clinically. However, purpura may be seen earlier and is distinguishable by haematological testing. Key features are summarised in Table 20.1.

Table 20.1   Kaposi's sarcoma — key features
● The most common type of oral sarcoma ● Most common in male homosexuals with AIDS ● Appears clinically as a flat or nodular purplish area ● Consists histologically of minute, proliferating blood vessels ● Good response to radio- or chemotherapy while localised ● May be widely disseminated when oral lesions appear ● Death more frequently from associated opportunistic infections

Other sarcomas of oral soft tissues

Neurofibrosarcomas, liposarcomas, leiomyosarcomas and even soft-tissue osteosarcomas and chondrosarcomas may be seen, but all are rare.

LYMPHOMAS

Lymphomas can arise from any type of lymphocyte, but most frequently from B cells. They are all malignant. They comprise Hodgkin's disease and the more common non-Hodgkin's lymphoma. Lymphomas relatively frequently involve the cervical lymph nodes but are rare in the mouth. However, in AIDS, lymphomas may account for 2% of oral neoplasms.

Non-Hodgkin's lymphomas

Adults are predominantly affected, and, within the mouth, lymphomas form nondescript, usually soft, painless swellings, which may become ulcerated by trauma.

Histologically, lymphomas frequently present difficulties of precise diagnosis. Non-Hodgkin's lymphomas may be *diffuse* and appear as solid sheets of lymphocytes, which may be predominantly small or large. Alternatively, they may have a *follicular* pattern. Most follicular lymphomas are low grade and have a better prognosis. The neoplastic lymphocytes show varying degrees of differentiation from mature small cells to large immunoblasts which may resemble histiocytes (Fig. 20.15). Most are of B cell origin (Fig. 20.16).

Invasion of adjacent tissues may be seen and helps to confirm the malignant nature of these tumours (Fig. 20.17). If traumatised, inflammatory cells can obscure the lymphomatous nature of the tumour. However, lymphoma cells are monoclonal and this can be recognised by immunohistochemistry by production of κ or λ light chains only.

Fig. 20.15 High-grade non-Hodgkin lymphoma. Neoplastic lymphocytes with large vescicular nuclei are packed in confluent sheets. Mitotic figures are numerous.

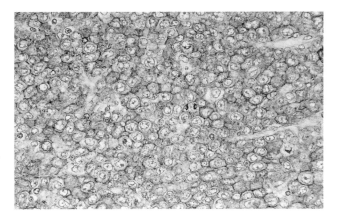

Fig. 20.16 High-grade lymphoma. Immunocytochemistry for a B cell marker produces a ring of positive brown stain on the membrane of virtually every tumour cell, indicating its B cell origin.

Fig. 20.17 High-grade non-Hodgkin lyphoma. Small darkly staining lymphoma cells infiltrating through muscle and fat.

Management

As well as biopsy, staging is necessary to determine the extent

Fig. 20.18 Burkitt's lymphoma. Small darkly staining neoplastic lymphocytes form sheets in which the macrophages containing cellular debris form round, pale holes (starry sky appearance).

of spread. In general, localised disease is treated by irradiation, while disseminated disease (the majority of patients) is treated by combination chemotherapy. Oral complications of treatment, such as ulceration and infection, are common.

Burkitt's lymphoma

This was the first lymphoma where an association with the Epstein–Barr virus (EBV) was shown. It is predominantly extranodal. It is unusual in that its onset is in childhood and it is endemic in East Africa. It is also unusual in that the jaw is the single most common initial site, and spread to the parotid glands is common. Over 95% of cases respond completely to single-dose chemotherapy.

Histologically, Burkitt's lymphoma is a small cell lymphoma containing scattered pale macrophages which give the dark sheets of cells a so-called 'starry sky' appearance (Fig. 20.18). Lymphomas resembling Burkitt's lymphoma microscopically can also be a complication of immunosuppressive treatment or AIDS but do not behave like African Burkitt's lymphoma.

Nasopharyngeal (T cell) lymphoma is a rare cause of midline granuloma syndrome (Ch. 28) and can cause swelling and ulceration of the palate as a presenting feature.

Hodgkin's disease

The cervical lymph nodes are frequently affected but lesions are exceptionally uncommon in the mouth. They are not clinically distinguishable from non-Hodgkin lymphoma.

Histologically, the characteristic features are the mixed cellular picture and occasional Reed–Sternberg giant cells with paired (mirror-image) nuclei.

Permanent cure of some types of Hodgkin's disease is possible as a result of irradiation of localised disease or combined chemotherapy, and the overall 5-year survival rate may be up to 80%.

SUGGESTED FURTHER READING

Cawson R A, Binnie W H, Eveson J W 1994 Color atlas of oral disease, 2nd edn. Mosby-Wolfe, London

Cawson R A, Langdon J D, Eveson J W 1996 Surgical pathology of the mouth and jaws. Wright, Oxford

Chen S-Y, Thakur A, Miller A S, Harwick R D 1995 Rhabdomyosarcoma of the oral cavity. Report of four cases. Oral Surg Oral Med Oral Pathol Oral Radiol Endod 80:192–201

Damm D D, Cibull M L, Geissler R H et al 1993 Investigation into the histogenesis of congenital epulis of the newborn. Oral Surg Oral Med Oral Pathol 76:202–212

DiCerbo M, Sciubba J J, Sordill W C, DeLuke D M 1992 Malignant schwannoma of the palate: a case report and review of the literature. J Oral Maxillofac Surg 50:1217–1221

El Naggar A K, Batsakis J G, Ordonez N G et al 1993 Rhabdomyosarcoma of the adult head and neck: a clinicopathological and DNA ploidy study. J Laryngol Otol 107:716–720

Enzinger F M, Weiss S W 1995 Soft tissue tumors, 3rd edn. Mosby, St Louis

Geist J R, Gander D L, Stefanac S J 1992 Oral manifestations of neurofibromatosis types I and II. Oral Surg Oral Med Oral Pathol 73:376–382

Greager J A, Reichard K, Campana J P, Das Gupta T K 1994 Fibrosarcoma of the head and neck. Am J Surg 167:437–439

Hajdu S I 1993 Peripheral nerve sheath tumours. Histogenesis, classification and prognosis. Cancer 72:3549–3552

Herdier B G, Kaplan L D, McGrath M S 1994 Pathogenesis of AIDS lymphomas. AIDS 8:1025–1049

Hirshberg A, Leibovich P, Buchner A 1993 Metastases to the oral mucosa: analysis of 157 cases. J Oral Pathol Med 22:385–390

Kraus D H, Dubner S, Harrison L B et al 1994 Prognostic factors for recurrence and survival in head and neck soft tissue sarcomas. Cancer 74:697–702

Mark R J, Sercarz J A, Tran L, Selch M, Calcaterra T C 1991 Fibrosarcoma of the head and neck. Arch Otolaryngol Head Neck Surg 117:396–401

Meehan S, Davis V, Brahim J S 1994 Embryonal rhabdomyosarcoma of the floor of the mouth. A case report. Oral Surg Oral Med Oral Pathol 78:603–606

Noel J-C, Hermans P, Andre J et al 1996 Herpesvirus-like DNA sequences in Kaposi's sarcoma. Cancer 77:2132–2136

Peszkowski M J, Larsson A 1990 Extraosseous and intraosseous oral traumatic neuromas and their association with tooth extraction. J Oral Maxillofac Surg 48:963–967

Regezi J A, MacPhail L A, Daniels T E et al 1993 Oral Kaposi's sarcoma: a 10-year retrospective histopathologic study. J Oral Pathol Med 11:292–297

Shapiro S D, Abramovitch K, Van Dis M L 1984 Neurofibromatosis: oral and radiographic manifestations. Oral Surg Oral Med Oral Pathol 58:493–498

Stewart C M, Watson RE, Eversole L R et al 1988 Oral granular cell tumors: a clinicopathologic and immunocytochemical study. Oral Surg Oral Med Oral Pathol 65:427–435

Tran L M, Mark R, Meier R, Calcaterra T C, Parker R G 1992 Sarcomas of the head and neck. Cancer 70:160–177

Wang M B, Strasnick B, Zimmerman M C 1992 Extranodal Burkitt's lymphoma of the head and neck. Arch Otolaryngol Head Neck Surg 118:193–199

Wolvius E B, van der Valk P, van der Wal J E et al 1994 Primary extranodal non-Hodgkin lymphoma of the oral cavity. An analysis of 34 cases. Oral Oncol Eur J Cancer 30B:121–125

Zuker R M, Buenchea R 1993 Congenital epulis: review of the literature and report of a case. J Oral Maxillofac Surg 51:1040–1043

Melanoma and other pigmented lesions

Melanoma is a highly malignant oral tumour. It usually appears as a pigmented patch which must be distinguished from many other pigmentations (Table 21.1).

Table 21.1   Oral pigmented lesions

Usually brown or black	Typically purple or red
Malignant melanoma	Amelanotic melanomas
Pigmented naevi	Erythroplasia (Ch. 16)
Amalgam tattoo	Haemangiomas (Ch. 20)
Addison's disease (Ch. 31)	Kaposi's sarcoma (Ch. 20)
Peutz–Jeghers syndrome	Purpura (Ch. 23)
Racial pigmentation	Other blood blisters
Lichen planus rarely (Ch. 13)	Telangiectases
	Lingual varices (Ch. 14)
	Pyogenic granuloma (Ch. 19)
	Pregnancy epulis (Ch. 19)
	Giant cell epulis (Ch. 19)
	Geographical tongue (Ch. 14)
	Erythematous candidosis (Ch. 12)
	Median rhomboid glossitis (Ch. 14)

Racial pigmentation

This is the most common cause of oral pigmentation. The gingivae are particularly affected (Fig. 21.1). The inner aspect of the lips is typically spared.

Fig. 21.1   Racial pigmentation. The distribution of melanotic mucosa around the gingival margin is characteristic.

Lesions of lichen planus can also become pigmented, often intensely in association with racial pigmentation (Fig. 21.2).

Amalgam tattoo

Fragments of amalgam frequently become embedded in the oral mucosa and form the most common pigmented patches, which may simulate melanomas clinically. They are usually close to the dental arch and typically 5 mm or more across (Fig. 21.3). Dense tattoos may be radiopaque.

Pathology

Amalgam is seen as brown or black granules, deposited particularly along collagen bundles and around small blood vessels (Fig. 21.4). There may be no inflammatory reaction or there may be a foreign body reaction with amalgam granules in the macrophages or giant cells.

Excision is necessary to exclude a melanoma.

Peutz–Jeghers syndrome

This autosomal dominant syndrome comprises intestinal poly-

Fig. 21.2   Pigmented lichen planus. Inflammatory conditions may become pigmented, especially in dark skinned races. Here melanin delineates mucosa affected by lichen planus.

Fig. 21.3 Amalgam tattoo. The colour ranges from light brown through dark blue to black and the floor of mouth and gingivae are common sites. There are almost always adjacent teeth with restorations (the lower second premolar is crowned).

Fig. 21.4 Amalgam tattoo. There are large fragments of amalgam surrounded by foreign body giant cells and macrophages and smaller particles dispersed in fibrous tissue. Silver leeching from the smaller fragments has stained the adjacent collagen brown.

posis and melanotic macules, particularly of the face and mouth.

There are multiple freckles on the lips and oral mucosa. Facial pigmentation (mainly around the mouth, eyes and nose) usually fades after puberty, but mucosal pigmentation persists (Fig. 21.5). Microscopy shows increased melanin in the basal keratinocytes.

Polyps may be present throughout the gastrointestinal tract (Ch. 29).

Oral melanotic naevi

Pigmented naevi are benign lesions of melanocytes which form

Fig. 21.5 Peutz–Jehgers syndrome. There are multiple flat, pigmented patches on the palate. Those on the lips are most characteristic but fade with age.

Fig. 21.6 Melanocytic naevi. These flat, pigmented patches are occasionally found on the lip and intraorally.

circumscribed brown to black patches about 5 or 6 mm across (Fig. 21.6). They are asymptomatic but should be excised and sent for microscopy to exclude early malignant melanoma.

Pathology

The main features are modest numbers of pigmented melanocytes in the basal cell layer but many clumps of melanocytes in the corium (Fig. 21.7). Rarely, intraepithelial foci of proliferating melanocytes project into the corium and appear to be dropping off the basal layer (junctional activity). Equally rarely, junctional activity is associated with circumscribed nests of melanocytes in a limited area of the upper corium (compound naevus).

Blue naevus

The epithelium is normal, but beneath and separate from it is a focus of spindle-shaped pigmented melanocytes.

All these types of naevi should be excised and sent for histology.

Fig. 21.7   Intramucosal naevus. A cluster of naevus cells lies in the connective tissue separated from the epithelium by a layer of normal fibrous tissue.

Fig. 21.8   Melanotic patch. There is poorly-demarcated pigmentation of varying density in the palate. All pigmented lesions such as this should be treated with the utmost suspicion and biopsied to exclude melanoma.

MALIGNANT MELANOMA

Intraoral melanomas are rare. They are usually dark brown or black or, if non-pigmented, red. The peak age incidence is between 40 and 60. They are macular or nodular and may ulcerate: the palate is most frequently affected (Fig. 21.8). They are typically firm and rubbery but asymptomatic at first. Hence melanomas may remain unnoticed until they cause soreness, bleeding or a neck mass, unless noticed by chance.

Early diagnosis by biopsy is essential.

Fig. 21.9   Superficial spreading melanoma. Numerous pigmented and atypical melanocytes form nests and clusters along the basement membrane and are present within the epithelium and superficial connective tissue.

Fig. 21.10   Melanoma. Malignant spindled and round melanocytes, often with bizarre nuclei and some with melanin pigment, invading deep tissue.

Pathology

Melanomas consist of neoplastic melanocytes, often surrounded by clear haloes, both within the epithelium and invading deeper tissues. These cells are round to spindle-shaped and typically speckled or intensely pigmented with melanin (Figs 21.9 and 21.10). However, in amelanotic melanomas the absence of pigment makes these cells more difficult to recognise. Melanomas of the superficial spreading type are rare in the mouth and are usually invasive unless recognised unusually early.

The prognosis of intraoral melanomas is poor as they are frequently unrecognised until there are symptoms or involvement of lymph nodes. Distant spread is to the lungs, liver, bones and other organs.

Treatment is by radical excision and usually chemotherapy or radiotherapy, or both. In a recent series the median survival for mucosal melanomas was less than 2 years. Key features are summarised in Table 21.2.

Table 21.2 Malignant melanoma — key features

- Peak incidence between 40 and 60 years
- Usually appear as black or brown patches
- Amelanotic melanomas appear red
- Later cause soreness and bleeding
- Histologically consist of neoplastic melanocytes, often surrounded by clear haloes, within the epithelium and invading deeper tissues
- Neoplastic melanocytes are round to spindle-shaped and typically speckled or intensely pigmented with melanin
- Should be widely excised but median survival probably not longer than 2 years

Melanotic neuroectodermal tumour of infancy

One of these tumours (Ch. 9) may rarely show through the palatal mucosa as an ill-defined pigmented area in a neonate or infant.

SUGGESTED FURTHER READING

Barrett A W, Bennett J H, Speight P M 1995 A clinicopathological and immunohistochemical analysis of primary oral malignant melanoma. Oral Oncol Eur J Cancer 31B:100–115

Buchner A, Hansen L S 1980 Amalgam pigmentation (amalgam tattoo) of the oral mucosa: a clinicopathological study of 268 cases. Oral Surg Oral Med Oral Pathol 49:139–147

Buchner A, Hansen L S 1987 Pigmented nevi of the oral mucosa: a clinicopathologic study of 36 cases and review of 155 cases from the literature. Oral Surg Oral Med Oral Pathol 63:566–572

Cawson R A, Binnie W H, Eveson J W 1994 Color atlas of oral disease, 2nd edn. Mosby-Wolfe, London

Cawson R A, Langdon J D, Eveson J W 1996 Surgical pathology of the mouth and jaws. Wright, Oxford

Eisen D, Voorhees J J 1991 Oral melanoma and other pigmented lesions of the oral cavity. J Am Acad Dermatol 24:527–537

Ficarra G, Shillitoe E J, Adler-Storthz K et al 1990 Oral melanotic macules associated with HIV. Oral Surg Oral Med Oral Pathol 70:301–307

Gazit D, Daniels T E 1994 Oral melanocytic lesions: differences in expression of HMB-45 and S-100 antigens in round and spindle cells of malignant and benign lesions. J Oral Pathol Med 23:60–64

Kaugars G E, Heise A P, Riley W T, Abbey L M, Svirsky J A 1993 Oral melanotic macules. A review of 353 cases. Oral Surg Oral Med Oral Pathol 76:59–61

Langford A, Pohle H D, Gelderblom H et al 1989 Oral hyperpigmentation in HIV-infected patients. Oral Surg Oral Med Oral Pathol 67:301–307

Patton L L, Brahim J S, Baker A R 1994 Metastatic malignant melanoma of the oral cavity. A retrospective study. Oral Surg Oral Med Oral Pathol 78:51–56

Strauss J E, Strauss S I 1994 Oral malignant melanoma: a case report and review of literature. J Oral Maxillofac Surg 52:972–976

Umeda M, Shimada K 1994 Primary malignant melanoma of the oral cavity — its histological classification and treatment. Br J Oral Maxillofac Surg 32:39–47

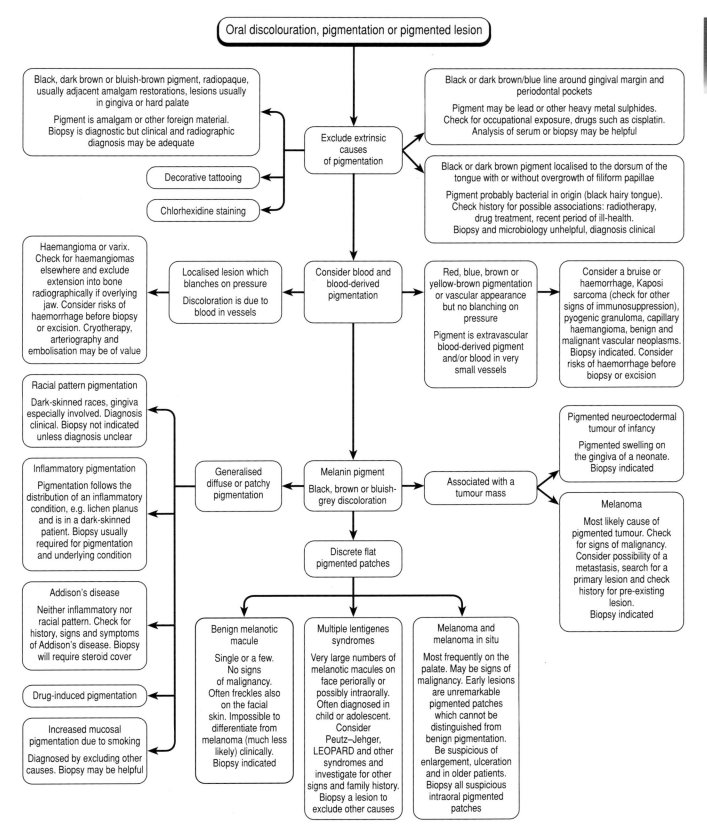

Summary 21.1   The common causes of oral pigmented lesions.

THE MEDICALLY-
COMPROMISED
PATIENT

Anaemias and leukaemias

Haematological disease is common and can cause serious complications or oral symptoms (Table 22.1).

Table 22.1 Important effects of haematological diseases

- Anaesthetic complications
- Oral infections
- Prolonged bleeding
- Mucosal lesions

Haemoglobin estimation and routine indices are informative and should be carried out when any patient has suspicious signs in the mouth or has to undergo oral surgery.

ANAEMIA

Causes and important types are summarised in Table 22.2.

Iron deficiency (microcytic) anaemia is the most common type and usually results from chronic menstrual blood loss. Women of child-bearing age or over, or men with peptic ulcer or haemorrhoids, are mainly affected.

Pernicious anaemia chiefly affects women of middle age or over and is the main cause of macrocytic anaemia. Unlike other anaemias it can cause neurological disease, particularly subacute combined degeneration of the cord. Folate deficiency also causes a macrocytic anaemia, often in younger patients, particularly in pregnancy. It must be firmly differentiated from pernicious anaemia because administration of folate in the latter can worsen neurological disease.

Leukaemia is an uncommon but frequently lethal cause of normocytic anaemia, but should be suspected in an anaemic child.

Sickle cell trait is most common in immigrants from the West Indies. Sickle cell anaemia is relatively uncommon.

Thalassaemia is mainly seen in immigrants from the Mediterranean littoral.

Clinical features

Anaemia, irrespective of cause, produces essentially the same

Table 22.2 Types and features of important anaemias

Type of anaemia	Causes or effects
1. Iron deficiency (microcytic, hypochromic anaemia)	Usually due to chronic blood loss
2. Folate deficiency (macrocytic)	Pregnancy, malabsorption, alcohol*, phenytoin-induced, etc.
3. Vitamin B_{12} deficiency (macrocytic anaemia)	Usually due to pernicious anaemia, occasionally to malabsorption
4. Leukaemia and aplastic anaemia (normochromic normocytic)	Raised susceptibility to infection and bleeding tendency often associated
5. Sickle cell disease (normocytic anaemia)	Genetic. Sickle cells seen in special preparations
6. β-Thalassaemia (hypochromic, microcytic)	Genetic. Many misshapen red cells
7. Chronic inflammatory disease (normochromic, normocytic)	Rheumatoid arthritis is a common cause
8. Liver disease (usually normocytic)	Haemorrhagic tendency may be associated

*Alcoholism should always be excluded when macrocytosis in the absence of anaemia is found — it is a characteristic sign of alcoholism.

clinical features (Table 22.3), particularly if severe, but some anaemias have distinctive features.

Table 22.3 General clinical features of anaemia

- Pallor
- Fatigue and lassitude
- Breathlessness
- Tachycardia and palpitations
- Glossitis or other mucosal lesions

The complexion is a poor indicator of pallor. The conjunctiva of the lower eyelid, the nail beds, and sometimes the oral mucosa, are more reliable. Cardiovascular signs (tachycardia or oedema of the ankles) result from severe anaemia. Glossitis and other mucosal diseases (Table 22.4), by contrast, can be the earliest signs, as discussed below.

Table 22.4 Features of anaemia important in dentistry

- Mucosal disease
    Glossitis
    Angular stomatitis
    Recurrent aphthae
    Infection, particularly candidosis
- Risks from general anaesthesia
    Shortage of oxygen can be dangerous
- Lowered resistance to infection
    Apart from candidosis, this is seen only in severe anaemia or
    when due to leukaemia

Mucosal disease

Glossitis

Anaemia is the most important, though not the most common, cause of a sore tongue. Soreness *can precede any fall in haemoglobin levels*, particularly when resulting from vitamin B$_{12}$ or folate deficiency, and can be their first sign. Later there may be obvious inflammation and atrophy of the filiform papillae (Fig. 22.1). Variants of sore tongue have been discussed in Chapter 14, but it is emphasised again that this symptom always requires careful haematological investigation, initially by means of a haemoglobin level and routine indices. Serum iron, ferritin and folate levels may be required. Even though the haemoglobin may be within normal limits, enlarged erythrocytes (mean corpuscular volume (MCV >96 fl) frequently indicate pernicious anaemia. If any deficiency is found, the underlying cause, such as gastrointestinal disease, must be investigated.

Recurrent aphthae

Aphthae are sometimes secondary to haematological deficiency, particularly of vitamin B$_{12}$ or folate, in patients whose aphthae start or worsen late in life.

Candidosis and angular stomatitis

Iron deficiency, in particular, is a predisposing factor for candidosis (Ch. 12). Angular stomatitis is also a classical sign of iron deficiency anaemia and due to candidosis.

Dangers of general anaesthesia

Any reduction of oxygenation can precipitate irreparable brain damage or myocardial infarction when there is significant anaemia. General anaesthesia should therefore be given in hospital. The dangers are particularly great in sickle cell disease, as discussed later.

Lowered resistance to infection

Oral candidosis is the main example but, in the past particularly, osteomyelitis could follow extractions in severe anaemia (Fig. 22.2). Currently, sickle cell disease is more important in this context.

Fig. 22.1 Iron deficiency anaemia. The tongue is slightly reddened, smooth and depapillated. There is also angular cheilitis as a result of candidal infection.

Fig. 22.2 Acute osteomyelitis in an anaemic patient. Widespread bone destruction followed straightforward extraction of the posterior teeth. The patient was found to have a haemoglobin level of 30%.

SICKLE CELL DISEASE AND SICKLE CELL TRAIT

Sickle cell anaemia mainly affects people of African, Afro-Caribbean, Indian, Mediterranean or Middle Eastern origin. About 5000 persons in Britain are estimated to have sickle cell disease (homozygotes), but many more have sickle cell trait (heterozygotes). The defect in sickle cell disease is an abnormal haemoglobin (HbS), with the risk of haemolysis, anaemia and other effects. In heterozygotes, sufficient normal haemoglobin (HbA) is formed to allow normal life with only rare complications.

Sickle cell disease. The complications arise from polymerisation of deoxygenated HbS, which is less soluble than HbA. This forms long fibres which deform the red cells into sickle shapes and makes them vulnerable to haemolysis. Chronic haemolysis causes chronic anaemia but patients, under normal circumstances, typically feel well, as HbS more readily releases its oxygen content to the tissues than HbA. Exacerbation of sickling raises blood viscosity, causing blocking of capillaries and sickling crises (Tables 22.5 and 22.6).

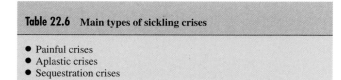

Table 22.5 **Factors that can precipitate sickling crises**

- Hypoxia, particulaly from poorly conducted anaesthesia
- Dehydration
- Infections (including dental)
- Acidosis and fever

These patients are also abnormally susceptible to infection, particularly pneumococcal or meningococcal, and osteomyelitis.

Table 22.6 **Main types of sickling crises**

- Painful crises
- Aplastic crises
- Sequestration crises

Painful crises are caused by blockage of blood vessels and bone marrow infarcts. Painful crises can affect the jaws, particularly the mandible, and mimic acute osteomyelitis. The infarcted tissue forms a focus susceptible to infection, and salmonella osteomyelitis is a recognised hazard.

Aplastic crises are caused by human parvovirus B19 infection and require immediate transfusion.

Sequestration crises result from sickle cells pooling in the spleen, liver or lungs. An acute chest syndrome, characterised by pain, fever and leucocytosis, is the most common cause of death.

Dental aspects of sickle cell trait and disease

Sickling trait should be suspected, particularly in those of Afro-Caribbean origin, and investigated if anaesthesia is anticipated.

If the haemoglobin is less than 10 g/dl the patient is probably a homozygote with sickle cell disease. Screening tests depend on the lower solubility of HbS which produces turbidity when a reducing agent is added. Confirmation is by electrophoresis.

In those with sickle cell trait the main precaution is that general anaesthesia should be carried out with full oxygenation. In sickle cell disease the oral mucosa may be pale or yellowish due to haemolytic jaundice. Radiographic changes can be seen in the skull and sometimes the jaws (Ch. 10).

Occasionally, crises may be precipitated by dental infections such as acute pericoronitis. Prompt antibiotic treatment is therefore important. Painful bone infarcts should be treated with non-steroidal anti-inflammatory analgesics, and fluid intake should be increased. Admission to hospital is required for severe painful crises not responsive to analgesics. Rigorous routine dental care is necessary because of the increased susceptibility to infection.

THE THALASSAEMIAS

α-thalassaemias mainly affect Asians, Africans and Afro-Caribbeans, while β-thalassaemias mainly affect those from the Mediterranean littoral, such as Greeks (thalassaemia — literally, 'sea in the blood').

Thalassaemias result from diminished synthesis of one or more of the globin chains of haemoglobin. The resulting relative excess of either the α- or β-globin chains, which are unstable, causes them to precipite in the red cells. Haemolysis can result.

The severity of the disease depends on the numbers of α- or β-globin genes affected. In simplified terms the diseases are thalassaemia minor in heterozygotes and thalassaemia major in homozygotes.

Thalassaemia minor causes mild but persistent microcytic anaemia but is otherwise asymptomatic, apart sometimes from splenomegaly. Iron therapy is ineffective and leads to iron deposition in the tissues.

Thalassaemia major (usually homozygous β-thalassaemia) causes severe hypochromic, microcytic anaemia, great enlargement of liver and spleen and skeletal abnormalities (Ch. 10) due to marrow expansion. There is failure to thrive and early death if regular transfusions are not given. These are life-saving and prevent the development of bony deformities, but lead to progressive iron deposition in the tissues. Haemosiderosis is the main cause of complications in survivors and leads to dysfunction of glands and other organs. Xerostomia can result from iron deposition in the salivary glands. Desferrioxamine, a chelating agent, may lessen the effects of iron overload, and folic acid treatment may ameliorate the haemolytic anaemia.

LEUKAEMIA

The effect of leukaemic overproduction of white cells is to suppress other cell lines of the marrow (Table 22.7). Leukaemia can affect virtually any of the white cell series but different types of acute leukaemia cannot be distinguished clinically.

Acute leukaemia

Acute lymphoblastic leukaemia is the most common leukaemia in children (usually between 3 and 5 years), while acute myeloblastic anaemia is the most common type in adults.

Table 22.7 Major effects of acute leukaemia
• Anaemia due to suppression of erythrocyte production
• Raised susceptibility to infection due to deficiency or abnormalities of granulocytes
• Bleeding tendency (purpura) due to suppression of platelet production

Splenomegaly or hepatomegaly or both, and lymphadenopathy, particularly in lymphoblastic leukaemia, are usually associated. Mucosal pallor or abnormal gingival bleeding, particularly in a child, strongly suggest acute leukaemia (Table 22.8). Diagnosis depends on the peripheral blood picture and marrow biopsy.

Table 22.8 Oral and perioral effects of acute leukaemia
• Gingival swelling
• Mucosal ulceration
• Leukaemic deposits
• Purpura
• Anaemia
• Cervical lymphadenopathy

Gingival swelling results from lack of healthy white cells to counter low-grade gingival infection. The gingivae become packed and swollen with leukaemic cells, particularly in acute myelogenous leukaemia in adults. The gingivae are often purplish and may become necrotic and ulcerate (Figs 22.3 and 22.4).

Mucosal ulceration is often a combined effect of immunodeficiency and cytotoxic drugs such as methotrexate. Herpetic infections and thrush are common, and ulceration may be caused by a variety of opportunistic microbes. Also as a result of the immunodeficiency, the first sign of acute leukaemia may occasionally be an infection such as acute osteomyelitis following routine extractions.

Leukaemic deposits are tumour-like masses of leukaemic cells which may occasionally form in the mouth or salivary glands (Fig. 22.5).

Purpura can appear as excessive gingival bleeding, purplish mucosal patches, blood blisters or prolonged bleeding after

Fig. 22.3   Acute monocytic leukaemia. The gingivae are grossly swollen and purplish; in addition there is ulceration along the palatal aspect of the anterior teeth resulting from the increased susceptibility to infection.

Fig. 22.4   Acute leukaemia. The gingivae and bone marrow of the interdental bone contain a confluent infiltrate of leukaemic cells.

surgery. Leukaemic infiltration of an extraction socket can delay healing (Fig. 22.6).

Anaemia can cause mucosal pallor and is an important sign in children, among whom anaemia is otherwise uncommon.

Cervical lymphadenopathy is particularly common in lymphocytic leukaemia but may be seen in other types or be secondary to opportunistic infections in the mouth.

Management

Biopsy of gingival swelling unresponsive to conventional treatment may lead to the diagnosis of leukaemia.

Fig. 22.5   Myeloid leukaemia. An ulcerated tumour mass formed by leukaemic cells emigrating into the tissues.

Fig. 22.6   Delayed healing of an extraction socket in acute leukaemia. The socket has become filled with a dense mass of leukaemic cells, and healing has not got beyond early organisation of the clot. The lamina dura has been resorbed, but there is no new bone formation.

Ideally, patients with leukaemia, or any others having cytotoxic treatment, should have vigorous oral hygiene to control the bacterial population *before* complications develop.

Mouth rinses (0.2% chlorhexidine or tetracycline and amphotericin) will often control severe gingival changes and superficial infections. Mucosal ulceration by Gram-negative bacilli or anaerobes may need specific antibiotic therapy, which is also necessary to prevent systemic spread of infection.

Oral ulceration caused by methotrexate may be controlled by giving folinic acid. Extractions should be avoided because of the risks of severe infections, bleeding or anaemia. If unavoidable, blood transfusion and generous antibiotic cover are required.

Chronic leukaemia

Chronic leukaemia is a slowly progressive disease of adults. Chronic lymphocytic leukaemia can be completely asymptomatic and may not even shorten life.

Oral manifestations (Table 22.9) are relatively uncommon or mild.

Table 22.9   Possible oral effects of chronic leukaemia
● Mucosal pallor ● Gingival or palatal swelling ● Purpura ● Oral ulceration*
*Ulceration may be due to infection or cytotoxic drugs or both.

Management

Routine dentistry can usually be carried out with normal care. If there is significant anaemia, bleeding tendencies or susceptibility to infection, similar precautions need to be taken to those for acute leukaemia.

LEUKOPENIA AND AGRANULOCYTOSIS

Leukopenia is a deficiency of white cells (fewer than $5000^3/l$) with many possible causes (Table 22.10). It is a peripheral blood manifestation of actual or incipient immunodeficiency.

Leukopenia can be a chance haematological finding and may cause no symptoms until it becomes so severe as to impair defences against infection. Thus lymphopenia in an apparently healthy person may be a sign of HIV infection.

Table 22.10   Important causes of leukopenia
● Leukaemia ● Aplastic anaemia ● Drugs (Table 22.11) ● Autoimmune ● HIV infection

Agranulocytosis

Agranulocytosis is the term given to the clinical effects of severe neutropenia, namely fever, prostration and mucosal ulceration, particularly of the gingivae and pharynx.

Table 22.11 Important causes of drug-induced leukopenia

- Analgesics, especially phenylbutazone*
- Antibacterial drugs, especially chloramphenicol or (rarely) co-trimoxazole
- Phenothiazine antipsychotic drugs
- Antithyroid drugs such as thiouracil
- Cytotoxic drugs

*Use now restricted as a consequence.

Table 22.12 Principles of general and dental management of leukopenia

General
Stop any drug which may be causative
Give antibiotics
Give blood transfusions if necessary

Dental
Optimise oral hygiene
Control oral infections (as for acute leukaemia)
Avoid extractions
Antibiotic cover and transfusions if necessary if surgery is unavoidable

Drug-induced leukopenia (Table 22.11)

Management (Table 22.12)

Aplastic anaemia

Aplastic anaemia is failure of production of all bone marrow cells (pancytopenia). The systemic and oral effects are not unlike those of acute leukaemia (purpura, anaemia and susceptibility to infection). Aplastic anaemia may be of unknown cause but is probably autoimmune. Otherwise drugs (see Table 22.11) are the main cause.

The management is to stop any drugs that may be responsi-ble and to give antibiotics and transfusions. Nevertheless, approximately 50% of patients die within 6 months, usually from infection or haemorrhage, but marrow transplantation has occasionally been successful. Dental management is as for acute leukaemia.

Cyclic neutropenia

In cyclic neutropenia there is a fall in the number of circulating neutrophils at regular intervals of 3–4 weeks. There have been only about 40 reported cases in 70 years and undue emphasis has been placed on the fact that cyclic neutropenia occasionally, but not necessarily, causes oral ulceration or rapidly progressive periodontitis.

SUGGESTED FURTHER READING

Banerjee A K, Layton D M, Rennie J A et al 1991 Safe surgery in sickle cell disease. Br J Surg 78:516–519

Cranfield T, Bunch C 1995 Acute leukaemias. Medicine UK 23:503–509

Field E A, Speechley J A, Rugman F R 1995 Oral signs and symptoms in patients with undiagnosed vitamin B_{12} deficiency. J Oral Pathol Med 24:468–470

Gregory G, Olujohungbe A 1994 Mandibular nerve neuropathy in sickle cell disease. Local factors. Oral Surg Oral Med Oral Pathol 77:66–69

Hatton C, Mackie P H 1996 Haemoglobinopathies and other congenital haemolytic anaemias. Medicine Int 24:14–19

Higgs D R 1993 The thalassaemia syndromes. Q J M ed 86:559–564

Luker J, Scully C, Oakhill A 1991 Gingival swelling as a manifestation of aplastic anaemia. Oral Surg Oral Med Oral Pathol 70:55–56

O'Connor N, Bunch C 1995 Laboratory diagnosis in haematology. Medicine Int 23:489–494

O'Rourke C, Mitropoulos C 1990 Orofacial pain in patients with sickle cell disease. Br Dent J 169:130–132

Pippard M J, Heppleston A D 1996 Microcytic and macrocytic anaemias. Medicine Int 24:4–10

Podlesh S W, Boyden D K 1996 Diagnosis of acute bone/bone marrow infarction of the mandible in sickle hemoglobinopathy. Report of a case. Oral Surg Oral Med Oral Pathol Oral Radiol Endod 81:547–549

Sansevere J J, Miles M 1993 Management of the oral and maxillofacial patient with sickle cell disease and related haemoglobinopathies. J Oral Maxillofac Surg 51:912–916

Haemorrhagic diseases

Purpura (usually platelet defects) and clotting defects are the main causes of haemorrhagic disorders.

Investigation of a history of excessive bleeding

A careful history (Table 23.1) is absolutely essential. Most of the severe haemorrhagic diseases such as haemophilia are hereditary and a positive family history should be carefully evaluated. Bleeding for up to 24 hours after an extraction is usually due to local causes or a minor defect of haemostasis manageable by local measures. More prolonged bleeding is significant. Even a *mild* haemophilic can bleed for weeks after a simple extraction.

Table 23.1 **Information required about haemorrhagic tendencies**

1. Results of previous dental operations? Have simple extractions lead to prolonged bleeding?
2. Has bleeding persisted for more than 24 hours?
3. Has admission to hospital ever been necessary for dental bleeding?
4. Have other operations or injuries caused prolonged bleeding?
5. Is there a family history of prolonged bleeding?
6. Are anticoagulants or other drugs being taken?
7. Is there any medical cause such as leukaemia or liver disease?
8. Does the patient carry a warning card or hospital letter about bleeding tendencies?

Clinical examination

Signs of anaemia and purpura should be looked for. Examination of the mouth shows how any operation should be planned. In the case of haemophilia, all essential extractions should be carried out at a single operation with factor VIII cover. Radiographs should be taken to anticipate possible difficulties in the extractions.

Laboratory investigations

Details of investigations are decided by the haematologist, but are summarised in Table 23.2.

Table 23.2 **Important investigations in haemophilia**

- Haemoglobin level and blood picture
- Assessment of haemostatic function, particularly:
  Bleeding time
  Prothrombin time (expressed as the INR)
  Activated partial thromboplastin time
  Thrombin time
- Blood grouping and cross-matching

It is essential to look for anaemia. It is an almost inevitable result of repeated bleeding and is worsened by any further bleeding as a result of surgery. Anaemia increases the risks of general anaesthesia and should be treated before any surgery. Anaemia is also an essential feature of some haemorrhagic diseases, particularly acute leukaemia.

Blood grouping is required as transfusions may be needed before operation to improve haemostasis, or afterwards if blood loss is severe.

PURPURA

Purpura is typically the result of platelet disorders (Table 23.3) and is relatively rarely caused by vascular defects. The bleeding time is prolonged but clotting function is normal. An exception is von Willebrand's disease, where there is an associated deficiency of a clotting factor.

General features of purpura

Purpura (bleeding into the skin or mucous membranes, causing petechiae or ecchymoses or 'spontaneous bruising') also causes prolonged bleeding after injury or surgery. Unlike haemophilia, haemorrhage immediately follows the trauma but, usually, bleeding in purpura ultimately stops spontaneously as a result of normal coagulation.

Many women will say that they bruise easily, but such bruises are usually only a few millimetres across. The most informative test of platelet function is the *bleeding time*, supplemented as necessary by tests of platelet aggregation and adhesion.

Table 23.3 Causes of purpura

Platelet disorders
- Idiopathic thrombocytopenic purpura
- Connective tissue diseases (especially systemic lupus erythematosus)
- Acute leukaemias
- Drug-associated
- HIV infection

Vascular disorders
- von Willebrand's disease
- Corticosteroid treatment
- Ehlers–Danlos syndrome
- Infective

Fig. 23.2 Systemic purpura.

Fig. 23.1 and 23.2 Systemic purpura. The lesions are due to spontaneous bleeding into the tissues and often form at sites of trauma.

Deficiency of platelets (fewer than 100 000 mm³) is termed thrombocytopenia, but spontaneous bleeding is uncommon until the count falls below 50 000 mm³.

A typical site of oral purpura is the palate where the posterior border of a denture presses into the mucosa. Excessive gingival bleeding or blood blisters are other signs (Figs 23.1 and 23.2).

Idiopathic thrombocytopenic purpura

The immediate cause is IgG autoantibodies which bind to platelets. The number of platelets in the peripheral blood is greatly reduced.

The disease may affect children or young adult women, and the first sign may be profuse gingival bleeding or postextraction

haemorrhage. More often there is spontaneous bleeding into the skin.

Management

Thrombocytopenic purpura frequently responds, at least in the short-term, to corticosteroids, which can be used for urgently needed surgery. Long-term use of corticosteroids is associated with their usual hazards. Some cases resolve spontaneously but persistent cases may respond to splenectomy. However, 10–20% of cases are unresponsive to any form of treatment, and, now that haemophilia is a manageable disease, such cases have become one of the most troublesome of the haemorrhagic diseases. For operative treatment, transfusions of platelet concentrates can be given, but immunosuppressive drugs may also have to be given to prevent platelet destruction by antibodies. As with other platelet disorders, aspirin and other anti-inflammatory analgesics should be avoided.

AIDS-associated purpura

Autoimmune thrombocytopenia can complicate HIV infection and can be an early sign. Purpuric patches in the mouth, particularly in a young male, should suggest this possibility and also need to be distinguished from oral Kaposi's sarcoma by tests of haemostasis and, if necessary, biopsy.

Drug-associated purpura

Many drugs, particularly aspirin, interfere with platelet function (Table 23.4). Others act as haptens and cause immune destruction of platelets or suppress marrow function, causing pancytopenia (aplastic anaemia), of which purpura is typically an early sign. The most frequent cause of aplastic anaemia in Britain has been phenylbutazone. If purpura develops, the drug should be stopped, but in the case of aplastic anaemia the process may be irreversible and fatal.

Table 23.4 Important causes of drug-associated thrombocytopenia

Chloramphenicol
Phenylbutazone
Indomethacin
Thiazide diuretics
Quinine and quinidine

Fig. 23.5 Localised oral purpura. A blood-filled space is seen immediately below the epithelium in this intact bulla.

Localised oral purpura

Blood blisters occasionally appear in the oral mucosa after minor or unnoticed trauma, but there is no haemostatic defect. Such blisters may form in the throat and cause a choking sensation ('angina bullosa haemorrhagica'). Rupture of a blood blister leaves an ulcer (Figs 23.3–23.5).

Systemic purpura should be excluded by haematological examination, and the patient can be reassured.

von Willebrand's disease

von Willebrand's disease is characterised both by a prolonged bleeding time and deficiency of factor VIII. It is usually inherited as an autosomal dominant trait. Both males and females are therefore affected.

The deficiency of factor VIII is usually mild compared with the platelet defect, so that purpura is the more common manifestation. However, some patients have factor VIII levels low enough to cause a significant clotting defect. The platelet defect is usually correctable with desmopressin, which may also be sufficient to correct any significant factor VIII deficiency. In unusually severe cases the deficiency of factor VIII is such that surgery has to be managed as for haemophilia A. However, factor VIII remains active in the blood for a considerably longer period.

CLOTTING DISORDERS

Important causes are shown in Table 23.5.

Fig. 23.3 Localised oral purpura. An intact blood blister on the soft palate and fauces.

Table 23.5 Important causes of coagulation defects

- Heritable deficiencies of plasma factors
  Haemophilia A (far the most important cause)
  Haemophilia B
  von Willebrand's disease with low factor VIII levels
- Acquired clotting defects
  Vitamin K deficiency
  Anticoagulant treatment
  Liver disease

Fig. 23.4 Localised oral purpura. A ruptured blood blister forming a large ulcer on the soft palate.

Haemophilia A

Haemophilia is the most common and severe clotting disorder. Haemophilia A (factor VIII deficiency) affects approximately

6 per 100 000 of the population and is about 10 times as common as haemophilia B (Christmas disease, factor IX deficiency). In the past, extractions in haemophiliacs have been fatal, and extractions are still common emergencies or occasions when haemophiliacs need specific treatment.

Severe haemophilia typically causes effects in childhood, usually as a result of bleeding into muscles or joints after minor injuries. By contrast, mild haemophilia (factor VIII level over 25%) may cause no symptoms until an injury, surgery or a dental extraction precipitates prolonged bleeding. This may not happen until adult life. Severe and prolonged bleeding deeply into the soft tissues can also follow local anaesthetic injections. Inferior dental blocks are most dangerous because of the rich plexus of veins in this area, from which blood can leak down to the glottis. Even a submucous infiltration can occasionally have severe consequences (Fig. 23.6).

Clinical features

As mentioned earlier, a positive family history is always significant. However, over 30% of haemophiliacs have a negative family history, and occasionally haemophilia is discovered only as a result of postextraction haemorrhage. By contrast, it is certain that a patient who has had extractions or tonsillectomy without serious bleeding is not haemophiliac.

Typically, bleeding starts after a short delay as a result of

normal platelet and vascular responses which provide the initial phase of haemostasis. There is then persistent bleeding which, if untreated, can continue for weeks or until the patient dies. Pressure packs, suturing or local application of haemostatics are ineffective.

Haemarthroses are well-recognised complications of uncontrolled haemophilia but most dangerous is intracranial haemorrhage. Deep tissue bleeding can also occasionally spread down from the neck and obstruct the airway. Many haemophiliacs are carriers of hepatitis B virus (HBV), hepatitis C virus (HCV) or HIV infection as a result of receiving untreated blood products. Formation of antibodies to factor VIII is another complication.

Principles of management (Table 23.6)

Before surgery, radiographs should be taken to forestall any complications resulting from unsuspected disease and to decide whether any other extractions are necessary. Arrangements must usually be made for admission to hospital. The number of occasions when replacement therapy has to be given should be kept to a minimum. When replacement therapy has been given, as much surgical work as possible should be done in that session. It is always wise to plan treatment with the possibility in mind that, the next time the patient needs surgery, he may be in a place where replacement therapy is unobtainable or he has developed antibodies to factor VIII.

Fig. 23.6 Haemophilia. This was a mild and unsuspected haemophiliac who had never had any previous serious bleeding episodes. This enormous haematoma developed after a submucous injection for extirpation of an incisor pulp. (By kind permission of Mr A J Bridge.)

Table 23.6 **Principles of dental management of haemophilia**

- History
- Laboratory findings
  Prolonged activated partial thromboplastin time
  Normal prothrombin time
  Normal bleeding time
  Low factor VIII levels
- Regular meticulous dental care to avoid the need for extractions
- Preoperative planning of unavoidable extractions or other surgery
- Preoperative replacement therapy
- Postoperative precautions

A factor VIII level between 50% and 75% is necessary for dental extractions, and factor VIII requirement depends on the serum level and the expected severity of the surgical trauma. It is usual also to give tranexamic acid or desmopressin to reduce the amount of factor VIII needed.

Postoperatively, an antibiotic such as oral penicillin (250 mg four times a day for 7 days) is usually given to reduce the chance of wound infection and secondary haemorrhage. The risks of bleeding are greatest on the day of operation and again from 4 to 10 days postoperatively. If bleeding starts at any time after the operation, factor VIII must be given, or it may be given prophylactically on the 4th or 5th postoperative day. Administration of tranexamic acid is usually continued for 10 days. Aspirin and related analgesics should be avoided.

For routine dentistry, relative analgesia is preferable for

sedation to avoid the risk from accidental damage to a vein. Now that haemophiliacs have a personal stock of factor VIII for use in emergencies, these problems have greatly declined. However, it may be necessary to check that the factor VIII has been taken.

Extractions in mild haemophilia may be managed by giving antifibrinolytic drugs, particularly tranexamic acid or desmopressin rather than factor VIII. For those with antibodies to factor VIII, factor VIII inhibitor bypassing fraction may be given.

Christmas disease (haemophilia B)

Christmas disease is inherited in the same way as, and is clinically identical to, haemophilia A. However, factor IX is more stable than factor VIII. Dried factor IX fraction is given for replacement.

Factor IX remains active in the blood for more than 2 days, so that replacement therapy can be given at longer intervals than for haemophilia A. All other aspects of management of haemophilia A and B are the same.

Acquired clotting defects

Overall, these are more common than the inherited defects (Table 23.7).

Table 23.7   **Important acquired clotting disorders**

- Vitamin K deficiency
- Anticoagulant drugs
- Liver disease

Vitamin K deficiency

Causes include obstructive jaundice, or, less commonly, malabsorption. Important causes of obstructive jaundice are hepatitis, gall stones and carcinoma of the pancreas.

Extractions or other surgery should preferably be delayed until haemostasis recovers. In an emergency, vitamin K can be given, preferably by mouth, and its effectiveness checked by the prothrombin time. If the latter does not return to normal within 48 hours there is probably parenchymal liver disease.

Anticoagulant treatment

Coumarin anticoagulants such as warfarin are used for thromboembolic disease, which can complicate atrial fibrillation or insertion of prosthetic heart valves. The underlying condition may therefore influence dental management more than the treatment. Anticoagulation should be checked regularly to maintain the prothrombin time. This is reported as the INR (international normalised ratio), at 2–3 in most cases but at 3–4.5 for those with prosthetic valves. Dental extractions can usually be carried out safely with an INR of 2–3, but the INR alone is not a completely reliable guide to haemostatic function.

As a precaution, only a few teeth should be extracted at one session; trauma should be minimal and the sockets can be sutured over a layer of oxidised cellulose. Because of the risk of rebound thrombosis, anticoagulation should not be stopped. For more major surgery, anticoagulant treatment may have to be stopped if the physician agrees. If serious bleeding starts, tranexamic acid can be given, but, if otherwise uncontrollable, vitamin K may be needed.

Short-term anticoagulation with heparin is given before renal dialysis. Heparin is effective only for about 6 hours. Extractions or other surgery can therefore be delayed for 12–24 hours after the last dose of heparin, when the benefits of dialysis are also maximal.

Liver disease

Haemorrhagic tendencies can result either from obstructive jaundice (infective hepatitis also has an obstructive component) or from extensive liver damage. In obstructive jaundice, vitamin K absorption may be severely impaired. Viral hepatitis or alcoholism are important causes of liver failure, which results in inability to metabolise vitamin K and to produce most clotting factors. Haemorrhage can be severe and difficult to control. In mild liver disease vitamin K may be effective. In more severe cases it is valueless, but tranexamic acid and fresh plasma infusions may control bleeding.

SUGGESTED FURTHER READING

Ascher L F, Ord R A 1992 Pseudothrombocytopenia in maxillofacial surgery patients: a report of two cases. J Oral Maxillofac Surg 50:1108–1110

Association of Hemophilia Clinic Directors of Canada 1995 Hemophilia and von Willebrand's disease: 2. Management. Can Med Assoc J 153:147–157

Beatty C 1995 The patient with easy bruising and bleeding. Medicine UK 23:514–517

Capitano A M, Secco R, Mannucci P M 1991 Pseudopathologies of haemostasis and dental surgery. Oral Surg Oral Med Oral Pathol 71:184–186

Chesterman C N, Chong B H 1995 Acquired haemostatic failure. Medicine UK 23:518–524

Durham T M, Hodges E D, Harper J et al 1993 Management of traumatic oral–facial injury in the hemophiliac patient with inhibitor. Pediatr Dent 15:282–287

Giles A R, Lillicrap D P 1995 Haemophilia A and related disorders. Med Int 23:525–530

Lethagen S R 1995 Pathogenesis, clinical picture and treatment of von Willebrand's disease. Ann Med 27:641–651

Ludlam C A, Steel C M 1993 Haemostasis: von Willebrand's variants. Lancet 341:997

McLaughlin P, Chen S, Phillips J G 1994 Disseminated intravascular coagulation presenting as perioral haemorrhage. Br J Oral Maxillofac Surg 32:94–95

Manabe M, Tsujimaki M, Kakuta S, Nagumo M 1993 Acquired factor X deficiency: an experience with multiple tooth extraction. J Oral Maxillofac Surg 51:922–924

SUGGESTED FURTHER READING (*cont'd*)

Marshall D A S, Berry C, Brewer A 1993 Fatal disseminated intravascular coagulation complicating dental extraction. Br J Oral Maxillofac Surg 31:178–179

Morrison A E, Ludlam C A 1994 Acquired heamophilia and its management. Br J Haematol 89:231–236

Rakocz M, Mazar A, Varon D et al 1993 Dental extractions with bleeding disorders: the use of fibrin glue. Oral Surg Med Oral Pathol 75:280–282

Saulnier J, Marey A, Horellou M-H et al 1994 Evaluation of desmopressin for dental extractions in patients with haemostatic disorders. Oral Surg Oral Med Oral Pathol 77:6–12

Steinberg M J, Moores J F 1995 Use of INR to assess degree of anticoagulation in patients who have dental procedures. Oral Surg Oral Med Oral Pathol Oral Radiol Endod 80:175–177

Todd D, Galbraith D 1993 Management of an orthognathic surgery patient with factor XI deficiency: review and case report. J Oral Maxillofac Surg 51:417–420

Wahl M J, Howell J 1996 Altering anticoagulant therapy: a survey of physicians. J Am Dent Assoc 127:625–638

Wood G D, Deeble T 1993 Warfarin: dangers with antibiotics. Dent Update October: 350–353

Immunodeficiency diseases and the acquired immune deficiency syndrome

Immune deficiencies can be primary or acquired (Table 24.1) and affect B or T lymphocytes, or both. T lymphocytes regulate B lymphocyte activity, T cell defects may therefore impair antibody production as well as cell-mediated immunity. There can also be failures of production of individual immunoglobulins, such as IgA, or of complement components.

Any patient who develops recurrent infections, particularly if they respond poorly to treatment or are caused by otherwise harmless microbes (opportunistic infections), is likely to be immunodeficient (Fig. 24.1).

Table 24.1 Important causes of immunodeficiency

- Primary (genetic)
    T or B lymphocyte defects (Swiss type agammaglobulinaemia,
        DiGeorge's syndrome, etc.)
    IgA deficiency
    Complement component deficiencies
    Down's syndrome (multiple defects)
- Secondary (acquired)
    Infections (HIV, other severe viral or bacterial
        infections, malaria, etc.)
    Drug-induced (immunosuppressive and anticancer treatment)
    Malnutrition (worldwide a major cause)
    Cancer (particularly lymphoreticular)
    Diabetes mellitus

The main causes of *severe* immunodeficiency are human immunodeficiency virus (HIV) infection and immunosuppressive treatment, particularly for organ transplants. Many cancer patients are also severely immunodeficient as a result of both the neoplasm and the cytotoxic drugs used for treatment. The severe primary immunodeficiencies are rare and, unless a marrow transplant can be given, are usually fatal in childhood.

Oral manifestations of immunodeficiencies

The main effect, as mentioned earlier, is abnormal susceptibility to infections, particularly candidosis or viral infections such as herpes zoster, as in AIDS (see below).

Fig. 24.1 Thrush. In immunodeficiency there may be widespread mild and chronic signs of candidal infection, as here, with erythema but only occasional white flecks or plaques.

SELECTIVE IgA DEFICIENCY

Selective IgA deficiency is common and potentially relevant for the mouth. Selective IgA deficiency may affect about 1 in 600 of the population and has varied possible effects (Table 24.2).

Table 24.2 Possible effects of selective IgA deficiency

- Normal health
- Enhanced susceptibility, especially to respiratory tract infections
- Atopic disease
- Connective tissue disease, especially lupus erythematosus

Susceptibility to oral infections

Evidence regarding the effect of IgA deficiency on dental caries and periodontal disease is conflicting. Both high and low prevalences of dental caries have been reported. Compensatory secretion of other immunoglobulins into the mouth may explain these variable findings. Gingivitis may be less severe than normal, but even this may be the result of antibiotic treatment for respiratory infections. There is no evidence of any significant association between oral mucosal infection and IgA deficiency.

Atopic disease. IgA deficiency may facilitate absorption of allergens: asthma, eczema or any of the related diseases may be the first sign. However, this has no oral effects unless allergic angio-oedema involves the floor of mouth or lips.

HEREDITARY ANGIO-OEDEMA

The familial form of this disease results from Cl esterase inhibitor deficiency. Pedantically speaking, it is an immunodeficiency but there is no abnormal susceptibility to infection.

Since C1 esterase inhibitor is an inactivator of the first complement component, its absence leads to uncontrolled activation of the classical pathway. In the process, C4 is consumed and its persistently low level in the serum during asymptomatic periods is a useful diagnostic test. Alternatively serum C1 esterase inhibitor titration may be necessary for diagnosis of genetic variants.

As a result of stimuli such as minor injuries (including dental trauma), episodes of increased capillary permeability cause gross but localised oedematous swelling. Visceral angio-oedema can cause acute abdominal pain but, more important, oedema of the head and neck region can cause respiratory obstruction, and there is a significant mortality. Treatment of an acute attack is with purified C1 esterase inhibitor concentrate. Prophylaxis and maintenance treatment is with the synthetic androgen stanozolol which, if taken daily, maintains C1 esterase inhibitor at normal levels. Hereditary angio-oedema must be distinguished from allergic angio-oedema (which can also threaten the airway) by the latter's history of allergic disease and, usually, raised IgE levels.

BONE MARROW TRANSPLANTATION

Bone marrow transplantation is used, if suitable donors can be found, for such conditions as some severe primary immunodeficiency diseases, some leukaemias, aplastic anaemia, and some lymphomas and other neoplasms. Preoperatively, total immunosuppression by cytotoxic chemotherapy and, sometimes, total body irradiation is required to prevent graft rejection.

Oral sources of infection should be eliminated and the mouth brought to as near perfect health as possible. Elimination of oral infection (particularly periodontal disease) has a significant effect on lessening post-transplant complications and also lessens the need for dental treatment during the difficult post-transplant period.

Possible complications after transplantation are numerous (Table 24.3), particularly during the initial intensive phase of immunosuppression.

Table 24.3 Possible complications of bone marrow transplantation

- Oral complications
  Mucositis, mucosal ulceration, infections, haemorrhage, dry mouth, parotitis
  Gingival hyperplasia if cyclosporin is used
  In children, dental hypoplastic defects may develop
- Graft-versus-host disease
- Systemic infections (sometimes by oral bacteria). These are the chief cause of death

Graft-versus-host disease results from an attack on an immunosuppressed host by transplanted immunocompetent cells. It is in effect a graft rejection reaction in reverse. It most frequently follows bone marrow transplantation, both because of the deep immunosuppression and because of the many immunologically active cells in the implanted marrow.

The oral effects of graft-versus-host disease are lichen planus, a Sjögren-like syndrome with xerostomia, and a condition resembling systemic sclerosis (Ch. 25) with limited oral opening.

Graft-versus-host disease can be acute and self-limiting or responsive to treatment, or chronic. The last is the chief cause of morbidity and mortality.

Post-transplant management

The main considerations are maintenance of meticulous oral hygiene, use of fluorides to control caries, and prompt treatment of any infections that develop.

In successful cases deep immunosuppression is maintained for up to a year after transplantation. The implanted marrow then takes over normal haematological and immune functions. Any oral surgery should preferably therefore be postponed until this happens.

OTHER ORGAN TRANSPLANTS

Transplantation of other organs, most frequently kidneys, is associated with similar complications to those of bone marrow transplantation. The main differences are that immunosuppression is less complete but has to be maintained indefinitely.

The chief problems are therefore the enhanced susceptibility to infections and the greater risk of lymphomas. Gingival hyperplasia due to cyclosporin may be difficult to control and can lead to progressive periodontal destruction.

THE ACQUIRED IMMUNE DEFICIENCY SYNDROME (AIDS)

A great variety of oral diseases can arise in AIDS (see

Table 24.6). They sometimes form the first sign of the disease and some of them herald rapid deterioration, and sometimes early death.

AIDS has spread worldwide and several millions have been infected. It is epidemic in parts of the USA and Africa. By June 1994, more than 22 000 cases and over 14 000 deaths from AIDS had been reported in Britain, despite the fact that the infection rate is the lowest in Europe. In the USA, cases exceeded half a million by 1995. Many times these numbers of persons in all parts of the world have acquired the infection and may be able to transmit it, but have not yet had any clinical effects.

AIDS is transmissible to health care personnel, particularly surgeons, dental surgeons and nurses, via needles or other sharp instruments. However, the risk of acquiring HIV infection by such means is considerably smaller than that of hepatitis B.

Aetiology

AIDS is caused by a retrovirus, the human immunodeficiency virus (HIV), mainly HIV-1. HIV-2 is as yet only widely prevalent in West Africa.

The chief mode of transmission is by male homosexual activity, which accounts for over 70% of cases in Britain. Intravenous drug abusers are also a high-risk group. Heterosexual transmission is far less common in the Western world than in Africa. Nevertheless, as a result of spread of the virus in the population, heterosexual transmission (though still uncommon in Britain) has become *relatively* more frequent. Once infected, pregnant women can transmit the infection to the fetus. Many haemophiliacs have acquired the disease from infected blood products but heat treatment of clotting factor concentrates should have eliminated this risk.

The incubation period of AIDS is highly variable. In male homosexuals it averages approximately 5 years, but is sometimes as long as 10 years. Testing of infected persons also shows deterioration of immune function long before clinically apparent disease and it is still not clear whether all those who develop prodromal signs will develop the full, lethal syndrome.

In 5–15% of cases, HIV infection shows no clinical progress for periods up to 10 years, possibly because of variations in pathogenicity of HIV strains, or stronger host immune responses.

Immunology

The human immunodeficiency virus directly infects lymphocytes and other cells, such as some macrophages, which carry the CD4 marker. However, the virus appears only to be able to fuse with and enter CD4 cells via a coreceptor termed *fusin*. A second coreceptor, CC-CKR-5, has also been identified and there may be others. The virus kills T helper (CD4) cells and reverses the ratio of helper to suppressor lymphocytes.

Antibody is produced in response to the virus but is not protective. Antibodies to HIV indicate only that infection has been acquired and all seropositive persons must be assumed to be capable of transmitting it. Detection of these antibodies is often misnamed 'the AIDS test', but it cannot predict the development of symptomatic disease. It has been useful for detecting HIV-infected persons, particularly among blood donors.

Detection of viral antigens, such as p24 protein in the blood, provides a more direct and reliable indicator of infection. Minute amounts of provirus DNA can be detected by the polymerase chain reaction in lymphocytes. Haematological markers indicating progression to AIDS include viral antigens in the serum, high β_2-microglobulin levels and failure of or greatly depressed antigen-induced interferon γ production. T helper (CD4) lymphocyte counts of less than $0.2 \times 10^9/l$ or a total lymphocyte count of less than $1 \times 10^9/l$ represent advanced disease.

Clinical indicators of a poor prognosis are oral thrush, *Herpes zoster* or other persistent or recurrent infections, hairy leukoplakia, unexplained constitutional symptoms, cutaneous anergy and lymphadenopathy. Between approximately 20% and 70% of such patients can be expected to deteriorate within less than 5 years.

The main effect of depletion of T helper cells is deepening depression of cell-mediated immunity. Thus there are declining responses of lymphocytes to antigens in vitro, and impaired or absent delayed hypersensitivity responses long before any clinical signs of the disease appear. Apparently paradoxically, there is also polyclonal B lymphocyte activation, resulting in hypergammaglobulinaemia and autoantibody production. The main effect of the immunodeficiency and chief cause of death is infection by a great variety of microbes.

The human immunodeficiency virus also attacks the central nervous system, cells of which carry receptors for the virus.

Clinical aspects

Possible major events after infection by HIV are shown in Fig. 24.2 but, as mentioned earlier, it is still uncertain whether any symptomless carriers will ultimately remain healthy.

Usually there is a latent period of several years before signs of immunodeficiency appear. Within 10 years, approximately 50% of infected persons will probably have developed AIDS and the remainder will usually have prodromal disease or laboratory markers of immune deficiency. Severe infectious complications are to be expected and are usually the chief cause of death.

The earliest clinical manifestation of HIV infection can be a transient illness resembling glandular fever, associated with antibody production. Thereafter, in progressive cases, markers of declining cell-mediated immunity eventually become detectable and, later, there are various clinical syndromes.

Generalised lymphadenopathy syndrome (GLS), with widespread persistent enlargement of lymph nodes, is a typical early

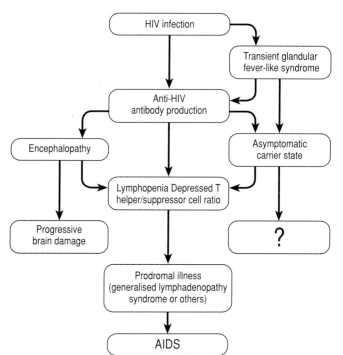

Fig. 24.2 Outcomes of HIV infection. The fate of currently asymptomatic carriers is unknown.

sign. However, the course of AIDS is highly variable and none of the prodromal symptoms appear to be inevitable.

The full syndrome of AIDS is characterised by multiple infections by bacteria, fungi, parasites and viruses. Many of these infections, such as *Pneumocystis carinii* pneumonia, are opportunistic and almost unknown in immunocompetent persons.

Though infections are the main cause of death, there is also a greatly raised incidence of tumours, particularly Kaposi's sarcoma and lymphomas, which frequently affect the oral or perioral tissues. In normal persons these tumours are not merely uncommon or rare but are particularly rare in the oral tissues.

Sometimes the first clinical sign of AIDS can be *Pneumocystis carinii* pneumonia or Kaposi's sarcoma.

Neuropsychiatric disease in AIDS can range from depression, to dementia and death. Opportunistic infections or tumours can also involve the central nervous system, These neurological disorders may be associated with, but can develop in the absence of, immunodeficiency.

A lesser manifestation of AIDS in some patients is autoimmune disease, particularly thrombocytopenic purpura or, less frequently, a lupus erythematosus-like disease.

Once AIDS has developed, the outcome is usually fatal within 2–3 years, though the course of the disease may be modified to some degree. Currently, combination chemotherapy with zidovudine plus didanosine or zalcitabine appears to be the most effective means of reducing viral load. Novel nucleoside and non-nucleoside reverse transcriptase inhibitors and protease inhibitors offer the possibility of even more effective treatment. Vigorous treatment of opportunistic infections and other complications is also essential.

In the terminal stages of AIDS, the patient may be emaciated, with persistent diarrhoea, suffering a multiplicity of infections, disfigured by skin disease, breathless from *Pneumocystis carinii* pneumonia, frequently with a malignant tumour, and sometimes also blind and demented.

AIDS assessment and staging

Staging of HIV infection is important for selecting patients for treatment and assessing prognosis, and for epidemiological studies. The Centers for Disease Control/World Health Organization classification (Table 24.4) takes both clinical and laboratory findings into account.

Table 24.4 CDC/WHO classification of HIV infection

I Clinical	
Category A	Primary clinical HIV infection (seroconversion illness)
	Asymptomatic HIV infection
	Persistent generalised lymphadenopathy
Category B	Indicative of HIV-associated cellular immune deficiency not listed in Category C, such as:
	Bacterial pneumonia or meningitis
	Pharyngeal or vaginal candidosis
	Cervical dysplasia or carcinoma
	Oral hairy leukoplakia
	Recurrent or multidermatomal herpes zoster
	Pulmonary tuberculosis
	Idiopathic thrombocytopenic purpura
	Unexplained constitutional disturbance
Category C	(Old CDC stages IV B, C1, C2, D & E)
	B Neurological disease
	C Severe clinical immunodeficiency
	C1 CDC AIDS definition
	C2 Severe infection outwith AIDS
	D Secondary cancers within AIDS definition:
	Kaposi's sarcoma
	Non-Hodgkin lymphoma
	E Other conditions

II Laboratory CD4 cells ($\times 10^9/l$)	Total lymphocyte count ($\times 10^9/l$)
[1] >0.5	>2
[2] 0.2–0.9	1–1.9
[3] <0.2	<1

General aspects of dental management

The possibility of transmitting HIV infection during dental treatment inevitably causes anxiety but the risk is considerably lower than that of acquiring viral hepatitis. Oral infections and other features of AIDS or its prodromes may enable patients to be recognised. A young adult male who develops thrush for no apparent reason is likely to have AIDS, but if he has oral Kaposi's sarcoma, it is virtually pathognomonic. However, there are many more patients with nothing to suggest that they are infective. At the time of writing there are tens of thousands of antibody-positive, potentially infective persons in Britain, and the number rises each month.

All patients must now, therefore, be regarded as potentially infective and treated with full infection control, as for hepatitis B. A few nurses and others have become infected as a result of needle-stick injuries causing accidental injection of a significant amount of infected blood. By contrast, many other needle-stick injuries where little blood has been tranferred have failed to transmit the virus. Most health care workers who have developed AIDS have not acquired it as a result of their occupation.

As to the risk to general surgeons, at least two in the Western world are known to have died from the disease, acquired at operation. By contrast, only one dental surgeon is as yet known to have acquired the disease occupationally. He was working in New York (by far the highest incidence area in the Western world), did not practise a high standard of infection control and had had many needle-stick injuries. No other dental surgeons, even in high incidence areas, are known to have acquired the disease occupationally.

Infection control, as discussed earlier, and awareness of the patient's low resistance to secondary infection are the major management considerations. Key features are summarised in Table 24.5.

Table 24.5   AIDS — key features

- Caused by a retrovirus — usually HIV 1
- Transmitted sexually or by intravenous drug abuse and by blood or blood products
- Progressive deterioration mainly of cell-mediated immunity
- Immunodeficiency leads to opportunistic infections such as *Pneumocystic carinii* pneumonia
- Common oral lesions include candidosis and hairy leukoplakia
- Greatly increased frequency of Kaposi's sarcoma and lymphomas, often in oral regions
- Neurological and psychological disorders may be associated
- Deaths mainly due to opportunistic infections

ORAL LESIONS IN AIDS

More than 75% of patients with AIDS have orofacial disease (Table 24.6). Among 2235 HIV-positive, homosexual or bisexual men in San Francisco, the most frequent oral lesions were hairy leukoplakia (18.7%), thrush (6.6%) or erythematous candidosis (2.1%), Kaposi's sarcoma (1.6%) and oral ulcers (2%). However, the frequency of such lesions varies in other groups. Kaposi's sarcoma and hairy leukoplakia, for example, are disproportionately frequent in homosexual men.

Table 24.6   Oral disease in HIV infection

More common diseases	Less common
Infections	*Infections*
• Fungal	• Fungal
Thrush and other forms of candidosis	Deep mycoses
	Cryptococcosis
	Histoplasmosis
	Aspergillosis
	Geotrichosis
• Viral	• Viral
Herpes simplex	Human papilloma virus
Varicella zoster	Cytomegalovirus
EB virus, including hairy leukoplakia	
• Bacterial	• Bacterial
HIV-associated gingivitis and periodontitis	*Mycobacterium tuberculosis* and non-tuberculous ('atypical') mycobacterioses
Necrotising gingivitis	Klebsiella pneumonia
	Salmonella enteritidis, *Escherichia coli* and *Enterobacter cloacae* infections
	Sinusitis
	Exacerbations of apical periodontitis
	Submandibular cellulitis
Tumours	*Tumours*
Kaposi's sarcoma	Non-Hodgkin lymphoma (squamous cell carcinoma)
Lymphadenopathy	*Neurological disease*
	Paraesthesiae
	Hyperaesthesia
	Facial palsy
	Dysphagia
	Miscellaneous
	Recurrent aphthae
	Progressive necrotising ulceration
	Delayed wound healing
	Purpura
	Pigmentation

Oral candidosis

Oral thrush or other forms of candidosis may be seen in over 70% of patients at some stage. It indicates declining immunity, and other infections may be associated or are likely to follow. Appoximately 50% of patients with HIV-associated thrush are likely to develop AIDS within 5 years.

Most other types of candidosis, such as angular stomatitis, palatal erythema or hyperplastic candidosis may also be seen in AIDS patients (Fig. 24.3).

Viral mucosal infections

Herpetic stomatitis is less common than might be expected but can cause atypical or chronic ulceration (Fig. 24.4). Severe orofacial zoster may indicate a poor prognosis.

Fig. 24.3 Erythematous candidosis. An extensive red patch on the palate without white flecks which appears as denture stomatitis but without any denture being worn. Such a presentation is characteristic of immunodeficiency. (By kind permission of Mr G Palmer.)

Fig. 24.4 Herpes simplex ulceration in immunodeficiency. There is extensive ulceration along the midline of the dorsal tongue and separate ulcers towards the lateral margins. In immunodeficiency the ulcers may be chronic and their clinical appearance does not suggest viral infection. Biopsy is required for diagnosis.

Cytomegalovirus can be found in some oral ulcers, and the Epstein–Barr virus may be the cause of hairy leukoplakia.

Papillomaviruses have been isolated from proliferative lesions, such as verruca vulgaris, condyloma acuminatum and focal epithelial hyperplasia.

Bacterial infections

Infections by bacteria which rarely involve the oral tissues, such as *Klebsiella pneumoniae*, *Enterobacter cloacae* and *Escherichia coli*, can develop.

In the later stages, there may be oral lesions secondary to systemic infections, particularly mycobacterial ulcers.

Fig. 24.5 Hairy leukoplakia. The characteristic appearance on the lateral margin of the tongue. Posteriorly the vertical ridging pattern of the lateral tongue is enhanced.

Deep mycoses

Histoplasmosis or cryptococcosis can give rise to proliferative or ulcerative lesions.

Hairy leukoplakia

Hairy leukoplakia is highly characteristic of HIV infection (Ch. 15 and Fig. 24.5).

Tumours

Nearly 50% of patients with AIDS have a malignant tumour at the time of presentation. By far the most frequent are Kaposi's sarcoma and non-Hodgkin lymphomas. Unlike non-AIDS patients, these tumours are particularly frequent in the head and neck region.

Among patients with AIDS, Kaposi's sarcoma is mainly seen in male homosexuals, and in some areas of the USA, for example, it has become the most common malignant tumour of the oral cavity. It is also occasionally seen in immunosuppressed organ transplant patients.

Kaposi's sarcoma in the mouth, particularly in a young male who is not receiving immunosuppressive treatment, is virtually pathognomonic of AIDS. It is usually associated with a CD4 lymphocyte count of less than 200/μl and frequently associated with other effects of HIV infection such as candidosis, hairy leukoplakia or HIV-associated gingivitis. Though oral Kaposi's sarcoma may be the cause of early symptoms, the tumour is usually multifocal, with lesions affecting skin, lymph nodes and viscera. At autopsy most organs are frequently found to be involved.

The site may be oropharyngeal, cutaneous or in the cervical lymph nodes. Within the mouth the palate is the most frequent site and the tumour typically produces a flat or nodular purplish

Fig. 24.6 Bacillary angiomatosis. A small red-purple nodule on an edentulous ridge in an HIV-infected individual. This condition occurs rarely in the mouth, but should be considered and excluded by biopsy when Kaposi's sarcoma is suspected becase it may be effectively treated by antibiotics.

Fig. 24.7 Purpura. Purpura and petechiae are common intraorally at sites of trauma when thrombocytopenia develops.

lesion. The clinical differential diagnosis is from oral purpura, bacillary angiomatosis and pyogenic granulomas, from which it can be distinguished by biopsy (Ch. 20).

Epithelioid bacillary angiomatosis

Bacillary angiomatosis (Fig. 24.6) can mimic Kaposi's sarcoma clinically, and to some extent histologically, but is a vascular proliferative disease caused by *Bartonella henselae*. It affects the skin more frequently than the oral cavity but should respond to antimicrobial therapy. Biopsy is essential to exclude Kaposi's sarcoma.

Lymphomas

AIDS-related lymphomas can develop in intraoral sites or salivary glands far more frequently than in HIV-negative persons. Typical sites within the mouth are the palate or gingiva, where the tumours form soft painless swellings which ulcerate when traumatised.

Microscopically, most lymphomas in AIDS are high-grade B cell lymphomas of large cell or immunoblastic type. Epstein–Barr virus is associated in about 50%.

Burkitt's lymphoma is 1000 times more common than in HIV-negative persons in the Western world.

Lymphadenopathy

Lymphadenopathy is characteristic of AIDS and its prodromes. Cervical lymphadenopathy is probably the most common head and neck manifestation of HIV infection.

Microscopy. Typical findings are smaller numbers of T helper cells in the paracortical region, associated with greater numbers of T suppresssor cells there and in the follicles.

Follicles may initially be hyperplastic but later undergo involution. The lymph nodes become virtually or entirely functionless.

Enlarged cervical lymph nodes can also be due to lymphomas.

Autoimmune disease

The most common autoimmune phenomenon in AIDS is thrombocytopenic purpura (Fig. 24.7). This can give rise to oral purple patches which may be mistaken for Kaposi's sarcoma, petechiae or blood blisters.

Other autoimmune diseases reported in AIDS are lupus erythematosus and a Sjögren-like salivary gland disease.

Gingivitis and periodontitis

HIV-related periodontal disease includes necrotising gingivitis and accelerated periodontitis (Ch. 5). Necrotising ulcerative periodontitis (NUP) indicates immunological deterioration and a poor prognosis (Fig. 24.8).

Salivary gland disease

Chronic parotitis, possibly due to Epstein-Barr virus or cytomegalovirus, appears to affect children with AIDS particularly.

A Sjögren-like syndrome with xerostomia, but lacking the characteristic autoantibodies (particularly SS/A and SS/B), can affect adults.

Parotid swellings due to lymphoepithelial lesions are frequently cystic, bilateral and identifiable by CT or ultrasound.

Recognition of parotid cysts or microscopic diagnosis of

Fig. 24.8 Necrotising periodontitis. A small lesion of chronic necrotising gingivitis has progressed to involve the palate, forming a deep crater with bone destruction. Despite the tissue loss such lesions often respond suprisingly well to treatment.

Fig. 24.10 Oral ulceration in HIV infection. Extensive irregular ulcers indistinguishable from major aphthous ulcers form most commonly on the soft palate and in the pharynx.

biopsied as they may be amenable to treatment if specific agents such as herpes virus, cytomegalovirus or mycobacteria are identified. Major aphthae may respond dramatically to thalidomide but this can only be used when other causes have been excluded.

Oral hyperpigmentation

Occasionally, pigmentation may be secondary to Addison's disease due to fungal destruction of the adrenals. Alternatively, it may be a complication of treatment with zidovudine or due to unknown mechanisms.

Neurological disease

Orofacial effects include facial palsy and trigeminal neuropathy.

Fig. 24.9 Oral ulceration in HIV infection. Large ulcers indistinguishable from major aphthous ulcers on the soft palate are very painful, interfere with eating and add to the patient's disability. (By kind permission of Professor W H Binnie.)

Sjögren-like changes, particularly in a young adult male, are important indicators of HIV infection of which surgeons should be aware when dealing with a tumour-like lesion of salivary glands.

Miscellaneous oral lesions

Mucosal ulcers. Major aphthae (Fig. 24.9) can be troublesome, interfere with eating and accelerate deterioration of health. Necrotising oral ulceration of an ill-defined nature and aphthae-like lesions are common oral signs (Fig. 24.10). In the floor of these ulcers, cytomegalovirus can sometimes be seen.

Oral ulcers associated with HIV infection should always be

RESTRICTIONS ON TYPE OF WORK THAT MAY BE PERFORMED BY INFECTED DENTAL CLINICIANS

Current regulations require that dental clinicians who have become, or think that they have become, infected by HIV, hepatitis or other blood-borne viruses should seek counselling and appropriate medical supervision.

If infection is confirmed, changes to clinical practice may mean cessation of work involving exposure-prone procedures. These procedures are those where there is a risk of exposing the patient's open tissues to the blood of the worker and include procedures where clinicians' gloved hands may come into contact with sharp instruments or tissues (spicules of bone or teeth) inside patients' open body cavities.

In practice this may mean that infected clinicians may be restricted to carrying out prosthetic dentistry.

SUGGESTED FURTHER READING

Barrett A P 1986 Oral complications of bone marrow tranplantation. Aust N Z J Med 16:239–240

Berkowitz R J, Strandford S, Jones P et al 1987 Stomatological complications of bone marrow transplantation in a pediatric population. Pediatr Dent 9:105–110

Chaushu G, Itzkovitz-Chaushu S, Yefenof E et al 1995 A longitudinal follow-up of salivary secretion in bone marrow transplant patients. Oral Surg Oral Med Oral Pathol Oral Radiol Endod 79:164–169

Dahllof G, Heimdahl A, Modeer T et al 1989 Oral mucous membrane lesions in children treated with bone marrow transplantation. Scand J Dent Res 97:268–277

Greenspan D, Greenspan J S 1996 HIV-related oral disease. Lancet 348:729–733

Greenberg M S, Dubin G, Stewart J C B et al 1995 Relationship of oral disease to the presence of cytomegalovirus DNA in the saliva of AIDS patients. Oral Surg Oral Med Oral Pathol Oral Radiol Endod 79:175–179

Kline M W 1996 Oral manifestations of pediatric human

immunodeficiency virus infection: a review of the literature. Pediatrics 97:380–388

Lin R Y, Goodhart P 1993 The role of oral candidiasis in survival and hospitalization patterns: analysis of an inner city hospital human immunodeficiency virus/acquired immune deficiency registry. Am J Med Sci 305:345–353

Rosen F S, Cooper M D, Wedgwood R J P 1995 The primary immunodeficiencies. N Engl J Med 333:434–440

Scully C, Laskaris G, Findborg J et al 1991 Oral manifestations of HIV infection and their management. Oral Surg Oral Med Oral Pathol 71:158–171

Silverman S 1996 Color atlas of oral manifestations of AIDS, 2nd edn. Mosby, St Louis

Sim T C, Grant J A 1990 Hereditary angioedema: its diagnostic and management perspectives. Am J Med 88:656–665

Weinert M, Grimes R M, Lynch D P 1996 Oral manifestations of HIV infection. Ann Intern Med 125:485–496

Summary 24.1   Types of gingivitis and periodontitis seen in HIV infection

Immunologically-mediated diseases

Many endocrine diseases are immunologically mediated and most of the immunologically-mediated diseases have some dental relevance (Table 25.1).

Table 25.1 Aspects of immunologically-mediated diseases affecting dental management

- Systemic effects affecting dental management
- Immunologically-mediated oral diseases
- Risks of abnormal reactions to drugs (e.g. penicillin anaphylaxis)

Immunologically-mediated diseases fall into two main groups (Table 25.2). By far the most common are atopic disease and contact dermatitis, which are abnormal reactions to exogenous antigens. The autoimmune diseases, by contrast, are mediated by immune reactions directed against host tissues.

ATOPIC DISEASE

Atopic disease is the common type of allergy and affects approximately 10% of the population. It is mediated by IgE and susceptibility is genetically determined.

There are no oral manifestations of atopic disease itself, and there is no such entity as oral eczema. However, acute angio-oedema (sometimes a drug reaction) can indirectly involve the mouth by causing oedematous swelling of the floor of the mouth or lips. In such cases the airway may be endangered. It must be distinguished from hereditary angio-oedema due to C1 esterase deficiency (Ch. 24).

Acute severe asthma has a significant mortality and is a potential cause of an emergency in the dental surgery. Drugs (Table 25.3) used to treat it and other atopic diseases may complicate dental treatment.

Contact dermatitis

Contact dermatitis resembles eczema clinically, but is a cell-mediated (type 4) reaction. There is no convincing evidence of any oral counterpart to contact dermatitis (Figs 25.1 and 25.2).

Table 25.2 Important immunologically-mediated diseases

- Atopic disease and related allergies (reactions to exogenous antigens)
    - Asthma, eczema, hay fever, urticaria, food allergies
    - Some drug reactions
    - Anaphylaxis and acute allergic angio-oedema
    - Contact dermatitis
- Autoimmune diseases (reactions to endogenous antigens causing autoantibody production)
    - Connective tissue diseases
        - Rheumatoid arthritis
        - Sjögren's syndromes*
        - Lupus erythematosus*
        - Systemic sclerosis*
    - Autoimmune diseases with specific autoantibodies
        - Pernicious anaemia*
        - Idiopathic and drug-associated thrombocytopenic purpura*
        - Drug-associated leukopenia*
        - Autoimmune haemolytic anaemia
        - Addison's disease*
        - Hypothyroidism (Hashimoto's thyroiditis)
        - Hyperthyroidism
        - Idiopathic hypoparathyroidism*
        - Pemphigus vulgaris*
        - Mucous membrane pemphigoid*

*Can give rise to characteristic oral changes.

Table 25.3 Effects of drugs used for atopic disease

- Antihistamines (for minor allergies)
    - Drowsiness
    - Potentiation of sedating drugs
    - Dry mouth
- Corticosteroid inhalers
    - Oropharyngeal thrush
- Systemic corticosteroids for severe asthma (see Table 31.8)

Contact dermatitis of the hands to dental materials is a hazard to dentists and especially to laboratory technicians. Methyl methacrylate monomer in particular is a sensitising agent, but contact dermatitis to it is a surprisingly rare occupational hazard of dentistry.

Fig. 25.1 Allergic rash triggered by impression material. There is generalised facial erythema and slight oedema.

Fig. 25.2 Hypersensitivity to impression material. The same patient as in Figure 25.1, showing the site of the impression photographed at the same time. No allergic response is evident intraorally.

Latex allergy

The necessity for gloving for all clinical work has resulted in a growing frequency of latex allergy. In one dental school the prevalence of latex allergy was 9%, while 22% complained of chronic glove dermatitis. For those with latex allergy, gloves made from other plastics are required, but as yet there is no completely satisfactory alternative.

Occasionally also patients may react to a dentist's gloves with a perioral rash.

Rarely, reactions to latex can be severe and anaphylactoid in character, and have been fatal.

Mercury allergy and toxicity

The dangers of mercury are either from systemic absorption, particularly of organic mercury compounds such as methyl mercury, or from the development of hypersensitivity (contact dermatitis). Mercury intoxication is frequently confused with allergy by the public and the media.

Fig. 25.3 Patch testing for dental materials. Four panels of 12 patches impregnated with different dental materials have been in contact with the skin for 48 hours. Erythema, oedema and a palpable nodule indicate reaction to mercury but amalgam restorations provoked no intraoral reaction.

Hypersensitivity to mercury or its salts causes an inflammatory and sometimes vesiculating reaction when it is in contact with skin. This can readily be confirmed by patch testing, but even those with proven sensitivity can tolerate mercury amalgams in the mouth (Fig. 25.3). Nevertheless, in practical terms it is usually simpler to use composite materials to obviate the precautions necessary to prevent mercury coming into contact with their skin. If a dentist develops sensitivity, gloving and covering the arms (as required for infection control) should provide adequate protection during preparation and insertion of amalgams.

Systemic mercury toxicity is another possible occupational hazard of dentistry. Mercury, and particularly methyl mercury, are neurotoxic. To what extent the metal is converted to organic compounds in the body is unclear, but care should be taken in handling mercury and preventing it from being spilt or scattered in fine particles during amalgam mixing. Drilling out old amalgams also gives off traces of mercury vapour if the bur is poorly cooled. Serious pollution arises from spilling a substantial quantity of mercury, particularly on to carpeted or wooden flooring. Decontamination can then be difficult. Even worse is when (as has happened) a dental surgery assistant spills mercury behind an autoclave but fails to report the accident. As a result of the rapid evaporation, mercury absorption by the dental staff can then rise to alarming levels.

Nevertheless, many dentists have had decades of exposure to mercury and absorbed significant amounts but do not appear to have been significantly harmed.

Though mercury and particularly its organic compounds are undoubtedly toxic, public anxiety about mercury-containing dental amalgams has been aroused by unscrupulous practitioners, scaremongers and others. It was conspicuous, for example, that the alleged dangers of mercury toxicity ('allergy') achieved sudden publicity when a new and expensive composite restorative material was introduced.

Minute traces of mercury can be absorbed through the oral mucosa from amalgams and may occasionally give rise to mucosal lichenoid reactions. Otherwise there is no convincing evidence that dental amalgams are toxic or the cause of vague symptoms such as poor memory, lassitude and depression, from which most people seem to suffer from time to time. It has also been shown that patients who complain of vague symptoms from 'mercury allergy' tend also to suffer from a variety of complaints (such as irritable bowel syndrome) which have no clear organic basis. In one group of 20 patients complaining of amalgam-related symptoms, none was found to be hypersensitive to mercury. It also, incidentally, cannot be shown that alternative materials such as composites, of which there is much less experience, are necessarily safer. Some of them give off traces of formaldehyde, which is suspected of carcinogenicity.

A few patients with multiple sclerosis have been persuaded that their disease had been caused by their amalgam restorations and demanded their replacement. There is no medical justification for so doing, apart from offering the patient some temporary emotional comfort.

Despite the high risks of litigation in the USA, the Council on Dental Therapeutics of the American Dental Association has stated that, 'there is insufficient evidence to justify claims that mercury from amalgam restorations has an adverse effect on the health of the patients.'

THE AUTOIMMUNE DISEASES

This blanket term is used for a variety of diseases due to defective modulation of immune responses and production of autoantibodies which can damage host tissues. By no means all of their mechanisms are clearly understood. The autoimmune diseases have many features in common (Table 25.4). All of those listed in Table 25.2 are likely to show these features. Those with particular dental relevance have been discussed in other chapters and only the connective tissue diseases are described here.

Table 25.4 Autoimmune disease — typical features

- Significantly more common in women
- Onset often in middle age
- Family history frequently positive
- Levels of immunoglobulins (autoantibodies) usually raised
- Circulating autoantibodies frequently also detectable in unaffected family members
- Circulating autoantibodies to several tissues but not all attacked (e.g. antithyroid antibodies are common in Sjögren's syndrome)
- Often an increased risk of developing other autoimmune diseases (e.g. greater risk of patients with thyroiditis developing pernicious anaemia)
- Immunoglobulin and/or complement often detectable at sites of tissue damage (e.g. pemphigus vulgaris)
- Often associated with HLA-B8 and -DR3
- Immunosuppressive treatment frequently limits tissue damage

---

The connective tissue diseases

The main connective tissue diseases are rheumatoid arthritis, lupus erythematosus, systemic sclerosis, primary biliary cirrhosis and Sjögren's syndrome, which can be associated with any of them or develop in isolation.

A characteristic feature is the multiplicity of autoantibodies, none of which is specific to the tissues under attack and which frequently also are not specific to the disease either. Thus in rheumatoid arthritis the most constantly found autoantibody (rheumatoid factor) is not directed against the joint tissues but against an immunoglobulin. Moreover, rheumatoid factor is frequently detectable in other diseases of this group in the absence of arthritis. The connective tissue diseases are probably mediated by immune complex (type 3) reactions causing inflammation and tissue damage.

Rheumatoid arthritis

Rheumatoid arthritis is by far the most common connective tissue disorder and affects at least 3% of the population. Arthritis is the main feature but it is a multisystem disease. The temporomandibular joints are frequently involved in the more severe cases, but clinical effects are frequently insignificant (Ch. 11).

The chief importance of rheumatoid arthritis in dentistry is its association with Sjögren's syndrome. Drugs used for rheumatoid arthritis (particularly aspirin and other anti-inflammatory drugs, corticosteroids, antimalarials, gold and penicillamine) can also affect dental management or occasionally cause oral reactions. Many patients with rheumatoid arthritis are anaemic as a result of the disease itself, or as a result of gastric blood loss induced by analgesics.

Sjögren's syndrome (see Ch. 18)

Systemic lupus erythematosus

Systemic lupus erythematosus (SLE) can affect almost any body system, which may affect dental management. Oral mucosal lesions are seen in about 20%.

The most important of the many autoantibodies seen in SLE are antinuclear factors. Only antibodies against double-stranded DNA (anti-dsDNA) are peculiar to SLE but many other antinuclear factors are found in other connective tissue diseases.

Clinically the features vary according to the main organ systems affected (Table 25.5). Joint pains and rashes are the most common manifestations but the 'classical' picture of a young woman with a butterfly rash across the mid-face is uncommon, and not peculiar to SLE. Corticosteroids and other immunosuppressives or antimalarials are the main forms of treatment.

Dental aspects. Oral lesions somewhat resemble lichen planus (Ch. 13). However, they are more difficult to treat and may not respond to the doses of systemic corticosteroids which control more major manifestations of the disease.

Table 25.5 Organs and tissues affected in systemic lupus erythematosus

Organ/tissue	Clinical feature
Joints	Joint pains and arthritis
Skin	Rashes
Mouth	Stomatitis, Sjögren's syndrome
Serous membranes	Pleurisy, pericarditis
Heart	Endocarditis, myocarditis
Lungs	Pneumonitis
Kidneys	Nephritic syndrome
Central nervous system	Neuroses, psychoses, strokes, cranial nerve palsies
Eyes	Conjunctivitis, retinal damage
Gastrointestinal tract	Hepatomegaly, pancreatitis
Blood	Anaemia, purpura

Antimalarials used in treatment can also cause oral lichen planus. Otherwise dental management may be affected according to the pattern of systemic involvement, but frequently the treatment is likely to affect dental management more than the disease itself. The chief dental considerations are summarised in Table 25.6.

Table 25.6 Features of lupus erythematosus affecting dental management

- Corticosteroid and other immunosuppressive drugs
- Painful oral lesions
- Sjögren's syndrome
- Bleeding tendencies (antiplatelet antibodies or anticoagulants)
- Anaemia
- Cardiac disease and risk of endocarditis

Discoid lupus erythematosus

Discoid lupus erythematosus mainly causes mucocutaneous lesions essentially similar to those of SLE but without the latter's serological changes and systemic disorders.

Systemic sclerosis (scleroderma)

Systemic sclerosis is rare but causes subcutaneous and visceral fibrosis. It has a poor prognosis. The pathogenesis of the progressive fibrosis and stiffening of the skin and often the gastrointestinal tract, lungs, heart and kidneys is unclear.

Inflammatory changes are minimal. Circulating antinuclear antibodies are detectable in about 50% of patients but their role is also unclear.

Clinically, the most common early sign is Raynaud's phenomenon and joint pains. Later the skin becomes thinned, stiff and pigmented and the facial features become smoothed out and mask-like. Fibrosis of viscera is liable to cause dysphagia, dyspnoea and pulmonary hypertension. Later there may be renal involvement, hypertension and cardiac failure.

Immunosuppressive drugs appear to be ineffective and the 5-year survival rate is only about 50%. Oral features are summarised in Table 25.7.

Table 25.7 Systemic sclerosis — possible oral features

- Sjögren's syndrome
- Limited oral opening
- Widened periodontal ligament shadow in 7%
- Gross resorption of the jaws, rarely
- Firm whitish-yellow fibrotic mucosal plaques, very rarely

Localised scleroderma (morphoea)

Morphoea is characterised by localised fibrosis resembling that of scleroderma but without the latter's systemic involvement of serological changes. The face is frequently the chief site and the area of fibrosis resembles the scar from a sabre cut (coup de sabre). Childhood morphoea is a possible cause of facial hemiatrophy.

SUGGESTED FURTHER READING

Black C 1994 Scleroderma (systemic sclerosis). Medicine UK 22:70–75
Hall F C, Walport M J 1994 Systemic lupus erythematosus. Medicine UK 22:58–64
Herrström P, Högstrom B 1993 Clinical study of oral galvanism: no evidence of toxic mercury exposure but anxiety disorder an important background factor. Scand J Dent Res 101:232–237
Katelaris C H, Widmer R P, Lazarus R M 1996 Prevalence of latex allergy in a dental school. Med J Aust 164:711–714
Mjör I A 1994 Side effects of dental materials. No evidence that dental restorations are hazardous to health (editorial). BMJ 309:621–622
Smart E R, Macleod R I, Lawrence C M 1992 Allergic reactions to rubber gloves in dental patients: report of three cases. Br Dent J 172:443–445
Walls R S 1996 Latex allergy: a real problem (editorial). Med J Aust 164:707–708

chapter 26

Cervical lymphadenopathy

Dental and periodontal infections are by far the most common causes of cervical lymphadenopathy (Fig. 26.1). Other possible causes include life-threatening diseases such as lymphomas. Lymphadenopathy is one of the most common features of HIV infection. Cervical lymphadenopathy without an obvious cause is therefore a warning sign that must not be ignored.

Important causes of cervical lymphadenopathy are summarised in Table 26.1, but many have been discussed in previous chapters.

Table 26.1 Important causes of cervical lymphadenopathy

Infections
- Bacterial
  Dental, tonsils, face or scalp infections
  Tuberculosis
  Syphilis
  Cat-scratch disease
  Lyme disease
- Viral
  Herpetic stomatitis
  Infectious mononucleosis
  HIV infection
- Parasitic
  Toxoplasmosis
- Possibly infective
  Mucocutaneous lymph node syndrome (Kawasaki's disease)

Neoplasms
- Primary
  Hodgkin's disease
  Non-Hodgkin lymphoma
  Leukaemia especially lymphocytic
- Secondary
  Carcinoma — oral, salivary gland or nasopharyngeal
  Malignant melanoma
  Other mesenchymal tumours

Miscellaneous
Sarcoidosis
Drug reactions
Connective tissue diseases

Investigation

The most common cause of persistent cervical lymphadenopathy is a recent viral illness. No cause may then be identifiable but the lymphadenopathy resolves after some months.

Fig. 26.1 Enlarged submandibular lymph node with incipient drainage to the skin.

Investigations for cervical lymphadenopathy of which the cause is not obvious are summarised in Table 26.2.

TUBERCULOUS CERVICAL LYMPHADENOPATHY

Tuberculous infection of the cervical lymph nodes is a primary infection which accounts for less than 10% of tuberculosis in Britain. *Mycobacterium tuberculosis* (human) accounts for over 90% of isolates. Patients are mostly adults, mainly immigrants of Asian or Afro-Caribbean origin. Non-tuberculous ('atypical') mycobacteria, particularly *M. avium-intracellulare* or *M. scrofulaceum*, are now the major cause of cervical mycobacterial lymphadenitis in immunocompetent children. As discussed earlier, the incidence of mycobacterial infections is growing and multiply-resistant strains are emerging.

Clinical features (Table 26.3)

Pathology

Diagnosis depends on finding granulomas in which mycobacteria should be demonstrable by Ziehl–Neelsen staining or by

Table 26.2 Investigation of cervical lymphadenopathy

History
- Is there a history of a systemic illness?
- Has there been any contact with infectious disease (e.g. HIV or syphilis)?
- Has there been an animal scratch?
- Are there recurrent fever, lassitude, sweats or anaemia to suggest Hodgkin's disease?
- Do any symptoms (e.g. epistaxis or hoarseness) suggest a nasopharyngeal cause?
- Are any drugs (especially phenytoin) being taken?

Examination
- Check the temperature
- Identify the node and its drainage area
- Check carefully for dental, other oral, pharyngeal or skin causes in the area
- If a possible primary cause is found (e.g. an oral ulcer) it should be biopsied
- If no local cause is found, consider ENT referral for a nasopharyngeal cause
- Examine the other side of the neck. Bilateral lymphadenopathy suggests a systemic cause

Special investigations (as appropriate)
- Blood picture (leukaemia? glandular fever?)
- Chest radiograph for mediastinal nodes (e.g. Hodgkin's disease, sarcoidosis)
- Serology (glandular fever, toxoplasmosis, HIV)
- Angiotensin-converting enzyme and calcium levels (sarcoid)
- Kveim test (sarcoid) or Mantoux (tuberculosis)
- Fine needle aspiration (primary or metastatic neoplasm, tuberculosis)
- Thyroid scan and function tests for unsuspected thyroid tumour
- Blind biopsy of nasopharynx and tonsils if needle biopsy of the node shows malignancy
- Biopsy of node itself is a last resort. Send fresh material for mycobacterial culture

Table 26.3 Tuberculous lymph nodes typical clinical features

- Firm swelling, usually of a group of nodes
- Nodes typically become matted
- Abscess or sinus formation, if neglected
- Calcified nodes from past, healed disease (Fig. 26.2)

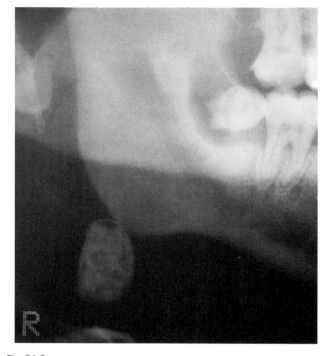

Fig. 26.2 Tuberculosis. Calcified cervical lymph node seen in a panoramic tomogram. Calcified nodes are often multiple and indicate past rather than active infection. (By kind permission of Mr E J Whaites.)

Fig. 26.3 Tuberculosis. Lymph node contains numerous granulomas of pink staining macrophages, in the centre of which there are multinucleate Langhans-type giant cells.

immunofluorescence using auramine-rhodamine. However, infection by non-tuberculous mycobacteria, even in immunocompetent children, is likely to give rise to poorly-defined or irregular granulomas without palisading, or to ill-defined aggregates of epithelioid histiocytes (Fig. 26.3). Caseation may be absent but there may be areas of necrosis with numerous neutrophils. Ziehl–Neelson staining is also negative.

Mycobacterial culture or detection of mycobacterial DNA is required. The tuberculin skin test should be positive unless the patient is severely immunodeficient.

Management

The clinical picture is variable and the diagnosis is usually only made after fine needle aspiration or excision of a node. If a tuberculous ('cold') abscess and sinus form, incision is con-traindicated and affected nodes should be excised intact. A course of isoniazid should also be given.

SYPHILIS

The cervical lymph nodes are enlarged, soft and rubbery when the primary chancre is in the mouth or on the lip. They are also involved in the widespread lymphadenopathy of the secondary stage.

Diagnosis is by finding *Treponema pallidum* in a direct smear from the oral lesion in the primary stage, and thereafter by the serological findings (Ch. 12).

Management

Antibiotic treatment, usually with penicillin, is required.

CAT-SCRATCH DISEASE

This infection is common in the USA, and though rare in Britain is increasingly frequently found. Typical features are summarised in Table 26.4.

Table 26.4   Cat-scratch disease — typical features

- Frequently a history of a scratch by a cat or other animal
- Formation of papule which may suppurate, at the site of inoculation
- Mild fever, malaise and regional lymphadenitis 1–3 weeks after exposure
- Lymph nodes soften and typically suppurate
- Conjunctivitis may be associated. Encephalitis is a rare complication

---

Pathology

There is destruction of lymph node architecture, necrosis and lymphocytic infiltration, formation of histiocytic granulomas and central suppuration (Fig. 26.4).

These appearances can readily be mistaken for one of the deep mycoses. However, it may be possible to show the usual causative organism, *Bartonella henselae*. It is a small Gram-negative bacillus demonstrable with a silver (Warthin–Starry) stain (but not H & E) at the site of inoculation or in the lymph nodes.

Fig. 26.4   Cat-scratch disease. There is necrosis in larger more irregular foci than tuberculosis and giant cells.

Management

Diagnosis depends on a history of a scratch, particularly by a cat, clinical features and exclusion of other causes for lymphadenopathy. The histological findings are confirmatory if *B. henselae* can be identified.

The disease is typically mild and self-limiting but may lead to suppuration and sinus formation. The response to antibacterials is variable. Trimethoprim-sulphamethoxazole has been recommended but some cases resolve spontaneously.

LYME DISEASE

Lyme disease is caused by a spirochaete, *Borrelia burgdorferi*, which is transmitted by insects, particularly deer ticks. The disease is worldwide but far more common in the USA than in Britain. Typical features are summarised in Table 26.5.

Table 26.5   Lyme disease — typical features

- A rash spreading outwards from the insect bite
- Enlarged regional lymph nodes
- Fever and often other systemic symptoms
- Arthritis (the main chronic effect) particularly of the knees, rarely of the temporomandibular joints
- Neurological complications (in about 15% of patients) include facial palsy or other cranial nerve lesions

---

Management

Diagnosis is by the history and clinical picture. It is confirmed serologically or sometimes, by demonstration of the spirochaete by silver staining, in a skin biopsy.

The spirochaete is sensitive to penicillin or tetracycline which should be given as early as possible. However, joint pains may recur or destructive arthritis may develop later.

INFECTIOUS MONONUCLEOSIS

The Epstein–Barr virus (EBV) is the main cause of this self-limiting lymphoproliferative disease with polyclonal activation of B lymphocytes. Typical features are summarised in Table 26.6. The clinical features are usually distinctive, but rarely there is more persistent lymphadenopathy which may mimic a lymphoma both clinically and histologically.

Management

The diagnosis is confirmed by a peripheral blood picture showing the atypical (monocyte-like) lymphocytes. A heterophil antibody (Paul–Bunnell) test and, if necessary, demonstration

Table 26.6 Infectious mononucleosis — typical features

- In children especially
  Generalised lymphadenopathy, typically with conspicuous
  enlargement of the cervical nodes
  Sore throat
  Fever
- In adolescents
  Lymphadenopathy often less conspicuous
  Vague illness with fever
- In the anginose type of disease
  Sore throat, tonsillar exudate and pharyngeal oedema
  Palatal petechiae (Fig. 26.5)

Fig. 26.5 Petechiae on the palate are frequently seen in infectious mononucleosis.

of a raised titre of EBV antibodies are confirmatory. If these tests are negative in an otherwise typical case, cytomegalovirus infection or toxoplasmosis should be considered.

There is no specific treatment but infection is usually self-limiting.

Ampicillin or amoxycillin should be avoided. They are prone to cause irritating macular rashes unrelated to penicillin allergy.

THE ACQUIRED IMMUNE DEFICIENCY SYNDROME

Lymphadenopathy is one of the most frequent manifestations of HIV infection (Ch. 24). Soon after infection there may be a transient glandular fever-like illness. Later there may be widespread and persistent lymphadenopathy (generalised lymphadenopathy syndrome, GLS), which is likely to progress to AIDS in over 50% within less than 4 years. Lymphadenopathy in AIDS may also be due to lymphomas.

TOXOPLASMOSIS

Toxoplasma gondii is a common intestinal parasite of many domestic animals, particularly cats. It is a low-grade pathogen but can affect previously healthy persons, particularly young

women. Infection can be acquired by ingestion of oocytes and three main types of disease can result (Table 26.7).

Table 26.7 Possible effects of toxoplasmal infection

- *Acute toxoplasmosis in normal children or adults*
  Disease resembling infectious mononucleosis, with cervical lymphadenopathy
  Atypical lymphocytes present in the blood but heterophil antibody production is absent
  Infection usually self-limiting
- *Toxoplasmosis in immunodeficient patients*
  Disseminated disease, particularly encephalitis
- *In pregnant women*
  An important cause of fetal abnormalities
- *Toxoplasmal chorioretinitis*
  Impairment or loss of sight
  Usually due to congenital infection
  Rarely, results from severe infections in previously healthy adults

Management

The diagnosis is confirmed serologically by a high or rising titre of antibodies or by other immunological methods.

Antimicrobial treatment is required only for severe infections and is with pyrimethamine and a sulphonamide.

MUCOCUTANEOUS LYMPH NODE SYNDROME (KAWASAKI'S DISEASE)

Kawasaki's disease is endemic in Japan and there have been outbreaks in Hawaii and the USA, where it has surpassed rheumatic fever as the leading cause of childhood-acquired heart disease. In Britain, it causes approximately 100 deaths per annum.

The distribution of cases suggests an infectious cause, but no agent has been identified with certainty.

Typical clinical features are summarised in Table 26.8.

Table 26.8 Kawasaki's disease — typical features

- Children under 5 years old affected
- Fever persisting for more than 5 days
- Generalised, often morbilliform rash
  Palms and soles become red, swollen and indurated
- Erythematous stomatitis
  Swelling and cracking of the lips and pharyngitis
- Unilateral mass of cervical lymph nodes
- Abdominal symptoms frequently
- Deterioration of mood ('extreme misery')
- Heart disease in approximately 20%

The overall mortality is 1–3%, from heart failure secondary to coronary artery disease or dysrhythmias secondary to myocardial ischaemia.

Management

The diagnosis usually depends on the clinical and, particularly, electrocardiographic findings.

There is no specific treatment, but aspirin, despite the possible risk of Reye's syndrome, is frequently given to lessen vascular damage and thromboses. However, a single large dose of intravenous γ-globulin given with aspirin in the early, acute stages appears to be the most effective means of reducing the risk of coronary artery damage.

LANGERHANS' CELL HISTIOCYTOSIS

Cervical lymph nodes can be enlarged, sometimes massively, in isolation, or more frequently in association with multisystem disease (Ch. 9).

PHENYTOIN AND OTHER DRUG-ASSOCIATED LYMPHADENOPATHIES

Lymphadenopathy is an occasional toxic effect of long-term treatment with the antiepileptic drug, phenytoin. Phenytoin lymphadenopathy (unlike that caused by many other drugs) is not usually associated with serum sickness-like symptoms of fever, rashes and joint pains. Moreover, the histopathology of phenytoin-associated lymphadenopathy can mimic a lymphoma.

Lymphadenopathy frequently first affects the neck but usually becomes widespread.

Management

Substitution of phenytoin with another anticonvulsant such as carbamazepine should allow the lymphadenopathy to subside and confirm the diagnosis.

Other drugs which can cause lymphadenopathy include penicillin (rarely), phenylbutazone (virtually obsolete), some other non-steroidal anti-inflammatory drugs, and some antimalarials. As mentioned earlier, lymphadenopathy with these drugs is typically associated with serum sickness-like features.

SUGGESTED FURTHER READING

Collip P J 1992 Cat-scratch disease: therapy with trimethoprim-sulphamethoxazole. Am J Dis Child 146:397–399

Ogden G R, Kerr M 1989 Mucocutaneous lymph node syndrome (Kawasaki disease). Oral Surg Oral Med Oral Pathol 67:569–572

Pinder S E, Colville A 1992 Mycobacterial cervical lymphadenitis in children: can histological assessment help differentiate infections by nontuberculous mycobacteria from *Mycobacterium tuberculosis*? Histopathology 22:117–119

Stansfeld A G, d'Ardenne A J (eds) 1992 Lymph node biopsy interpretation, 2nd edn. Churchill Livingstone, Edinburgh

Steiner M, Gould A, Wilkie W, Porter K 1994 Cat-scratch disease in the submandibular region: report of a case. J Oral Maxillofac Surg 52:614–618

Terezhalmy G T 1979 Mucocutaneous lymph node syndrome. Oral Surg Oral Med Oral Pathol 47:26–30

Cardiovascular disease

Cardiovascular disease is common and the most frequent single cause of death in Britain. Many patients with heart disease require dental treatment. Heart disease becomes more frequent and severe in later life, but younger patients can also be affected. Infective endocarditis is one of the few ways in which dental treatment can lead to death of a patient, but fortunately only very rarely. Myocardial infarction is a cause of major emergencies in the dental surgery and initial measures by the dental surgeon may be life-saving (Ch. 37).

In terms of dental management, patients fall into three main groups (Table 27.1) but a few may fall into more than one, and drug treatment may create additional problems (Table 27.2). It must be appreciated therefore that the following management suggestions are generalisations and each case must be considered on its own merits.

Table 27.1 **Dental management in major types of cardiac disease**

- Valvular or related defects (congenital or due to past rheumatic fever) or those patients who have a prosthetic replacement, susceptible to infective endocarditis
  Prophylactic antibiotic cover, particularly before extractions, is mandatory
- Ischaemic heart disease with or without severe hypertension
  Routine dentistry presents little hazard but the risk of dangerous arrhythmias must be minimised
  Local anaesthetics in normal dosage have only theoretical dangers, but pain and anxiety must be minimised
  The main risk is from general anaesthesia
- Cardiac failure
  The main risk is also from general anaesthesia

Table 27.2 **Some dental implications of drugs used for heart disease**

Drugs	Implications for dental management
Methyldopa, captopril	Stomatitis (Ch. 13)
Nifedipine (and analogues), diltiazem	Gingival hyperplasia (Fig. 27.4)
Anticoagulants	Risk of prolonged postoperative bleeding
Antihypertensives	Potentiated by general anaesthetics
Digoxin	Enhanced risk of dysrhythmias with halothane

General aspects of management

Patients chiefly at risk are severe hypertensives and those who have angina or have had a myocardial infarct. Anxiety or pain can cause outpouring of adrenaline, which can both greatly increase the load on the heart and also precipitate dangerous dysrhythmias.

There is some evidence that dental infections are a risk factor for coronary artery disease.

To die of fright is not a figure of speech but can sometimes result from severe dysrhythmia. The first essential for these patients is therefore to ensure painless dentistry and to alleviate anxiety.

Patients should be asked whether routine dental treatment under local anaesthesia is acceptable. In any session of treatment as little or much should be done as they feel able to tolerate.

Oral temazepam may be helpful (5 mg on the preceding night and again half an hour before treatment, and the patient accompanied by a responsible adult). If sedation is required, relative analgesia is safer because nitrous oxide has no cardiorespiratory depressant effects and is more controllable, but it should be administered by an expert.

For local anaesthesia, an effective surface anaesthetic should be applied and the injection given very slowly to minimise pain. The most effective agent is 2% lignocaine with adrenaline and, after decades of use, no local anaesthetic has been shown to be safer. The adrenaline content can theoretically cause a hypertensive reaction in patients receiving β-blocker antihypertensives, because of an unopposed α-adrenergic effect, but only if doses are very large.

Though patients with cardiovascular disease need to be treated with care, the risks of routine dental treatment under local anaesthesia (despite many statements to the contrary) and of adverse reactions are very low.

In Britain, all three deaths associated with dental local anaesthesia during the 10 years, 1980–1989, were related to the use of prilocaine. This does not of course mean that prilocaine is necessarily dangerous but it hardly suggests that it is safer than the more widely used lignocaine with adrenaline. However, doses of local anaesthetics need to be kept to a minimum and no more than two or three cartridges should be given (or be necessary) for an acceptable session of treatment. If larger doses have to be given, for example for multiple extractions, then continuous cardiac monitoring is necessary.

If general anaesthesia is unavoidable, it should be given by a specialist anaesthetist in hospital, especially as some of the drugs used for cardiovascular disease increase the risks. Cardiovascular disease is the chief cause of sudden death under anaesthesia.

Patients with left-sided cardiac failure are also at risk from dangerous pulmonary oedema if placed supine.

Patients at risk from infective endocarditis

Normally, bacteria entering the bloodstream are rapidly cleared by circulating leucocytes, but if there is a cardiac defect which can be colonised, infective endocarditis can develop.

There are many other sources of bacteraemias, such as cardiac surgery, intravenous catheterisation and intravenous drug addiction. Bacteraemias can also be detected in over 80% of persons after extractions and even after toothbrushing, but the numbers of bacteria released are often very small. Even in a patient with a heart lesion, infective endocarditis does not necessarily follow.

Relatively few bacteria inhabit the oral mucosa, and most are being constantly washed away by the saliva. By contrast, vast numbers of bacteria inhabit the gingival margins when oral hygiene is poor, and even greater numbers occupy periodontal pockets. These bacteria are in close contact with dilated, thin-walled blood vessels (Fig. 27.1). Movement of teeth

in their sockets repeatedly compresses and stretches or ruptures these vessels, so that bacteria can be pumped into the bloodstream.

Fewer than 15% of cases of infective endocarditis can be reliably related to dental operations but in these cases extractions have been the precipitating factor in over 95%. Viridans streptococci, such as those which colonise the teeth, are of low virulence but may be able to colonise heart valves because of attachment mechanisms (Ch. 3) which also enable them to cause dental disease.

Factors determining susceptibility to infective endocarditis are difficult to identify. For example, children with Down's syndrome, who are prone to severe periodontal disease, have multiple immune defects and, frequently, congenital cardiac defects, are not particularly susceptible to infective endocarditis.

Currently, advanced age, especially if there is periodontal sepsis, is the main risk factor (Fig. 27.2). Infective endocarditis is rare in children; the peak incidence and mortality is after the age of 60 years.

Once infective endocarditis develops, vegetations of bacteria and fibrin form on the valves, which are progressively destroyed (Fig. 27.3). Cardiac failure is the main cause of death but emboli and bacteria released into the bloodstream can also cause renal or cerebral damage.

Prevention is all-important. Patients who have valvular defects (congenital or due to past rheumatic fever) or some other congenital anomalies, such as septal defects, or who have prosthetic heart valves, should receive antibiotic prophylaxis (Appendix 27.1) before extractions (the highest risk), scaling and periodontal surgery. These are likely to release significant numbers of bacteria from the gingivae or, particularly, periodontal pockets.

Other dental procedures such as fitting metal bands which extend deep to the gingival margins, though they may cause bacteraemias, have rarely been followed by infective endocarditis, and antibiotic cover is not officially recommended. However, if the clinician considers the patient to fall into a high-risk group, then it may be prudent to give cover. Otherwise, orthodontic procedures are not in general recommended for antibiotic cover, particularly because most of these patients are children, in whom infective endocarditis is relatively rare.

Fig. 27.1 Subgingival plaque. The area of pocket wall in contact with plaque is large and the tissue contains numerous thin-walled blood vessels near the surface. This illustration serves to remind how easily microrganisms may be transferred into the circulation.

Fig. 27.2 Poor oral hygiene and severe pocketing such as this constitutes a risk to life, particularly in an elderly patient with a cardiac valve defect.

Fig. 27.3 Heart valve in subacute infective endocarditis. The free edge of the valve lies to the left of the picture and is covered by vegetations; centrally the valve is inflamed and thickened; and to the right the normal thickness of the valve at its attachment to the heart is seen.

Endodontic treatment rarely if ever leads to infective endocarditis and the risks of antibiotic prophylaxis exceed any benefits.

Infective endocarditis does not appear to be a risk after myocardial infarction or coronary artery bypasses, or for wearers of cardiac pacemakers, and antibiotic cover is not recommended for dental procedures.

It should be noted that the onset of infective endocarditis is typically very insidious. Even when antibiotic cover has been given, patients must be made to understand that they should report to the dentist if they develop any mild, unexplained, febrile illness within 3 months of the dental treatment. Delay in diagnosis is the main factor affecting survival in infective endocarditis.

For cardiac transplantation, patients are deeply immunosuppressed and might be considered to be at high risk of infective endocarditis after dental operations. However, data are limited and there is no agreed protocol for such patients.

Cardiac pacemakers

Pacemakers provide a stimulus to cardiac contraction when the normal rhythm is disturbed by disease of the sinoatrial node or conducting tissues, as a result, for example, of myocardial infarction.

Any ultrasonic scalers or electrosurgical equipment that interferes with pacemaker function should be avoided but pulp testers are safe.

Fig. 27.4 Drug-induced gingival hyperplasia resulting from treatment of hypertension with nifedipine. These swellings are centred on the interdental papillae.

Kawasaki's disease (mucocutaneous lymph node syndrome)

As noted earlier (Ch. 12) Kawasaki's disease is the only form of serious heart disease with specific orofacial manifestations, namely mucositis and cervical lymphadenopathy.

Cardiac damage is the result of vasculitis, which may result in coronary artery aneurysm formation, myocardial infarction and a mortality of over 5%.

Aspirin (80–100 mg/kg daily) has been the standby of treatment but is more effective if supplemented with intravenous γ-globulin.

APPENDIX 27

Antibiotic prophylaxis of infective endocarditis for dental patients

Prophylaxis is recommended for dental extractions, scaling or periodontal surgery*

Under local or no anaesthesia

- Patients not allergic to the penicillins and who have not received penicillin more than once in the previous month

Amoxycillin

Adults 3 g single oral dose taken under supervision, 1 hour before dental procedure
Children 5–10 years Half adult dose
Children under 5 years Quarter adult dose.

- Patients allergic to penicillins or who have received penicillin more than once in the previous month

Clindamycin

Adults 600 mg single oral dose taken under supervision, 1 hour before dental procedure
Children 5–10 years Half adult dose
Children under 5 years Quarter adult dose

Antibiotic prophylaxis may be supplemented with chlorhexidine gluconate gel 1% applied to the gingival margins.

Under general anaesthesia

- Patients not allergic to the penicillins, who have not received penicillin more than once in the previous month and who are not special risk patients (see below)

Amoxycillin

Adults 1 g intravenously or 1 g in 2.5 ml 1% lignocaine hydrochloride intramuscularly *or* 3 g orally 4 hours before induction then 3 g orally as soon as possible after recovery
Children 5–10 years Half adult dose
Children under 5 years Quarter adult dose *or* 3 g orally plus oral probenicid 1 g, 4 hours before procedure

Special risk patients who should be referred to hospital

1. Patients who have had a previous attack of infective endocarditis (whether or not general anaesthesia is to be given), and patients with prosthetic valves requiring a general anaesthetic but not allergic to penicillin.
Adults, AMOXYCILLIN 1 g i.v. or i.m. plus GENTAMICIN 120 mg i.v. or i.m. at induction
Children 5–10 years Amoxycillin half adult dose plus gentamicin 2 mg/kg
Children under 5 years Amoxycillin quarter adult dose plus gentamicin 2 mg/kg

2. Similar patients who are allergic to penicillins *either* VANCOMYCIN i.v., 1 g given over at least 100 minutes, then i.v. GENTAMICIN 120 mg at induction or 15 minutes before dental procedure
Children under 10 years Vancomycin i.v. 20 mg/kg, gentamicin 2 mg/kg

or TEICOPLANIN i.v., 400 mg plus GENTAMICIN 120 mg at induction or 15 minutes before dental procedure
Children under 14 years Teicoplanin 6 mg/kg, gentamicin 2 mg/kg

or CLINDAMYCIN i.v., 300 mg given over at least 10 minutes, at induction or 15 minutes before dental procedure, then oral or i.v. clindamycin 150 mg, 6 hours later
Children 5–10 years Half adult dose
Children under 5 years Quarter adult dose

Precautions

1. When clindamycin is used, periodontal or other multi-stage procedures should not be repeated at intervals of less than 2 weeks.

2. Whatever antibiotic cover has been given, patients must be instructed to report to the dentist any mild, unexplained, febrile illness developing within 3 months of the dental treatment.

---

*Prophylaxis is not considered necessary for other procedures such as orthodontic manipulations unless there is likely to be significant damage to the gingival margins.

SUGGESTED FURTHER READING

Aitken C, Cannell H, Sefton A M et al 1995 Comparative efficacy of oral doses of clindamycin and erythromycin in the prevention of bacteraemia. Br Dent J 178:418–422

Blinder D, Shemesh J, Taicher S 1996 Electrocardiographic changes in cardiac patients undergoing dental extractions under local anaesthesia. J Oral Maxillofac Surg 54:162–165

Durack D T 1995 Prevention of infective endocarditis. N Engl J Med 332:38–45

Findler M, Galili D, Meidan Z et al 1993 Dental treatment in very high risk patients with active ischaemic heart disease. Oral Surg Oral Med Oral Pathol 76:298–300

Findler M, Mazor Z, Galili D, Garfunkel A A 1993 Dental treatment in a patient with malignant phaeochromocytoma and severe uncontrolled high blood pressure. Oral Surg Oral Med Oral Pathol 75:290–291

Glick M 1995 Intravenous drug abusers: a consideration for infective endocarditis in dentistry? Oral Surg Oral Med Oral Pathol 80:125

Lockhart P B 1996 An analysis of bacteremias during dental extractions. Arch Intern Med 156:513–520

Mattila K J, Valtonen V V, Neiminen M, Huttunen J K 1995 Dental infection and the risk of new coronary events: prospective study of patients with documented coronary artery disease. Clin Infect Dis 20:588–592

Rahn R, Schneider S, Diehl O et al 1995 Preventing post-treatment bacteremia. J Am Dent Assoc 126:1145–1148

Smith A J, Adams D 1993 The dental status and attitudes of patients at risk from infective endocarditis. Br Dent J 174:59–64

Uyemura M C 1995 Antibiotic prophylaxis for medical and dental procedures. Postgrad Med 98:137–152

Van der Meer J T M, van Wilk W, Thompson J et al 1992 Awareness of need and actual use of prophylaxis: lack of patient compliance in the prevention of bacterial endocarditis. J Antimicrob Chemother 29:187–194

Working Party of the British Society for Antimicrobial Chemotherapy 1992 Antibiotic prophylaxis of infective endocarditis. Lancet 339:1292–1293

28 CHAPTER

Respiratory tract disease

SINUSITIS

Nasal congestion, purulent nasal discharge, some fever and malaise usually follow an upper respiratory infection such as a cold. Pain and facial tenderness are felt over the involved antrum. However, pain may be felt in teeth with roots close to the antral floor. Several adjacent molars may then be tender, but there should be little difficulty in distinguishing sinusitis from periodontitis. Radiographs show absence of periodontitis but opacity of the antrum.

Sinusitis can also result from dental infection or damage to the antral floor. A radiographic survey has shown antral disease to be twice as frequent in patients with periodontal disease as in matched controls.

Dental damage to the maxillary antrum

The floor of the antrum may be damaged during dental extractions which cause an oroantral fistula. If the antrum is opened during an extraction, a displaced root or bacteria from the mouth can introduce infection. There is also damage to the ciliated lining and loss of normal mucociliary transport which carries foreign material out of the cavity. If sinusitis becomes established and the fistula has not been closed, the walls of the passage may become epithelialised and the opening becomes permanent.

Displacement of a root or tooth into the maxillary antrum

A whole tooth can be driven into the antrum if the tooth is conical and considerable upward force has been used. More frequently, a root is driven into the antrum when an attempt is made to dig it out via the socket, particularly when a thin antral floor extends down into the alveolar ridge.

Clinical features

Displacement of a tooth or root into the antrum can give rise to signs (Table 28.1), partly depending on the size of the opening.

Table 28.1 Signs suggesting a tooth or root displaced into the antrum

- The root or tooth suddenly disappears during the extraction
- Blowing the nose may force air into the mouth or cause frothing of blood from the socket
- The patient may notice air entering the mouth during swallowing, or fluid from the mouth escapes into the nose
- Bleeding from the nose on the affected side, occasionally
- Later, a salty taste or unpleasant discharge
- Facial pain if acute sinusitis develops
- Rarely, antral lining may prolapse into the mouth

Management

The position of the root or tooth should be confirmed. Sometimes it is still within the alveolar process or outside the antrum and between its lining and bony floor.

A periapical radiograph should be supplemented with occlusal intraoral views. If the root has been displaced far, antral views should be taken with the head in two different positions to determine whether the tooth is mobile.

A root displaced into the antrum usually causes sinusitis, but it may cause no more than mucosal thickening. Severe sinusitis is less common. The root should be removed from the antrum and any oroantral opening closed. Several measures are important (Table 28.2).

Table 28.2 Principles of management of a root displaced into the antrum

- Explain to the patient how the accident has happened, and give the necessary reassurance
- Do not try to retrieve the lost root immediately by digging through the socket opening and damaging the antral floor and lining further
- If a root or tooth has been displaced into the antrum, it should be removed by elective surgery (see below)
- If the tip of a root causes a minimal antral reaction or lies between the bony floor and the mucosal lining, removal may not be essential but there is a risk of infection later

After any acute sinusitis has been treated, the surgical

approach depends on the position of the root and whether there is a wide oroantral opening. The usual method is to reflect a mucoperiosteal flap in the labiobuccal sulcus and to open the antrum in the canine fossa (Caldwell–Luc approach). The tooth or fragment may then be removable on a sucker nozzle small enough to prevent it from disappearing into the suction apparatus and being lost from confirmation of its removal.

Oroantral fistula

Rarely the antrum may be accidentally opened during extractions if the antral floor is damaged. If the fistula is not obvious, its presence should be verified by telling the patient to blow gently while blocking the nose by pinching the nostrils together. Air (detectable with a tuft of cotton wool held in tweezers), blood, pus or mucus will then be expelled from the opening into the mouth. Occasionally an opening may be blocked by prolapsed lining which is purplish red (Fig. 28.1) and, if the opening is large enough, it may sometimes be pushed gently back into the antrum, thus confirming its origin. Alternatively a silver probe can be gently insinuated beside the mass into the antral cavity to detect the opening.

Usually, a large oroantral fistula gives adequate drainage, but a pinhole fistula blocks drainage and is often associated with recurrent attacks of sinusitis. If the patient is not seen until late after the accident, there is typically chronic antral infection, persistent discharge and proliferation of granulation tissue. The inflamed antral lining is usually much thickened, and polyps may fill part of the cavity.

Principles of management are summarised in Table 28.3.

ASPIRATION OF A TOOTH, ROOT OR INSTRUMENT

A tooth or root can rarely slip from extraction forceps but is more frequently swallowed than inhaled. The patient should be reassured but should be sent for an abdominal radiograph and, if necessary, a chest radiograph and bronchoscopy. Small

Table 28.3	Principles of management of an oroantral fistula

The 'fresh' fistula
- Reflect a mucoperiosteal flap and suture to give an air-tight seal over the opening

The established infected fistula
- Control chronic sinusitis by removal of any polyps, usually via a Caldwell–Luc approach or through the oral opening if the fistula is sufficiently large
- Excise the entire epithelialised fistula
- Close the opening by advanced a mucoperiosteal flap over it

Postoperatively
- Give penicillin, for 5 days and a 10-day course of decongestant nose drops and inhalations
- Warn the patient against blowing the nose for 2 weeks

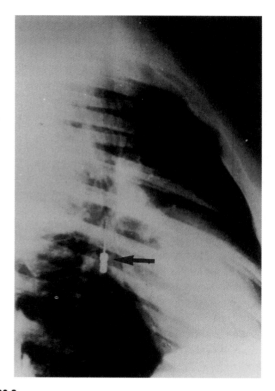

Fig. 28.2   Radiograph of the chest used to localise an inhaled reamer.

instruments such as reamers can also occasionally be inhaled (Fig. 28.2).

If left, a tooth in a bronchus can cause collapse of the related lobe and a lung abscess.

COMMON VIRAL UPPER RESPIRATORY TRACT INFECTIONS ('COLDS')

Colds often precede sinusitis. They are a contraindication to

Fig. 28.1   Antral polyp. A polyp of inflamed antral mucosa has prolapsed through an oroantral fistula left untreated after the extraction of an upper first permanent molar.

general anaesthesia. Transmission to the dentist is also a hazard.

TUBERCULOSIS

Open pulmonary tuberculosis can occasionally cause lingual ulceration as a result of coughed-up mycobacteria in the sputum (Ch. 12).

Dentists are likely to be non-immune, and are at significant risk from acquiring tuberculosis from such patients. This can be particularly dangerous if the mycobacteria are multiply resistant.

Rigorous infection control must therefore be maintained.

SARCOIDOSIS

Sarcoidosis is a chronic disease of unknown cause, in which granulomas form particularly in the lungs, lymph nodes (especially the hilar nodes), salivary glands and other sites such as the mouth (Fig. 28.3).

Oral lesions, usually painless swellings, may be seen. The most frequently affected sites are the gingivae (Fig. 28.4), lips, palate and buccal mucosa. In over 50% of patients with bilateral hilar lymphadenopathy, biopsy of a labial salivary

Fig. 28.4   Sarcoidosis. Gingival swelling is not clinically distinguishable from several other possible causes, but biopsy showed granuloma formation.

Fig. 28.5   Sarcoidosis. There is a scattered lymphoplasmacytic infiltrate in the gland and granulomas are scattered through the tissue. Here a granuloma contains several large, multinucleate giant cells.

gland shows typical granulomas and is a valuable diagnostic aid (Fig. 28.5).

Clinical involvement of major salivary glands is uncommon but can cause tumour-like swellings (Fig. 28.6). Parotid swelling due to sarcoidosis, with xerostomia, uveitis and often facial palsy, is known as *Heerfordt's syndrome*. Many minor abnormalities of immune responses, for example anergy to some antigens such as tuberculin and, frequently, hypergammaglobulinaemia, are detectable, but patients are not unusually susceptible to infection.

Pathology

Sarcoid granulomas are non-caseating, contain multinucleated giant cells and are surrounded by lymphocytes (Fig. 28.7). In an

Fig. 28.3   Sarcoidosis. Prominent hilar lymphadenopathy is the main radiological finding, though granuloma formation may be widespread.

Fig. 28.6 Bilateral parotid swelling in a case of sarcoidosis.

Fig. 28.7 Sarcoidosis. Microscopically the granulomas are compact with heavy peripheral lymphocytic infiltrate. However, they are not distinguishable by microscopy alone from other granulomatous diseases such as tuberculosis.

oral biopsy, sarcoid granulomas have to be distinguished from other granulomatous diseases (Table 28.4).

Management

Diagnosis depends on combined clinical and laboratory findings, particularly signs of pulmonary involvement, biopsy of affected tissue and a positive Kveim test. Labial gland biopsy showing granulomas may greatly facilitate diagnosis.

Treatment with systemic corticosteroids is indicated for pulmonary fibrosis, cerebral lesions or hypercalcaemia.

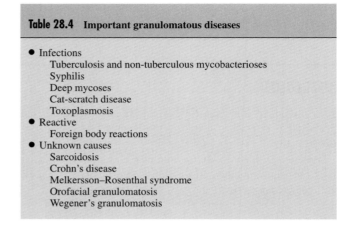

Table 28.4 Important granulomatous diseases

- Infections
    Tuberculosis and non-tuberculous mycobacterioses
    Syphilis
    Deep mycoses
    Cat-scratch disease
    Toxoplasmosis
- Reactive
    Foreign body reactions
- Unknown causes
    Sarcoidosis
    Crohn's disease
    Melkersson–Rosenthal syndrome
    Orofacial granulomatosis
    Wegener's granulomatosis

CHRONIC OBSTRUCTIVE AIRWAYS DISEASE (COAD)

Chronic obstructive airways disease is typically caused by smoking and recurrent respiratory infections. Patients are hypoxic and may be cyanotic. COAD is a contraindication to intravenous sedation because of its respiratory depressant effect, and to general anaesthesia except in specialised hands.

ASTHMA

Asthma is a common, potentially lethal disease which accounts for at least 2500 deaths a year. Rarely, acute severe asthma precipitates an emergency in the dental surgery and calls for immediate attention (Ch. 36).

'LETHAL MIDLINE GRANULOMA SYNDROME' (WEGENER'S GRANULOMATOSIS AND NASOPHARYNGEAL T CELL LYMPHOMA)

The main features of these formerly ill-defined diseases are variable degrees of destruction of the central facial tissues and a fatal outcome.

They start in the upper respiratory tract and are not clinically distinguishable in their early stages but are now recognised to result from either Wegener's granulomatosis or a peripheral (nasopharyngeal) T cell lymphoma.

Wegener's granulomatosis

Wegener's granulomatosis is a potentially lethal but uncommon systemic vasculitis; its features are summarised in Table 28.5.

Clinically, granulomatous inflammation of the nasal tissues and discharge is typically the first sign and can result in destruction of the nasal septum and a saddle nose deformity.

Occasionally, a characteristic proliferative gingivitis appears

Table 28.5 Wegener's granulomatosis — important features

- Granulomatous inflammation of nasal tract
- Cavitation of the lungs
- Potentially fatal glomerulonephritis
- Proliferative gingivitis occasionally
- Oral ulceration occasionally
- Antineutrophil cytoplasmic antibodies (ANCAs) typically present
- Histologically, granulomatous inflammation with giant cells and vasculitis

Fig. 28.9 Wegener's granulomatosis. There is epithelial hyperplasia with deeply penetrating irregular broad rete processes. In the connective tissue there is a mixed inflammatory infiltrate in which eosinophils are prominent and there may be occasional scattered giant cells.

Fig. 28.8 Wegener's granulomatosis. There is irregular gingival hyperplasia affecting a few teeth and redness extending the full breadth of the attached gingiva. The distribution is not related to plaque.

first. The changes initially resemble pregnancy gingivitis but the gingivae become swollen with a granular surface (Fig. 28.8) and dusky or bright red ('strawberry gums'). The changes can be widespread or patchy. Alternatively, mucosal ulceration may be widespread but appears at a later stage.

Pathology

Biopsy of affected gingivae typically shows a finely nodular surface, epithelial proliferation, a dense inflammatory infiltrate and collections of giant cells (Figs 28.9–28.11). In deeper tissues, vasculitis with destruction of small arteries is seen but granulomas are frequently inconspicuous.

Management

Early diagnosis by biopsy of any gingival changes is important. Early cytotoxic treatment, usually with cyclophosphamide, may then be life-saving, but haematuria suggests glomerulonephritis and a poor prognosis.

Nasopharyngeal T cell lymphomas

These rare lymphomas start in the nasal cavity and can cause extensive destruction of the centre of the face. As in Wegener's

Fig. 28.10 Wegener's granulomatosis. Gingival biopsy showing clusters of giant cells.

granulomatosis, nasal obstruction, discharge and crusting are typical early signs.

Extension of the disease through the palate can cause a small oral ulcer which may extend until the whole of the palate becomes necrotic. A deep biopsy is necessary to obtain lesional tissue not obscured by necrosis.

Histological diagnosis is difficult as these lymphomas are cellularly pleomorphic. They attack blood vessels, and thus simulate vasculitis (Fig. 28.12). Secondary inflammation may also obscure the lymphoma cells.

Fig. 28.11 Wegener's granulomatosis. At higher power a giant cell is visible centrally surrounded by an infiltrate of lymphocytes, plasma cells and neutrophils with occasional eosinophils.

Fig. 28.12 Nasopharyngeal T cell lymphoma. Obliteration and infiltration of vessel by lymphoma cells deep in the tissues from a biopsy of a non-healing palatal ulceration which extended into the nasal cavity.

In the past, death could result from infection secondary to massive facial necrosis. Usually now, death results from dissemination of the lymphoma, but this may be delayed by radiotherapy.

Key features are summarised in Table 28.6.

Table 28.6 Nasopharyngeal T cell lymphoma — key features
• Onset typically indistinguishable from Wegener's granulomatosis
• Downward extension may cause central ulceration or necrosis of the palate enabling early diagnosis
• Histologically, the cellular picture is pleomorphic but damage to blood vessels mimics vasculitis
• T cell markers confirm the diagnosis
• Spread of disease is similar to that of other lymphomas, and there is usually a fatal outcome
• Spread may be limited or delayed by radiotherapy

Fig. 28.13 Antral carcinoma. Occasionally an antral carcinoma will present intraorally, either after eroding the maxilla or through an extraction socket.

CARCINOMA OF THE ANTRUM

Carcinoma of the antrum is rare. As with cancer of the mouth, pain is not an early symptom. Later, anaesthesia in the distribution of any sensory nerves involved is almost as common as pain.

Oral and dental symptoms from carcinoma of the antrum result from involvement of its floor. This may cause pain in the teeth or under a denture. As the disease advances, teeth may become loose and a swelling becomes obvious (Fig. 28.13).

Radiographs should be taken for signs of destruction of the bony antral walls. It is a general rule that an opaque maxillary antrum in a person over 40 years of age without obvious underlying dental or nasal disease should have the antrum explored. If a mass is found, biopsy must be carried out.

MYCOPLASMAL (PRIMARY ATYPICAL) PNEUMONIA

Mycoplasmal pneumonia occasionally triggers bullous erythema multiforme (Ch. 13).

CYSTIC FIBROSIS (MUCOVISCIDOSIS)

Obstruction of the airways by the viscid sputum causes recurrent respiratory infections in childhood. Development and eruption of the teeth may be delayed and hypoplastic defects may be seen. Salivary gland swelling is another possible effect. Administration of tetracycline during dental development may cause staining of teeth.

SUGGESTED FURTHER READING

Abrahams J J, Glassberg 1966 Dental disease: a frequently unrecognised cause of dental sinus abnormalities? AJR 166:1219–1223

Bartlett J G A 1996 Antibiotic selection in sinusitis. Arch Otolaryngol Head Neck Surg 122:422–423

Benatar S R 1994 Sarcoidosis. Medicine Int 22:43–50

Brook I, Frazier E H, Gher M E 1996 Microbiology of periapical abscesses and associated maxillary sinusitis. J Periodontol 67:608–610

Calverley P M A 1995 Management of COPD. Medicine UK 23:308–312

Cawson R A 1965 Gingival changes in Wegener's granulomatosis. Br Dent J 118:30–32

Davies K J, Herbert A-M, Westmoreland D, Bagg J 1994 Seroepidemiological study of respiratory virus infections among dental surgeons. Br Dent J 176:262–263

Davies P D O 1995 Tuberculosis. Medicine UK 23:325–332

Devaney K O, Travis W D, Hoffman G, Leavitt R, Lebovics R, Fauci A S 1990 Interpretation of head and neck biopsies in Wegener's granulomatosis. A pathologic study of 126 biopsies in 70 patients. Am J Surg Pathol 14:555–564

Eufinger H, Machtens E, Akuamoa-Boateng E 1992 Oral manifestations of Wegener's granulomatosis. Int J Oral Maxillofac Surg 21:50–53

Fernald G W, Roberts M W, Boat T F 1990 Cystic fibrosis: a current review. Pediatr Dent 12:72–78

Harrison B 1995 Acute severe asthma in adults. Medicine UK 23:298–301

Hoffman G S, Kerr G S, Leavitt R Y et al 1992 Wegener granulomatosis: an analysis of 158 patients. Ann Intern Med 116:488–498

Johns C J 1995 Pulmonary sarcoidosis. Medicine UK 23:405–408

Landau L 1995 Cystic fibrosis. Medicine UK 23:400–404

Mahaney M C 1986 Delayed dental development and pulmonary disease in children with cystic fibrosis. Arch Oral Biol 31:363–367

Nachbar F N, Classen V, Nachbar T et al 1996 Orificial tuberculosis detection by polymerase chain reaction, Br J Dermatol 135:106–109

Parsons E, Seymour R A, Macleod R I et al 1992 Wegener's granulomatosis. A distinct gingival lesion. J Clin Periodontol 19:64–66

Smith W H R 1982 Intraoral and pulmonary tuberculosis following dental treatment. Lancet i:842–844

Gastrointestinal and liver disease

Though the mouth is the entry to the gastrointestinal tract, few gastrointestinal diseases directly affect the oral cavity.

GASTRIC REGURGITATION

Chronic vomiting of gastric acid contents, due to such causes as hypertrophic pyloric stenosis, can lead to erosion of the palatal aspect of the anterior teeth particularly (Fig. 29.1). This type of dental erosion is an important diagnostic sign of self-induced vomiting in bulimia.

CROHN'S DISEASE

Crohn's disease is of unknown aetiology. It most frequently affects the ileocaecal region, causing thickening and ulceration. Effects include abdominal pain, variable constipation or diar-rhoea, and sometimes obstruction and malabsorption.

Orofacial involvement (Table 29.1) may occasionally precede abdominal symptoms. Oral lesions such as these (Figs 29.2–29.4), particularly when associated with abdominal symptoms, can lead to the diagnosis of Crohn's disease.

Table 29.1 Crohn's disease — typical orofacial features
● Diffuse soft or tense swelling of the lips, or mucosal thickening
● Cobble-stone thickening of the buccal mucosa, with fissuring and hyperplastic folds
● Gingivae may be erythematous and swollen
● Sometimes, painful mucosal ulcers, linear or resembling aphthae
● Mucosal tags in sulcuses sometimes present
● Glossitis due to iron, folate or vitamin B_{12} deficiency can result from malabsorption

Fig. 29.2 Oral Crohn's disease. Gross irregular soft-tissue swelling of the buccal mucosa with linear ulcers at the base of some clefts is strongly suggestive of Crohn's disease, even if gastrointestinal signs are absent.

Histologically, the granulomas are typically small, loose and with few multinucleate giant cells. They are often deep in the corium and may be difficult to find. A biopsy may need to extend unusually deeply (Figs 29.5–29.7)

Management

Oral symptoms may resolve when intestinal Crohn's disease is

Fig. 29.1 Erosion of the palatal surfaces of the upper teeth due to repeated vomiting.

Fig. 29.3 Crohn's disease. There is lip swelling, clinically identical to that seen in orofacial granulomatosis, with cracking of the lips. Angular cheilitis is frequent in untreated disease because of anaemia resulting from malabsorption.

Fig. 29.4 Crohn's disease. The gingivae are hyperplastic and irregular and erythematous. These changes are florid, but more subtle signs are easily missed. The appearances are identical to those in sarcoidosis in the gingivae.

controlled, or may respond to oral sulphasalazine or to intralesional injections of a corticosteroid.

MALABSORPTION SYNDROMES

Malabsorption syndromes (Table 29.2) can cause haematological deficiencies which can contribute to development or exacerbation of recurrent aphthae, sore tongue or other symptoms.

Table 29.2 Important causes of malabsorption syndrome

- Coeliac disease
- Crohn's disease
- Resection of stomach or ileum
- Pancreatic insufficiency
- Liver disease (failure of bile secretion into the gut)
- Some parasitic and other chronic gut infections

Fig. 29.5 Crohn's disease. The granulomas are frequently isolated and loose in texture with scanty peripheral lymphocytic infiltrate, as here.

Fig. 29.6 Crohn's disease. The granulomas are frequently deep in the mucosa and widely dispersed. Here granulomas are present in muscle, showing the importance of adequate biopsy depth.

OROFACIAL GRANULOMATOSIS

The term *orofacial granulomatosis* has been given to swellings of such sites as the gingivae or lips (Fig. 29.8) due to granulomatous reactions (Fig. 29.9), but none of the recognised diseases (see Table 28.4) are involved. Some of these patients develop Crohn's disease or sarcoidosis later, but many others remain healthy.

In some, the granulomatous reaction appears to result from common food additives such as cinnamon or tartrazine. Such

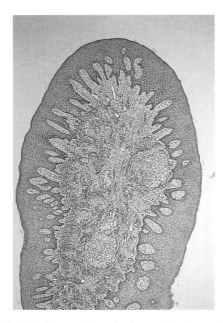

Fig. 29.7 Crohn's disease. A hyperplastic tag of gingiva contains several large round granulomas.

Fig. 29.9 Orofacial granulomatosis. Below the epithelium is a patchy inflammatory infiltrate and scattered granulomas containing large multinucleate giant cells.

Fig. 29.8 Orofacial granulomatosis. There is conspicuous swelling of the upper lip with eversion of the vermilion border. The lip is thickened and tense.

causes can only be confirmed by an exclusion diet which, if faithfully maintained, may greatly lessen the swellings.

When no cause can be found, regular follow-up should be maintained to ensure that any underlying condition, such as Crohn's disease or sarcoidosis, is recognised at an early stage.

The term 'orofacial granulomatosis' should not incidentally be confused with *midfacial granulomas* which are lethal diseases (Ch. 28).

PEUTZ–JEGHERS SYNDROME

In this disorder, pigmented macules, particularly oral, are markers for intestinal polyposis (Fig. 21.5).

Polyps may be present throughout the gastrointestinal tract, and in the small bowel can cause recurrent abdominal pain and minor intestinal obstruction. Malignant transformation is rare but not unknown.

LIVER DISEASE

Common types of liver disease are infections (particularly viral hepatitis), obstructive jaundice, cirrhosis (often due to alcohol) and tumours. Rarely, liver disease has followed dental treatment when halothane has been given or as a result of transmission of hepatitis B, and there are other aspects of liver disease relevant to dentistry (Table 29.3).

Table 29.3 **Important aspects of liver disease relevant to dentistry**

- Haemorrhagic tendencies (Ch. 26)
- Impaired drug metabolism
- Transmission of hepatitis B, particularly
- Drug-dependent patients are frequently viral hepatitis carriers
- Rarely a toxic effect of halothane

Impaired drug metabolism

Most drugs are metabolised in the liver, and no drugs should be given to patients with liver disease without first consulting the *British National Formulary*. Causes of parenchymal liver disease and liver failure are shown in Table 29.4. Cirrhosis is frequently the result of alcoholism but often of unknown cause. Halothane is a rare cause of severe liver damage and its use in dentistry has greatly declined.

Table 29.4   **Important causes of liver failure**

- Idiopathic cirrhosis
- Alcoholic cirrhosis
- Viral hepatitis
- Drugs, including halothane

VIRAL HEPATITIS

The main types of hepatitis relevant here are B, C and D. Hepatitis B is the chief risk to dental personnel but hepatitis C can also be transmitted during dentistry. The hepatitis B virus can also carry within it the delta agent, which can cause a particularly virulent infection (hepatitis D).

Hepatitis B

Hepatitis B can be readily transmitted during dentistry and, despite the outbreak of AIDS, is currently the greatest infective hazard to dental staff (Table 29.5).

Table 29.5   **Special hazards to dental staff from hepatitis B**

- The virus is widespread
- A chronic infective carrier state is common
- Minute traces of body fluids can transmit infection
- The virus survives well outside the body
- The virus is relatively resistant to disinfection
- Hepatitis B infection can cause serious complications (Table 29.6)

The risk of transmission of hepatitis B is emphasised by its previous name, 'syringe jaundice'. In the past particularly, countless patients were infected via imperfectly sterilised syringes and needles. The effects of hepatitis B infection vary widely (Table 29.6).

Clinical aspects

The incubation period is at least 2–6 months. The majority of infections are subclinical (anicteric) but 5–10% of patients, particularly those who have had no overt illness, become carriers and can transmit the infection. A minority develop acute hepatitis with loss of appetite, muscle pains, fever, jaundice and often a swollen, painful liver. The illness is often severe and debilitat-

---

Table 29.6   **Possible results of hepatitis B infection**

- Complete resolution
- Asymptomatic carrier state
- Acute hepatitis (rarely fatal)
- Chronic active hepatitis
- Cirrhosis
- Liver failure
- Liver cancer

---

ing but usually followed by complete recovery and long-lasting immunity. Overall mortality from clinical infection is probably about 1%. Occasionally it has been as high as 30%, probably as a result of co-infection by the delta agent.

Biochemical markers of infection are raised serum levels of liver transaminases, such as alanine aminotransferase (ALT), aspartate aminotransferase (AST) and γ-glutamyl transpeptidase (GGT), along with raised levels of bilirubin and often of alkaline phosphatase. However, confirmation of the diagnosis is by serology.

Serological markers of hepatitis B

The hepatitis B virus (HBV) is a DNA virus termed the Dane particle which consists of a central core and an outer shell. The core contains DNA, an enzyme (DNA polymerase, DNA-P) and the hepatitis B core antigen (HBcAg). The protein shell contains the hepatitis B surface antigen (HBsAg). Serological markers of hepatitis B are summarised in Table 29.7.

The carrier state and complications

Most patients with acute hepatitis B recover completely within a few weeks. Approximately 5–10% fail to clear the virus within 6–9 months and become chronic carriers.

Chronic carriage of HBsAg but not HBeAg has a low risk of severe liver damage. Persistent carriage of both HBsAg and HBeAg is associated with chronic active (aggressive) hepatitis. These patients have biochemical evidence of liver damage. They are chronically ill and at special risk from cirrhosis and, possibly, carcinoma of the liver.

Chronic active hepatitis with persistent malaise, and sometimes mild jaundice, is particularly likely to develop in the very young or old, and HIV-positive patients. Cirrhosis can result and lead to liver failure or hepatocellular carcinoma.

Risks to dental staff

The carriage rate of hepatitis B virus in the general population of Britain is 0.1–0.2%. The rate in British dentists is probably double that in the general population.

In hot climates, such as in Asia and Africa, it may be 5–40%, and dental staff there are at high risk. There are also high-risk groups (Table 29.8), and the hazard of infection is highest in

Table 29.7 Serological markers of hepatitis B and their significance

Serological marker	Relation to infection	Significance
Surface antigen (HBsAg)	HBsAg particles detectable in late incubation period, and during acute and chronic infections	HBsAg carriage indicates past infection, but confers little risk of transmitting infection, unless HBeAg is also present
Antibody to HB surface antigen (HBsAb)	Begins to appear when recovery starts but HBsAg may briefly disappear before anti-HBs becomes detectable. Both serological tests then become negative	During recovery, anti-HBs Abs usually appears and rises in titre; it usually implies persistent immunity. Anti-HBs also appears after hepatitis B immunisation
Hepatitis B core antigen (HBcAg)	Found only in liver cells, not serum	
Antibody to HB core antigen (HBcAb)	Anti-HBc appears at onset of disease. Quickly rises in titre and persists for many years	One of the most sensitive indicators of past infection
Hepatitis B e antigen (HBeAg)	Appears in the serum simultaneously with HBsAg but disappears earlier if there is full recovery	Indicator of high infectivity
Antibody to e antigen (anti-HBe, HBeAb)*	Usually appears in the serum soon after the e antigen and heralds recovery	Failure of development of anti-HBe indicates high infectivity
DNA polymerase (DNA-P)		Indicates high infectivity

*Carriers of both HBsAg and HBeAg but who lack anti-HBe are more likely to develop chronic active hepatitis and serious complications, and to transmit the infection.

inner urban areas and particularly for oral surgeons and periodontists. In the USA, 20% of American oral surgeons have serological evidence of previous infection and one of the highest infection rates of all health workers.

Table 29.8 Patients with higher risk of being hepatitis B carriers

- Promiscuous male homosexuals and STD (VD) clinic patients
- Intravenous drug addicts
- Patients and staff of dialysis and transplant units
- Patients (especially with Down's syndrome) and staff of institutions for the handicapped
- Immunosuppressed or immunodeficient patients
- Patients who have received unscreened blood or blood products
- Patients who have had acupuncture or tattooing, especially in tropical countries
- Consorts of patients with hepatitis B or of any of the above
- Patients with certain associated diseases, particularly AIDS, some chronic liver diseases and polyarteritis nodosa
- Immigrants, or travellers from high-risk areas, particularly tropical or subtropical countries

Transmission of HBV

Blood and blood products are most dangerous and can transmit infection in as little as 0.0000001 ml fluid, particularly when containing the e antigen. Many cases have followed needlestick injuries, injections and blood transfusions. Saliva can also contain hepatitis B antigens and, experimentally, can transmit the virus. Saliva is frequently also contaminated with blood, and when splashed on to the conjunctiva might transmit infec-

tion to a dentist. Hepatitis B can also be transmitted heterosexually, but more readily by male homosexual activity. Male homosexuals, particularly in the USA, are frequently also HIV-positive, and in London 30% of male prostitutes (many of them teenagers) are estimated to be HBV carriers and 20% of them to be HIV-positive.

As discussed earlier, the risk of infection is indicated by the serological markers. Infective carriers can only be suspected if they have a history of jaundice or are in a high-risk group. Nevertheless, it must be emphasised that only 1 in 4 carriers gives a positive medical history. In statistical terms, therefore, if a dentist treats 20 patients a day, one hepatitis B carrier will be encountered every 7 working days. Many infectious patients, as in the case of HIV carriers, will therefore be treated unknowingly.

Dental staff who are carriers of, or incubating, hepatitis B can also transmit infection to patients, some of whom have died as a consequence. The dangers to dentists have been emphasised by the death from hepatitis B of an unvaccinated male nurse after being bitten by a mentally handicapped carrier.

Prevention and management of hepatitis B

It is essential for dentists to have active immunisation. It is effective, safe and protects against both hepatitis B and delta infection. Three injections should be given at intervals into the deltoid muscle, but adequate protection may not develop until after 6 months. Side-effects are mild and rare, but a few people (particularly the obese) do not produce adequate antibody levels after a normal course of vaccination and need to have it repeated. Booster doses are needed at 3–to 5-year intervals, or more frequently in persons in whom the half-life of the vaccine is brief. Antibody levels should therefore be checked. Those who have not been immunised, but are wounded while treating a high-risk patient or known carrier, should have immediate active immunisation. Passive immunisation with hepatitis B immunoglobulin as well has also been advised. Treatment of chronic active hepatitis is with interferon α which may prevent cirrhosis or other complications.

The delta agent: hepatitis D virus (HDV)

The delta agent is a defective RNA virus that can only replicate in the presence of HBsAg. Delta infection is mainly transmitted by blood or blood products. It is widespread among intravenous drug abusers and in endemic areas such as the Mediterranean region. Delta infection causes acute hepatitis. This usually resolves, but fulminant liver disease can follow and the mortality rate is high. A few dental patients have acquired delta hepatitis and some have died. Immunisation against hepatitis B also protects against the delta agent, and this strengthens the need for immunisation.

Hepatitis C

The hepatitis C virus (HCV) was the most common cause of post-transfusion hepatitis but donors are now screened for both hepatitis C and B. Before such screening was available and blood products were inactivated, almost 100% of haemophiliacs became infected and remain carriers. Hepatitis C and B are similar in most respects but have some differences (Table 29.9).

Table 29.9 Important differences between hepatitis C and B
Hepatitis C
• is less widespread
• is less readily transmitted by needle-stick injuries
• is more vulnerable to antiseptics
• is rarely transmitted during dentistry
• acute hepatitis C is uncommon and usually mild
BUT
• no protective vaccine is as yet available
• infection persists in 80% of individuals
• infection more frequently leads to chronic active hepatitis
• there is a higher risk of cirrhosis and liver cancer

In the USA, 2% of oral surgeons and 0.7% of general dentists were found to be anti-HCV positive in 1996. This compares with 21% of oral surgeons and 8% of general dentists who were anti-HBV positive in the same group.

Chronic active hepatitis C is treated with interferon α but this frequently fails to clear HCV. Cirrhosis develops in approximately 20% of patients, 10% of whom may develop liver cancer.

Control of transmission of viral hepatitis

Because of the ease of transmission of hepatitis, the basic precautions are summarised in Table 29.10. Gloves, masks and eye-shields provide only partial protection. Double gloving is necessary for surgeons at high risk from acquiring or transmitting these infections. Immunisation is therefore the single most important protective measure, as it is virtually impossible completely to prevent transmission of hepatitis B by other means.

Table 29.10 Basic precautions against transmission of viral hepatitis
• Treat all patients as infectious ('universal precautions')
• Wear gloves for all clinical dental work
• Take special care to avoid needle-stick injuries
• Wear goggles for eye protection
• Use disposable instruments and autoclave all others
• Be immunised against hepatitis B

There is as yet no vaccine against hepatitis C and there are some strains of hepatitis B against which the current vaccine apparently confers no protection. Though the hazard from these is statistically small, the risk from them emphasises the need to maintain rigorous infection control.

Sterilisation and disinfection for viral hepatitis

Hepatitis B virus is tougher than HCV but sterilisation and disinfection measures (Table 29.11) apply to both. Dentists must ensure that infection control procedures are up to standard for their own protection. However, it is also a legal obligation under the Health and Safety at Work Act. Acquisition of viral hepatitis as a consequence of dental treatment could result in substantial claims for compensation. Restrictions on dentists who are viral hepatitis carriers have been summarised on page 297.

Table 29.11 Sterilisation and disinfection for hepatitis B and C
Sterilisation
• Autoclaving at 134°C for 3 minutes OR
• Hot air at 160°C for 1 hour (effective but automatic control necessary. Not widely used in UK)
Disinfectants
• Sodium hypochlorite, 1% of freshly diluted stock solution (0.1% + detergent for surface disinfection. HCV is also susceptible to solvent detergents)

Hepatitis A

Hepatitis A is the common form of infectious hepatitis. It is frequently acquired from contaminated food during a holiday abroad in the sun. There is little evidence that hepatitis A is transmitted during dentistry.

SUGGESTED FURTHER READING

Bowden D S, Moaven L D, Locarnini S A 1996 New hepatitis viruses: are there enough letters in the alphabet? Med J Aust 164:87–89

De Mitri M S, Poussin K, Baccarini P et al 1995 HCV liver cancer without cirrhosis. Lancet 345:413–415

Gross J B, Persing D H 1995 Hepatitis C: advances in diagnosis. Mayo Clin Proc 70:296–297

Hosey M T, Gordon G, Kelly D A et al 1995 Oral findings in children with liver transplants. Int J Paediatr Dent 5:29–34

Porter S R, Lodi G 1996 Hepatitis C virus (HCV) — an occupational hazard to dentists. Br Dent J 180:473–474

Sanchez-Tapias J M, Rodes J 1995 Interferon in chronic hepatitis C. Lancet 346:s11

Thomas D L, Gruninger S E, Siew C et al 1996 Occupational risk of hepatitis C infections among general dentists and oral surgeons in North America. Am J Med 100:41–45

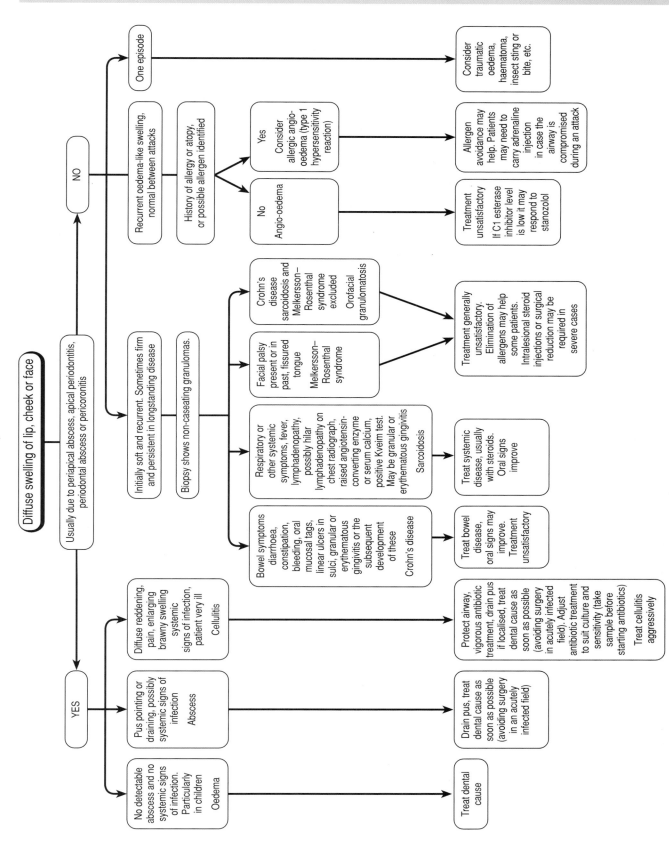

Summary 29.1 Causes and treatment of diffuse swelling of the lips and mucosa.

Nutritional deficiencies

Patients with nutritional deficiencies are rarely seen in Britain. Susceptible patients are the elderly living on a scanty diet, food cranks and severe alcoholics living on a grossly unbalanced diet. Malabsorption syndromes (Ch. 29) are another cause.

Several oral conditions of doubtful cause, such as periodontal disease or glossitis, have been ascribed to vitamin deficiencies, though patients have been otherwise healthy and well-fed. In such cases, giving vitamin preparations brings benefit only to the multibillion pound vitamin industry. Vitamin deficiencies are not a contributory cause of dental caries.

Vitamin deficiencies

The effects of specific deficiencies are summarised in Table 30.1.

Table 30.1   **Effects of specific vitamin deficiencies**

Deficiency	Systemic effects	Oral effects
Vitamin A	Night-blindness, xerophthalmia	Unconfirmed contribution to leukoplakia and cancer
Thiamin (B$_1$)	Neuritis and cardiac failure	None
Riboflavin (B$_2$)	Dermatitis	Angular stomatitis and glossitis
Nicotinamide	Dermatitis, CNS disease, diarrhoea	Glossitis, stomatitis and gingivitis
Vitamin B$_{12}$	Pernicious anaemia	Glossitis, aphthae
Folic acid	Macrocytic anaemia	Glossitis, aphthae
Vitamin C	Scurvy (purpura, delayed wound healing, bone lesions in children)	Gingival swelling and bleeding
Vitamin D	Rickets	Hypocalcification of teeth (severe rickets only)

Vitamin A deficiency

In rats, vitamin A deficiency has severe effects on secretory epithelium. Columnar cells become squamous in type and keratinised. Dental development is severely affected and secretory cells of salivary glands also become squamous and keratinised. However, there is no evidence that vitamin A deficiency causes such changes in humans.

Successful treatment of keratotic plaques (leukoplakias) with retinoids (vitamin A derivatives) has been claimed but not confirmed. The toxic effects of these drugs are severe and they are teratogenic. Epidemiological studies have suggested an association between low vitamin A intake and oral and other cancers, but there is growing doubt whether β-carotene is beneficial or harmful.

Riboflavin (B$_2$) deficiency

Riboflavin deficiency can occasionally result from a malabsorption syndrome. In severe cases there is typically angular stomatitis, with painful red fissures at the angles of the mouth, and shiny redness of the mucous membranes. The tongue is commonly sore. A peculiar form of glossitis in which the tongue becomes magenta in colour and granular or pebbly in appearance, due to flattening and mushrooming of the papillae, may be seen but is uncommon. The gingivae are not affected. Resolution follows within days when riboflavin (5 mg three times a day) is given.

Riboflavin is ineffective for the commonly seen cases of glossitis and angular stomatitis, which are rarely due to vitamin deficiency.

Nicotinamide deficiency (pellagra)

Pellagra, which affects the skin, gastrointestinal tract and nervous system, is rare in Britain but may occasionally result from malabsorption or alcoholism. Weakness, loss of appetite and changes in mood or personality are followed by glossitis or stomatitis and dermatitis. The tip and lateral margins of the tongue become red, swollen and, in severe cases, deeply ulcerated. The dorsum of the tongue becomes coated with a thick, greyish fur which is often heavily infected. The gingival margins also become red, swollen and ulcerated, and generalised stomatitis may develop.

Vitamin B$_{12}$ deficiency

This disease, unlike the others described in this section, is pri-

Fig. 30.1 Scurvy. There is gross periodontal destruction with deep pocketing and mobility of several teeth resulting from the combination of poor oral hygiene and deficiency of vitamin C.

marily a defect of absorption (Ch. 22). It is exceptionally rare for it to be caused by dietary deficiencies (veganism).

Folic acid deficiency

Deficiency can result from malnutrition but is more often seen in pregnancy, or as a result of malabsorption or drug treatment (particularly with phenytoin) (Ch. 25). Women are advised to take folic acid supplements preconceptually with the aim of reducing the risk of neural tube defects. In addition, it appears that multivitamin preparations containing folic acid also reduce the risk of orofacial clefts.

Vitamin C deficiency

Scurvy, once common among crews of sailing ships, is now exceedingly rare. In Britain scurvy may very occasionally be seen among elderly people with an inadequate income, or in those devoted to eccentric diets. The main features of scurvy are dermatitis and purpura and, in advanced cases, anaemia, delayed healing of wounds and swollen bleeding gums may develop (Fig. 30.1). In addition bone formation may be disturbed.

There is no evidence that deficiency of vitamin C plays any part in periodontal disease except in frank scurvy, and there is no correlation between low plasma ascorbic acid levels and gingivitis. There is no reason for giving ascorbic acid to healthy patients with periodontal disease.

Vitamin D deficiency

Deficiency of vitamin D during skeletal development causes rickets (Ch. 10).

A rich source of vitamin D is fish liver oils, but small amounts are also present in eggs and butter. In strong sunlight vitamin D can be synthesised in the skin. In Britain margarine is fortified with vitamins A and D, but requirements are small except during bone growth and pregnancy.

Rickets is now rare, but immigrants in the north of Britain are at risk. Contributory factors are lack of sunlight, a high-carbohydrate diet and possibly also the use of wholemeal flour (as in chupattis) containing factors which impair calcium absorption. However, there is no basis for the idea that dental caries is due to poor calcification of the teeth, and giving vitamin D and calcium for dental caries is valueless. There are also dangers associated with raising children's intake of vitamin D. Some are sensitive to this potent drug and hypervitaminosis D causes hypercalcaemia and renal calcinosis. Dental defects (hypocalcification) are a feature only of exceptionally severe rickets (Ch. 2).

Anorexia nervosa and bulimia

Anorexia nervosa is, in simple terms, an eating disorder particularly affecting young females, in which there is determined and persistent avoidance of food leading to emaciation and occasionally death. It is typically ascribed to fear of obesity and a distorted body image.

Bulimia is the term given to binge eating alternating with self-induced vomiting or purging to control excessive obesity but emaciation is not usually achieved. In a single eating binge up to 20 000 calories may be consumed and there may be addiction to drugs or alcohol also.

Oral and perioral effects of anorexia and bulimia are parotid swelling (sialadenosis) and dental erosion due to vomiting. Dentists may be able to identify such signs before medical intervention becomes imperative.

SUGGESTED FURTHER READING

Nowak R 1994 Beta-carotene: helpful or harmful? Science 264:500–501

Robb N D, Smith B G N 1996 Anorexia and bulimia nervosa (the eating disorders): conditions of interest to the dental practitioner. J Dent 24:7–16

Shaw G M, Lammer E J, Wasserman C R 1995 Risks of orofacial clefts in children born to women using multivitamins containing folic acid preconceptually. Lancet 346:393–396

Shelton R M 1992 Scurvy: a case in a young healthy woman. J Am Acad Dermatol 27:773–774

Siegal C, Barker B, Kunstadter M 1982 Conditioned oral scurvy due to megavitamin C withdrawal. J Periodontol 53:453–455

Endocrine disorders and pregnancy

Endocrine disorders, apart from diabetes mellitus and thyroid disease, are uncommon. They are rare causes of oral disease but occasionally, oral changes can lead to their diagnosis. Patients with Addison's disease, diabetes mellitus and thyrotoxicosis, in particular, may also need special care for dental surgery.

PITUITARY HYPERFUNCTION — GIGANTISM AND ACROMEGALY

Overproduction of growth hormone by the anterior pituitary during the period of skeletal growth causes *gigantism*. Overgrowth of the skeleton and soft tissues causes the patient to become a giant. Acromegaly usually develops later.

After the epiphyses have fused, an adenoma of growth hormone cells causes *acromegaly*. There is renewed growth, particularly of the jaws, hands and feet. The condylar growth centre becomes active and the mandible becomes enlarged and protrusive (Fig. 31.1). Radiographically, the whole jaw is lengthened and the angle more oblique (Fig. 31.2). The jaw and other bones are also made thicker by subperiosteal bone deposition. The teeth become spaced, or, if the patient is edentulous, dentures cease to fit the growing jaw. The hands and feet become spade-like (Fig. 31.3). Overgrowth of soft tissues causes thickening and enlargement of the facial features, particularly the lips and nose.

Headaches and visual disturbances due to the pituitary tumour are common. Later, weakness and, often, diabetes mellitus develop.

Irradiation or resection of the pituitary tumour may relieve the symptoms. Mandibular resection may be needed to improve the appearance.

THYROID DISEASE

Hyperthyroidism

Hyperthyroidism (Table 31.1) is most common in young adults,

Fig. 31.1 Acromegaly. The typical facial appearance of acromegaly resulting from excessive mandibular growth.

particularly women. Dental treatment of hyperthyroid patients may be affected by several factors (Table 31.2).

Table 31.1 Hyperthyroidism — important features

- Irritability and anxiety
- Loss of weight
- Exophthalmos (Fig. 31.4)
- Tachycardia
- Cardiovascular disease, particularly in untreated hyperthyroidism in older patients

Hyperthyroidism with excessive cardiac excitability is only a theoretical contraindication to lignocaine with adrenaline, and no other local anaesthetic has been shown to be safer.

Treatment of hyperthyroidism is by surgical removal of part

Table 31.2 Dental management of hyperthyroid patients

- Control of nervousness and excitability
- If clinical signs are seen but the patient is not under treatment, refer to a physician
- Avoid general anaesthesia in patients with long-standing thyrotoxicosis, particularly older patients

Fig. 31.3 Acromegaly. The jaw is enlarged and protrusive, the features thickened and the hands broad and spade-like.

Fig. 31.2 Acromegaly. The mandible is enlarged with an elongated ramus and increased obliquity of the angle. The pituitary fossa is also enlarged due to the tumour causing the disease.

of the gland, or by means of drugs such as thiouracil, carbimazole or iodine-131.

Hypothyroidism

Cretinism

Cretinism results from deficient thyroid activity at birth (Fig. 31.5). It is most common in areas of endemic goitre, but rare now that goitre is controlled with iodine.

A cretin is occasionally the offspring of a normal mother. The main features (Table 31.3) are particularly dwarfism and mental defect.

Treatment with thyroid extract must be begun early to provide normal physical development and improvement in the mental defect.

Adult hypothyroidism

Hypothyroidism (Table 31.4) is frequently autoimmune but can

Fig. 31.4 Thyrotoxicosis. Exophthalmos is typical but the enlarged thyroid is not conspicuous. The patient had not then started to lose weight.

Fig. 31.5 Cretinism in a child. The facial expression, excessive broadening of the features and the protruding tongue are characteristic.

Table 31.3 **Cretinism — typical features**

- Skeletal development and dental eruption greatly delayed
- Impaired mental development
- Broad, rather flat face partly due to defective growth of the skull and facial bones
- Overlarge, protrusive tongue
- Dull facial expression, dry thick skin
- Short stocky build and, often, umbilical hernia

---

follow removal of excessive thyroid tissue in the treatment of hyperthyroidism.

Table 31.4 **Adult hypothyroidism — typical features**

- Weight gain
- Slowed activity and thought
- Dry skin and hair loss
- Intolerance of cold
- Susceptibility to ischaemic heart disease

Aspects of dental management of hypothyroidism are summarised in Table 31.5.

Lingual thyroid

Thyroid tissue is occasionally present in the tongue as a result of imperfect descent of the anlage into the neck. Clinically, it usually causes a purplish soft swelling and may not be recognised for thyroid tissue until after biopsy. Scanning of the neck

---

Table 31.5 **Dental management of hypothyroidism**

- Avoid sedatives, including diazepam, opioid analgesics and general anaesthetics, because of the risk of myxoedema coma
- Anaemia or ischaemic heart disease may require dental treatment to be modified
- Local anaesthesia is always preferable
- Sjögren's syndrome is occasionally associated and requires to be treated

---

to ensure the presence of a thyroid gland is therefore essential before the lingual gland is removed. However, this may have to be done anyway if it is causing significant obstruction. Lifelong thyroid supplementation is then given.

PARATHYROID DISEASE

Hyperparathyroidism

This uncommon disease is usually caused by an adenoma of the parathyroids. Parathormone overproduction may cause decalcification of the skeleton and cyst-like areas of bone resorption (*osteitis fibrosa cystica*, Ch. 10).

Hypoparathyroidism

Postsurgical hypoparathyroidism. The most common cause of hypoparathyroidism is thyroidectomy. The resulting hypocalcaemia causes heightened neuromuscular excitability and tetany. These are controlled by giving the vitamin D analogue, 1, 25-dihydrocholecalciferol (DHCC), orally. Later, any residual parathyroid tissue undergoes compensatory hyperplasia.

Tetany. In mild cases tetany is latent but can be triggered by tapping on the skin over the facial nerve; this causes the facial muscles to contract. In more severe cases, muscle cramps and tonic contractions of the muscles may progress to generalised convulsions. An early symptom of tetany is paraesthesiae of the lip and extremities.

Tetany more frequently results from overbreathing, often neurotic in origin (*hyperventilation syndrome*).

Idiopathic hypoparathyroidism. Early onset hypoparathyroidism is rare. It sometimes forms part of the polyendocrinopathy syndrome, with autoantibodies to a variety of glandular tissues and deficiency states (particularly Addison's disease) and, frequently, mucocutaneous candidosis. Otherwise the disease and its treatment are similar to postsurgical hypoparathyroidism.

Effects on calcified tissues are summarised in Table 31.6.

ADRENOCORTICAL DISEASES

Adrenocortical insufficiency is rarely primary (Addison's disease) and more frequently secondary to corticosteroid therapy.

Table 31.6 Effects of hypoparathyroidism on calcified tissues

- Retarded new bone formation and diminished resorption are usually in equilibrium so that skeletal changes are rare
- Aplasia or hypoplasia of developing enamel*, which becomes deeply grooved
- Dentine may be incompletely mineralised but lamina dura may be thickened
- Short roots to teeth (Ch. 2)

*Results from associated ectodermal defects.

Addison's disease

Addison's disease results from atrophy of the adrenal cortices and failure of secretion of cortisol and aldosterone. The result is a severe disorder of electrolyte and fluid balance and serious clinical effects (Table 31.7). The disease is usually autoimmune, with organ-specific circulating autoantibodies. Tuberculous or fungal adrenal destruction are rare causes but can be secondary to AIDS.

Table 31.7 Addison's disease — typical clinical features

- Lassitude, anorexia, weakness and fatigue
- Abnormal oral and cutaneous pigmentation
- Gastrointestinal disturbances
- Loss of weight
- Low blood pressure
- Susceptibility to hypotensive crises

Pigmentation is often an early sign and, in the mouth, is patchily distributed on gingivae, buccal mucosa and lips (Figs 31.6 and 31.7). It is brown or almost black. However, Addison's disease is an exceptionally uncommon cause of oral pigmentation. The skin pigmentation looks similar to sun-tan but with a sallow appearance due to underlying pallor. Exposed and normally pigmented areas are most severely affected.

In an addisonian crisis there is a rapid fall in blood pressure,

Fig. 31.6 Addison's disease. A close-up shows the characteristic distribution of pigment rather patchily along the attached gingivae. It is a brownish black in colour.

Fig. 31.7 Addison's disease. Deep pigmentation of the buccal mucosa.

circulatory collapse (shock) and vomiting. These crises, which may be fatal, are often precipitated by such causes as infections, injuries, surgery or anaesthesia. Immediate treatment with intravenous hydrocortisone (several 100 mg) and fluid replacement may be life-saving.

Though Addison's disease is rare, it should be considered in a patient, other than a black individual, with pigmentation of the oral mucous membrane. A weak voice caused by general weakness and lassitude is also suggestive.

Long-term treatment of Addison's disease is usually by oral hydrocortisone which allows patients to live almost normal lives but with complications described below.

Corticosteroid treatment

Corticosteroids can have physiological effects resembling those of Cushing's disease (Table 31.8). Thus there may be sodium and water retention, a raised blood sugar and impaired protein metabolism. Hypertension and diabetes are possible complications, and a characteristic moon-face appearance is produced.

Table 31.8 Important side-effects of long-term use of corticosteroids

- Depression of adrenocortical function and risk of circulatory collapse
- Depression of inflammatory and immune responses
- Opportunistic infections
- Depressed protein metabolism
- Impaired wound healing
- Moon face
- Raised blood sugar
- Sodium and water retention
- Mood changes

Corticosteroids can also mask serious disease. The patient, for a time at least, can appear to be in perfect health with plump

Table 31.9 Cushing's disease — important features

- Obesity of trunk and face
- Bruisability and haematomas after venepuncture
- Hirsutism
- Headaches
- Hypertension
- Osteoporosis, especially of the skull
- Glycosuria

Fig. 31.8 Steroid collapse. This patient, taking only 5 mg prednisolone daily, was given brief sedation for an extraction. Adrenal suppression resulted in collapse and despite considerable doses of corticosteroid and fluid supplementation the patient did not recover fully for 48 hours.

rosy cheeks and often a sense of well-being to match. Thus, a young patient suffering from acute lymphocytic leukaemia taking corticosteroids can appear and feel well. However well a patient appears, the medical and drug history must therefore be carefully evaluated.

However, most important is the risk of circulatory collapse secondary to dental surgery or general anaesthesia (Fig. 31.8 and Ch. 37).

Adrenocortical hyperfunction (Cushing's disease)

Cushing's disease is usually due to an adrenocorticotrophic hormone-secreting pituitary adenoma which causes adrenocortical hyperplasia. The effects (Table 31.9) are rarely dentally important.

Rarely the moon-face of Cushing's disease has been mistaken for inflammatory swelling due to a dental infection.

DISEASES OF THE ADRENAL MEDULLA

Phaeochromocytoma

Phaeochromocytoma is a catecholamine-producing tumour of the adrenal medulla. The main effect is potentially lethal hypertension and dysrhythmias. Occasionally it is part of the multiple endocrine adenoma syndrome type III, when it is associated with hyperparathyroidism, thyroid medullary carcinoma and oral mucosal neurofibromas. Alternatively it may be associated with neurofibromatosis.

When an oral neurofibroma is found, the possibility of the presence of a phaeochromocytoma should be considered, especially if the patient is hypertensive.

DIABETES MELLITUS

Diabetes mellitus is a common endocrine disease and results from relative or absolute deficiency of insulin, causing a persistently raised blood glucose. Approximately 2% of the population are affected but probably at least 50% of diabetics with mild or early disease pass unrecognised. There are two clinical types.

Juvenile-onset (insulin-dependent) diabetes. Symptoms typically appear before the age of 25 and the disease is usually severe, with thirst, polyuria, hunger, loss of weight and susceptibility to infection.

Maturity-onset diabetes. Patients are typically over middle age and obese. The onset is insidious, often with deterioration of vision or pruritus or, sometimes, thirst, polyuria and fatigue. However, many cases are asymptomatic. The disease can be controlled by dietary restriction and, if necessary, oral hypoglycaemic drugs.

In terms of dental management it is usually said that the greatest problems are with 'uncontrolled' diabetes. However, 'uncontrolled' applies to several diabetic states. At one extreme there is the mild, unrecognised, and therefore untreated, diabetic. At the other there is the treated diabetic whose disease is difficult to control ('brittle' diabetes) or has been mismanaged. This last group is the one most likely to have oral complications and present difficulties in dental management (Table 31.10).

Rapidly destructive periodontal disease can result from severe untreated diabetes mellitus, but is rarely seen now. However, even treated diabetic children have slightly poorer periodontal health than controls. Diabetics also have higher DMFT levels (despite the sugar-free diet) and earlier loss of teeth than controls. Susceptibility to candidosis is another complication. Principles of dental management are summarised in Table 31.11.

Table 31.10 Complications of diabetes mellitus that can affect dental management

- Susceptibility to infection, particularly candidosis
- Hypoglycaemic coma
- Diabetic coma
- Ischaemic heart disease
- Acceleration of periodontal disease if control is poor
- Dry mouth secondary to polyuria and dehydration
- Oral lichenoid reactions due to oral hypoglycaemic drugs
- Sialadenosis

Table 31.11 Principles of dental management of diabetics

- Time treatment to avoid disturbance of routine insulin administration or meals
- Use local anaesthesia for routine dentistry — the amount of adrenaline in local anaesthetic solutions has no significant effect on the blood sugar
- Sedation can be given if required
- Dental operations under general anaesthesia should only be carried out in hospital under expert supervision
- Deal with any diabetic complications (Table 31.10)
- Manage hypoglycaemic coma as described in Chapter 36

Hypoglycaemic coma may be precipitated by dental treatment which delays a normal meal. Treatment should therefore be so timed as to avoid these risks — ideally, soon after the patient's breakfast.

Diabetic coma is a complication of poorly-controlled diabetes mellitus and much less likely to be seen.

PREGNANCY

Pregnancy (apart from other problems) can cause significant oral effects, and can affect dental management (Table 31.12). The chief oral effects are aggravation of gingivitis (Fig. 31.9) and possible development of a pregnancy epulis (Ch. 5). Occasionally, recurrent aphthae remit during pregnancy but may worsen due to iron or folate deficiency.

Table 31.12 Pregnancy — oral effects and management considerations

- Oral effects
    - Aggravated gingivitis and epulis formation
    - Variable effect on recurrent aphthae
- Management considerations
    - Risk of hypotension when laid supine
    - Possible hypertension of pregnancy
    - Possible iron or folate deficiency
    - Vomiting, especially with general anaesthesia

Fig. 31.9 Pregnancy gingivitis. A florid marginal gingivitis associated with poor oral hygiene during the first trimester of pregnancy.

A few women in late pregnancy become hypotensive when laid supine, when the swollen uterus impedes venous return. They should be treated in a sitting position. Respiratory reserve is diminished and there is a risk of fetal hypoxia. Neonatal respiration is further depressed by drugs such as general anaesthetics and sedatives, especially barbiturates, diazepam and opioids, all of which cross the placenta. Local anaesthesia is generally safe. There are also other risks to the fetus (Table 31.13).

Table 31.13 Possible hazards to a fetus from dental procedures

- X-rays hazardous, especially in first trimester
- Respiratory depression due to sedatives, including benzodiazepines
- Dental pigmentation due to tetracycline
- Theoretical risk of depressed vitamin B_{12} metabolism by nitrous oxide
- Prilocaine may rarely cause methaemoglobinaemia
- Theoretical risk of uterine contraction caused by felypressin
- Teratogenic risks of thalidomide, retinoids, azathioprine and possibly other drugs
- Aspirin may cause neonatal haemorrhage

The main risks of fetal abnormalities are from drugs and radiation: the hazard is greatest during organogenesis in the first trimester. Few drugs are known to be teratogenic for humans, and in many cases the risk is no more than theoretical or results only from prolonged high dosage. For example, no teratogenic risk from metronidazole for humans has ever been substantiated. Non-steroidal anti-inflammatory drugs in high dosage may cause premature closure of the ductus arteriosus and fetal pulmonary hypertension. Aspirin may also increase the risk of neonatal haemorrhage and paracetamol is the preferred analgesic. Systemic corticosteroids can cause fetal adrenosuppression. However, the only drugs known to be teratogenic are thalidomide (used occasionally for major aphthae), etretinate (used experimentally for leukoplakia) and possibly azathioprine (used occasionally for Behçet's syndrome and sometimes for connective tissue diseases). For details of drug usage in pregnancy, see the current *British National Formulary*.

The risks from dental radiography are small but only essential radiographs should be taken, the minimal radiation exposure should be given, and the patient should wear a lead apron.

SUGGESTED FURTHER READING

Cawson R A, Spector R G, Skelly A M 1995 Basic pharmacology and clinical drug use in dentistry, 6th edn. Churchill Livingstone, Edinburgh

Franklyn J A 1993 Hypothyroidism. Medicine UK 21:161–163

Franklyn J A 1993 Hypothyroidism. Medicine UK 21:164–169

Nathan D M 1993 Long-term complications of diabetes mellitus. N Engl J Med 328:1676–1685

Stephenson E, Haug R H, Murphy T A 1995 Management of the diabetic oral and maxillofacial surgery patient. J Oral Maxillofac Surg 53:175–182

Trainer P J, Howlett T, Besser E M 1993 Cushing's syndrome. Medicine Int 21:184–188

Trainer P J, Howlett T, Besser E M 1993 Addison's disease, Medicine Int 21:184–183

Williams J D, Slupchinsku O, Sclafani A P et al 1996 Evaluation and management of the lingual thyroid gland. Ann Otol Rhinol Laryngol 105:312–316

Renal disease

Renal disease has become important in dentistry because of the growing number of patients who, as a result of renal dialysis or transplantation, survive renal failure. Aspects of renal disease relevant to dentistry are summarised in Table 32.1.

Table 32.1   Aspects of renal disease affecting dental management

- Heparinisation before dialysis
- Possible hepatitis B or C carriage after chronic dialysis
- Permanent venous fistulae susceptible to infection
- Secondary hyperparathyroidism
- Immunosuppressive treatment for nephrotic or transplant patients
- Oral lesions due to drugs, particularly for immunosuppression
- Oral disease in chronic renal failure

Patients receiving regular dialysis remain otherwise in reasonably good general health. About 70% can return to full-time work. However, they are heparinised before dialysis and haemostasis is impaired for 6–12 hours.

These patients' permanent venous fistula for the dialysis lines is susceptible to infection, and antibiotic cover may be considered for dental surgical procedures. Drugs, including sedation, should not be given intravenously because of the risk of damage to superficial veins which are patients' lifelines. Dialysis patients also have a greater incidence of cardiovascular and cerebrovascular disease.

Renal osteodystrophy and secondary hyperparathyroidism

Prolonged dialysis or renal failure are now more common causes of giant cell lesions of bone than primary hyperparathyroidism. The jaws may be first affected (Chapter 6).

Renal transplant patients

Normal renal function and health can be restored by transplantation but it is associated with the complications of prolonged immunosuppressive treatment, such as susceptibility to infections or lymphomas. While awaiting a compatible donor these patients have often also been on dialysis, with its attendant complications.

Cyclosporin, which is widely used to help control graft rejection, can cause persistent gingival hyperplasia with false pocketing which readily progresses to periodontal destruction in some patients. If a calcium channel blocker, such as nifedipine, is also being given for hypertension, gingival hyperplasia is virtually inevitable and uncontrollable.

Hairy leukoplakia may develop.

Complications of graft rejection such as bone lesions due to secondary hyperparathyroidism may be seen (Ch. 10). It may be noted that graft rejection is frequently due to patients' non-compliance with immunosuppressive regimens.

Chronic renal failure

Some patients are unsuitable for, or unable to obtain, dialysis or a transplant. They can suffer a variety of oral effects (Table 32.2).

Table 32.2   Oral changes seen in renal failure

- Mucosal pallor (anaemia)
- Xerostomia
- Purpura
- Mucosal ulceration
- Thrush or bacterial plaques
- White epithelial plaques (Ch. 15)
- Giant cell lesions of the jaws (secondary hyperparathyroidism)

Dental management of patients with renal disease, but particularly chronic renal failure, may be affected by many factors (Table 32.3).

Table 32.3   Factors potentially affecting dental management of patients with renal disease

- Corticosteroid and other immunosuppressive treatment
- Haemorrhagic tendencies
- Anaemia
- Impaired drug excretion
- Hypertension
- Hepatitis B or C carriage
- Underlying causes of renal failure (e.g. diabetes mellitus, hypertension, or connective tissue disease)

SUGGESTED FURTHER READING

Cove-Smith R 1995 Drugs and the kidney. Medicine Int 23:165–173

King G N, Fullinfaw R, Higgins T J et al 1993 Gingival hyperplasia in renal allograft patients receiving cyclosporin A and calcium antagonists. J Clin Periodontol 20:286–293

King G N, Healy C M, Glover M T et al 1994 Prevalence and risk factors associated with leukoplakia, hairy leukoplakia, erythematous candidiasis and gingival hyperplasia in renal transplant recipients. Oral Surg Oral Med Oral Pathol 78:718–726

Mallick N P 1995 Presenting features of renal disease. Medicine Int 23:91–96

Mallick N P 1995 Renal transplantation. Medicine Int 23:156–158

Ziccardi V B, Siani J, Demas P N, Braun T W 1992 Management of the oral and maxillofacial surgery patient with end-stage renal disease. J Oral Maxillofac Surg 50:1207–1212

CHAPTER 33

Handicapping disorders

The term 'handicapped' usually refers to permanent mental, neurological or neuromuscular disabilities.

The prevalence of major handicaps is estimated at 1.5–2 per 1000 live births. Mental handicaps account for approximately 0.9 per 1000 and major physical handicaps for the remainder. The management of dental care is affected by the type of handicap and also parents' intelligence and attitudes. However, mental or physical handicap does not necessarily mean that dental care has to be compromised, though this may sometimes be inevitable.

Handicapped children present a wide variety of problems of dental management, but up to 90% of them can probably be managed by conventional means without a general anaesthetic. Nevertheless, handicapped children, especially those in institutions, are a dentally neglected group, even though valiant attempts have been made to overcome this deficiency in recent years.

Preconceptions that the handicapped are necessarily grimacing, drooling and uncooperative are seriously misplaced. In fact, those who manage handicapped children find the work more rewarding than dentistry in normal children. Such is the emptiness of handicapped children's lives, particularly when institutionalised, that dental treatment, which involves both relatively prolonged personal attention and a change from other endless dreary days, can be a pleasure for them. One Down's syndrome child, for instance, though well looked after by affectionate parents, was in a state of mysteriously eager expectation for days at the prospect (it was later found) of having a chest X-ray. Dental treatment may therefore be a real source of pleasure for those so deprived.

There is a welcome concern about the dental care of handicapped *children* but it should be remembered that these handicaps persist for life.

Difficulties with dental care of handicapped children are summarised in Table 33.1.

Major mental and physical handicaps particularly relevant to dentistry are summarised in Table 33.2.

Heart disease, haemorrhagic disease (particularly haemophilia), diabetes mellitus and other systemic diseases are discussed in Chapters 23 and 27–33.

Physical and mental defects are frequently combined, as in Down's syndrome and some cases of cerebral palsy. Mental

Table 33.1 Typical difficulties with dental care of the handicapped

- Inability to cooperate with normal dental treatment and to manage routine home oral hygiene
- Ability to accept normal dental treatment but inability to carry out normal home oral hygiene
- Associated systemic disease which may affect management
- Limited mobility preventing access to a dental surgery

Table 33.2 Major handicapping conditions affecting dental management

- Mental handicaps
    Psychiatric disorders
    Autism
    Subnormality
- Physical disorders
    Cerebral palsy
    Epilepsy
    Cleft palate (Ch. 2)
    Severe defects of the hands or arms
    Muscular dystrophies

handicap (often associated with physical disabilities) accounts for by far the largest group of handicapped children needing dental care. Three groups account for approximately 70–75% of handicapped children. These are patients with Down's syndrome, many spastics and some epileptics who are also mentally retarded. Conversely, many patients with cerebral palsy have normal intelligence but may be mislabeled as mentally handicapped because of communication difficulties.

Psychiatric disorders

These range from emotional disorders to psychotic personalities. Those with personality defects can sometimes be totally uncooperative. Like the severely mentally retarded, the best that can be done may merely be to repair severe dental disease under general anaesthesia.

Autism

Autism is a specific defect of mental development in which there is lack of emotional development, disordered use of language, defective communication and extreme 'aloneness'. At one extreme it may be impossible to communicate with or manage autistic children without heavy sedation or general anaesthesia. At the other, sympathy and patience may achieve all that is needed.

Subnormality (mental handicap)

Mental handicap, regardless of cause, is now classified by educational definitions and divided into progressive degrees of learning difficulty. These definitions reflect the fact that such patients are managed in special schools and also give some idea of the likely difficulties with dental care. Learning difficulties may be unassociated with any physical disorder, or physical defects may be severe, as in some cases of cerebral palsy.

Mental handicaps are not usually associated with any specific orofacial disorders, but in some uncommon genetic syndromes dental defects are associated with craniofacial anomalies.

Oral hygiene is usually poor and gross accumulation of plaque and gingivitis or destructive periodontal disease are common. Mildly subnormal children can usually be coaxed into accepting regular treatment and (if the parents are adequate) to maintain acceptable standards of oral hygiene. At the other extreme, all that may be possible, particularly for children with uncontrollable muscular activity such as jaw clenching, is first-aid dentistry under general anaesthesia. All intermediate grades exist, but the level of dental health that can be achieved depends greatly upon the level of the dentist's skill and devotion to the task (Fig. 33.1).

Down's syndrome

Down's syndrome is the most common clinically recognisable type of mental subnormality. The estimated incidence is 1 in 700 live births. It results from a chromosomal abnormality and is not usually hereditary. The total chromosome complement is 47 instead of the normal 46. This is usually the result of three chromosomes 21 (trisomy 21) instead of the usual two.

General features

Down's children have a characteristic facial appearance (Figs. 33.2 and 33.3), abnormalities of the skull and frequently of the dentition, abnormal susceptibility to infection (particularly viral) due to multiple immune defects and congenital cardiovascular disease in up to 50%.

The prominent medial epicanthic skinfold gives the eyes their readily recognisable appearance. There is hypoplasia of the mid-face, poorly developed paranasal sinuses and a malformed upper respiratory tract. Upper respiratory tract infections are common, and breathing is often snorting. Underdevelopment of the maxillae is usually associated with a protrusive mandible and class III malocclusion, with anterior open bite (Table 33.3).

The low caries activity has been ascribed to the form and spacing of the teeth and to the high bicarbonate content and pH of the saliva. Plaque accumulation and poor oral hygiene, due to the patient's disabilities and made worse by mouth breathing,

Fig. 33.1 Traumatic ulceration. This child with learning difficulties produced this deep and extensive ulcer after a local anaesthetic for dental treatment.

Fig. 33.2 Down's syndrome. This shows both the characteristic facial appearance and a cyanotic flush caused by associated congenital heart disease.

Fig. 33.3 Down's syndrome. This shows the characteristic anterior open bite together with gross gingival hyperplasia caused by phenytoin treatment for concomitant epilepsy.

Fig. 33.5 Down's syndrome. Very poor oral hygiene and malocclusion. (By kind permission of Professor C Scully.)

Table 33.3 Down's syndrome — typical oral features
• Malocclusion
• Protrusive, fissured tongue (Fig. 33.4).
• Everted, thick, dry and crusted lips
• Delayed eruption of teeth
• Hypodontia
• Morphological or hypoplastic dental defects
• Gross plaque accumulation
• Low caries activity
• Rapidly progressive periodontal disease

others are trainable to some degree. They are usually good-natured, cooperative within their ability, and affectionate. The success of dental treatment mainly depends on the level of care provided. The more intelligent ones can be treated normally in the dental chair, while the lowest grades, who are usually institutionalised, must be treated like any other severely retarded child. General anaesthesia may therefore be unavoidable.

Control of periodontal disease is usually difficult. However, the teeth should be retained as long as possible. Dentures are usually poorly tolerated and retained because of the large protrusive tongue, poor muscle tone and poor comprehension.

Antibiotic cover must be given, particularly before extractions, to those with cardiac defects (Ch. 27). The unstable atlantooccipital joint is at risk of dislocation with severe consequences if the head is manipulated, particularly during general anaesthesia or sedation.

Fig. 33.4 Macroglossia and fissuring of the tongue in Down's syndrome.

contribute to the early onset of periodontal disease and early tooth loss (Fig. 33.5). Acute ulcerative gingivitis is common and often recurs.

Cerebral palsy

Cerebral palsy is common and can be one of the most severe handicaps. These children, often loosely referred to as spastics, suffer various types of neuromuscular dysfunction (Table 33.4).

Table 33.4 Types of cerebral palsy
• Spastic
• Athetotic
• Ataxic
• Mixed

Management

All Down's children have learning difficulties, some severe, but

Neuromuscular dysfunction

Neuromuscular dysfunction can be so severe as to make speech unintelligible (dysarthria) and cause the children to appear mentally defective. Attempts at communication made by some persons with cerebral palsy can sometimes be understood by dentists prepared to spend time learning to comprehend them. Many cerebral palsy patients have visual speech-aids ('Bliss boards') or computerised devices to help them communicate.

Spasticity causes fixed contraction of the affected muscles and general stiffness. This may be so great that it may not even be possible to move an affected limb passively. Hemiplegia is the most common type: in such cases mental retardation is uncommon but other neurological disorders, such as epilepsy, are frequent. Quadriplegics, by contrast, are frequently mentally retarded but less often epileptic. Athetosis refers to involuntary jerking movements, often of a wriggling character, sometimes accompanied by grimacing.

Ataxia is characterised by lack of balance, an unsteady gait and poor control over voluntary movements. In addition to variants of these three main types of disease, different parts of the body may be affected to a greater extent than others.

Dental aspects

Wheel chair access to dental care is frequently difficult for those with cerebral palsy. Many have severe caries and often periodontal disease due to inability to maintain oral hygiene and their dental care is difficult, however willing they may be.

The first consideration is full assessment of the patient's capabilities. The child's ability to deal with dental disease can then be judged. If the child is uncontrollably anxious, sedation may help. If disabilities are not too severe, many of these children can be treated satisfactorily in the dental chair. The chief difficulty with athetotic children is the irregular movements. These may make it impossible to carry out good restorative work and also make it easy for the child to be injured with sharp dental instruments. Such children may need general anaesthesia. It is always essential to use a mouth prop with conscious athetotic patients, as the jaws may suddenly clench. Epilepsy, falls and sudden uncontrolled movements also render them prone to dental injury. Bruxism and masseteric hypertrophy are frequent and drooling may result from the open mouth posture and defective swallowing. These latter complaints often most trouble these patients. Key dental features are summarised in Table 33.5.

Table 33.5 Cerebral palsy — key dental features

- Frequently severe caries and periodontal disease
- Bruxism and masseteric hypertrophy
- Dental trauma
- Delayed eruption
- Drooling
- Malocclusion

Epilepsy

With modern treatment, epilepsy should present no special difficulties, unless associated with other handicaps. The development of fibrous gingival hyperplasia (Ch. 5) in those on long-term phenytoin should be minimised by high standards of oral hygiene or a change to carbamazepine or sodium valproate.

It is also important to be able to recognise and manage a major fit, should it happen in the dental surgery (Ch. 36).

Spina bifida

Spina bifida is failure of fusion of the vertebral arches. The mildest form (spina bifida occulta) is common but no more than a radiographic finding, sometimes with a tuft of hair overlying the defect. In the severe form (spina bifida cystica) there is a gross defect in the lower vertebral canal. The meninges, and often nerve tissue, protrude through it as a sac, which may be covered by skin. The consequences are paralysis and deformities of the lower limbs, with loss of sensation and reflexes, incontinence and other complications. Meningitis is an obvious hazard and epilepsy is frequently associated.

Since the upper part of the body is normal, the main difficulty in dental management is getting a chair adapted to the child's disability. Associated epilepsy may also affect dental management.

Hydrocephalus

Hydrocephalus may be seen in isolation or associated with spina bifida. Compression of the cerebral tissue can cause severe mental defect, but the intracranial pressure may be relieved by insertion of a catheter to shunt the cerebrospinal fluid directly into the right atrium or, sometimes, the peritoneal cavity. This shunt is susceptible to infection, and, for dental operations likely to cause bacteraemia, prophylactic antibiotics should be given as for infective endocarditis.

Severe hydrocephalus can also cause the skull to be so distended and heavy that the head has to be supported during treatment.

Severe limb defects

These are rare but have been brought to public notice by the thalidomide tragedy. One of the striking effects of this drug is absence of the proximal part of a limb (phocomelia). Thus the hands, often also defective, are attached close to the shoulder.

These children can receive normal dental care, but are totally dependent on parents for toothbrushing. Again, preventive measures to minimise caries activity are important.

The muscular dystrophies

Muscular dystrophies, of which the Duchenne type is the most common (approximately 1 in 5000 male births), are the main crippling diseases of childhood. Weakness of the muscles leads to progressively severe disability and is frequently associated with cardiomyopathy and respiratory impairment.

There appear to be no specific dental problems other than that of propping up a severely affected child in the chair. General anaesthesia is dangerous in the presence of cardiac disease or respiratory impairment.

SUGGESTED FURTHER READING

Hammond J 1996 Cerebral palsy. Medicine UK 24:82–84

Hollins S, Howlin P 1996 Learning disability and autism. Medicine UK 24:47–48

Moore R S, Hobson P 1989 A classification of medically handicapping conditions and the health risks they present in the dental care of children. Part I: Cardiovascular, haematological and respiratory disorders. J Paediatr Dent 5:73–83

Moore R S, Hobson P 1989 A classification of medically handicapping conditions and the health risks they present in the dental care of children. Part II: Neoplastic, renal, endocrine, metabolic, hepatic, musculoskeletal, neuromuscular, central nervous system and skin disorders. J Paediatr Dent 6:1–14

Pain, anxiety and neurological disorders

> ... within my private knowledge, two persons who had
> suffered alike from toothache and cancer, have
> pronounced the former to be on the scale of torture, by
> many degrees to be the worse.
>
> *Confessions of an English Opium Eater* Thomas de
> Quincey (1821)

Pain is the most common symptom for which patients seek help. Approximately 40% of the British population only visit a dentist for pain relief. Toothache can be so agonisingly severe that de Quincey claimed that it had made him dependent on opium. In the lay mind dentistry and pain are inseparable and there is the persistent belief that dental treatment is necessarily painful. This belief emphasises the important point that pain has strong emotional associations and these in turn may be determined to a varying degree by patients' preconceptions. Emotional disturbance itself can also produce the symptom of physical pain.

There are many causes of oral or maxillofacial pain (Table 34.1). Pulpitis and periapical periodontitis as sequels of dental caries are by far the most common. The source of such pain is usually obvious on examination but some sources of dental pain can be exceedingly difficult to identify (Table 34.2). These account for most causes of pain in this area. Disease of the teeth (usually the result of dental caries) and adjacent tissues must always be excluded in the investigation of pain.

Table 34.1 Causes of pain felt in the oral tissues

- Disease of teeth and/or supporting tissues
- Oral mucosal diseases
- Disease of the jaw
- Pain in the edentulous patient
- Postoperative pain
- Pain triggered by mastication
- Referred pain
- Neurological diseases
- Psychogenic (atypical) facial pain

Table 34.2 Causes of pain from the teeth or supporting tissues

- Pulpitis
- Dentine hypersensitivity, cracked tooth or cracked cusp syndrome
- Periapical periodontitis
- Lateral (periodontal) abscess
- Acute ulcerative gingivitis
- HIV-associated periodontitis
- Pericoronitis

Pulpitis

Pulpitis is usually the cause when hot or cold food or drinks trigger the pain. It is also the main cause of spasmodic, poorly localised attacks of pain which may be mistaken for a variety of other possible causes. The pain of acute pulpitis is of a sharp lancinating character peculiar to itself, impossible to describe but unforgettable once experienced. Recurrent attacks of less severe, subacute or chronic pain, often apparently spontaneous, suggest a diseased and dying pulp.

Investigation of pulpitis has been discussed earlier (Ch. 4). The only non-dental condition that is indistinguishable from pulp pain by the patient is the pain of *herpes zoster*. If no local cause can be found after the most careful search, it is important to look for early signs of the characteristic rash. Herpes zoster is an uncommon cause of toothache-like pain, but countless teeth have been extracted in patients with zoster under the mistaken impression that the pain was dental.

Acute periodontitis

Pain from acute periapical periodontitis should be readily identifiable as there is precisely localised tenderness of the tooth in its socket. Radiographs are of little value in the early stages but useful after sufficient destruction shows itself as loss of definition of the periapical lamina dura. In other cases, acute inflammation may supervene on chronic, and a rounded area of radiolucency is seen.

Acute maxillary sinusitis can rarely cause similar tenderness of a group of teeth, particularly upper molars, as discussed later.

Lateral, periodontal abscess

The tooth is tender in its socket but is usually vital and there is deep localised pocketing (Ch. 6). Occasionally both a periodontal and periapical abscess may form together on a non-vital tooth with severe periodontal disease, or a periodontal abscess may be precipitated by endodontic treatment when a reamer perforates the side of the root.

Acute ulcerative gingivitis and HIV-associated necrotising periodontitis

Acute ulcerative gingivitis usually causes soreness, but when it extends deeply and rapidly, destroying the underlying bone, there may be severe aching pain. In such cases the diagnosis is usually obvious clinically. HIV-associated periodontitis presents a somewhat similar picture and is painful.

Acute pericoronitis

Pericoronitis usually produces a characteristic clinical picture (Ch. 6).

Painful mucosal lesions

Ulcers generally cause soreness rather than pain, but deep ulceration may cause severe aching pain. Carcinoma, in particular, causes severe pain once nerve fibres become involved. It is important to emphasise again that early carcinoma is *painless*; pain is a late symptom. By the time that pain becomes troublesome the tumour is usually easily seen unless it is far back in the mouth.

Herpes zoster causes severe aching pain, sometimes indistinguishable from toothache, because of involvement of cervical ganglia (Ch. 12).

Painful jaw diseases

The salient feature of these conditions (Table 34.3) is that as well as the history and clinical presentation, the provisional diagnosis depends on the radiographic findings. Fractures and osteomyelitis should be recognisable by such means. Other lesions of the jaws, by contrast, sometimes have less clear-cut clinical and radiographic features, and the differentiation of (say) an infected cyst from a malignant tumour may be difficult.

With the exception of fractures and osteomyelitis, diagnosis then depends on biopsy and histological examination.

Pain in edentulous patients

These conditions (Table 34.4) differ from most others because dental causes can be excluded. The chief difficulty is to decide whether the pain is due to the dentures themselves, or to some condition of the mucosa or jaws on which a denture is pressing.

Table 34.3   Painful jaw diseases

- Fractures
- Osteomyelitis
- Infected cysts
- Malignant neoplasms
- Sickle cell infarcts

Table 34.4   Important causes of pain in edentulous patients

- Denture trauma
- Excessive vertical dimension
- Diseases (enumerated earlier) of the denture-bearing mucosa
- Diseases of the jaws (see Table 34.3)
- Teeth or roots erupting under a denture

Traumatic ulcers, usually the consequence of overextension, often cause trouble with a new denture. After the denture has been relieved, these ulcers heal within 24–48 hours. Persistent ulceration after adequate relief of the denture is likely to be due to some more serious cause, particularly a neoplasm. Biopsy is then essential. Later, dentures cause traumatic pain when the bone has become severely resorbed, allowing the denture to bear on the mylohyoid ridge or genial tubercles. These result from the patient's having worn the denture too long, and a well-designed replacement is necessary.

Lack of freeway space due to excessive vertical dimension of the dentures prevents the mandible and masticatory muscles from reaching their natural rest position. This causes the teeth to be held permanently in contact. Aching pain is usually felt in the fatigued masticatory muscles, but the excessive stress imposed on the denture-bearing area sometimes causes pain in this region. Very occasionally patients seem unable to tolerate dentures, however carefully they are constructed, and complain of such symptoms as gripping, burning or 'drawing' pain, particularly under the upper denture. These symptoms are not associated with any physical changes and are psychogenic.

It is usually straightforward to decide whether pain is caused by the dentures themselves or by some lesion under the dentures. Denture stomatitis is painless, but surprisingly few other mucosal diseases affect the denture-bearing area itself. Lichen planus can extend to the sulcus and impinge on the margin of the denture-bearing area. The most important condition to be excluded is *carcinoma*, either affecting the alveolar margin or in the labial or buccal sulcus or floor of the mouth. Persistent lesions, whether ulcerated or not, developing beneath or at the margins of dentures, must be biopsied without hesitation, as it is in the edentulous age-group that the incidence of carcinoma is highest. A carcinoma can persist for a long time with minimal symptoms, and the patient may notice no more than the fact that the fit of the denture has deteriorated.

Jaw lesions causing pain in the edentulous patient may be associated with a swelling or an area of radiolucency and have been discussed above. A painful swelling of the jaw in the edentulous patient is probably most often due to an infected residual cyst. Malignant tumours are very much less common but must be considered, as they cannot be reliably distinguished from cysts and other benign conditions by radiography alone. Histological examination is therefore essential. Osteomyelitis of the jaws in edentulous patients must be considered virtually only in those who have had radiotherapy to this region. In such patients denture ulceration can allow infection to penetrate and set up persistent painful chronic osteomyelitis of the ischaemic bone.

Retained roots, or, rarely, late eruption of buried teeth beneath a denture, become painful as they reach the surface, causing the mucosa to be pinched between them and the denture. This trouble will be obvious on clinical or radiographic examination, as are the late effects of a healed malaligned fracture.

Postoperative pain

Important causes are summarised in Table 34.5. By far the most common cause of pain after dental extractions is *alveolar osteitis (dry socket)*, which can usually be recognised on clinical examination (Ch. 6). Fracture of the jaw following operative treatment is rare but can also be recognised from the history, and by clinical and radiographic examination. Postoperative osteomyelitis *should* be a thing of the past, but forcible opening of the mouth under general anaesthesia, particularly for removing wisdom teeth, can damage the temporomandibular joint and lead to persistent pain on opening or during mastication.

Table 34.5 Postoperative pain

- Alveolar osteitis (dry socket)
- Fracture of the jaw
- Damage to the temporomandibular joint
- Osteomyelitis
- Damage to nerve trunks or involvement of nerves in scar tissue

---

Persistent postoperative pain is sometimes ascribed to damage to nerve fibres, either as a result of operative trauma or by involvement in scar tissue. However, if there is no objective evidence of disturbed sensation, there is little or nothing abnormal to be found. Operative intervention in the attempt to relieve such pain may do more harm than good. In some such cases there is complaint of persistent pain unresponsive to treatment but without any organic cause.

Rarely, damaged nerve tissue may proliferate to form a traumatic neuroma, which is tender to pressure. Its excision should lead to relief of the pain. However, meticulous investigation of postoperative pain is important as it is a major cause of medicolegal claims.

Pain induced by mastication

The common dental cause for pain on mastication is apical periodontitis, but any condition which causes the tooth to be tender in its socket, whether it be a lateral periodontal abscess or, occasionally, maxillary sinusitis, can cause this symptom (Table 34.6).

Table 34.6 Pain induced by mastication

- Diseases of teeth and supporting tissues
- Pain dysfunction syndrome
- Diseases of the temporomandibular joint
- Temporal arteritis
- Trigeminal neuralgia
- Salivary calculi

The least common cause of pain during eating is organic disease of the temporomandibular joint. Pain during eating comes much more frequently from the many other structures involved.

Fractures and dislocations of the temporomandibular joint are usually obvious from the history, their effects on the occlusion and the radiographic changes (Ch. 11).

Pain dysfunction syndrome usually causes dull, aching pain, often associated with clicking sounds from the joint, episodes of locking and some limitation of opening, in varying combinations. Young women are predominantly affected and there is typically a strong neurotic element.

The typical manifestation of temporal (giant cell) arteritis is headache. However, it is also a cause of masticatory pain and should be considered particularly in patients over middle age with this symptom. The pain is due to ischaemia of the masticatory muscles, caused by the arteritis, and is comparable to intermittent claudication (Ch. 11). Corticosteroids are effective in controlling the disease and relieving symptoms. They should be given when there is headache or masticatory pain associated with a tender other scalp artery and a high ESR.

The characteristic pain of trigeminal neuralgia is occasionally triggered by mastication. Trigeminal neuralgia may then be misdiagnosed as dental or due to pain dysfunction syndrome. However, the quality of these types of pain is quite different, as discussed later.

Calculi, particularly when obstructing the parotid duct, can cause pain when salivation is triggered by eating. Hence the history of the relationship of the pain to stimulation of salivation is distinctive.

Pain from extraoral disease

Extraoral causes of pain are summarised in Table 34.7.

Antral disease can cause pain felt in the upper teeth but a sinus radiograph should provide the diagnosis. Salivary gland and ear diseases typically cause preauricular pain. They may simulate temporomandibular joint symptoms but are rarely mistaken for a dental problem.

Table 34.7   Pain from extraoral disease

- Diseases of the maxillary antrum
  - Acute sinusitis
  - Carcinoma, particularly when it involves the antral floor
- Diseases of salivary glands
  - Acute parotitis
  - Salivary calculi (see above)
  - Sjögren's syndrome
  - Malignant neoplasms
- Diseases of the ears
  - Otitis media
  - Neoplasms in this region
- Myocardial infarction

Table 34.8   Painful intracranial and psychological disorders

- Trigeminal neuralgia
- Multiple sclerosis
- Herpes zoster
- Postherpetic neuralgia
- Migrainous neuralgia
- Intracranial tumours
- Bell's palsy
- Psychogenic pain (atypical facial pain)

Table 34.9   Trigeminal neuralgia — typical features

- Pain is confined to distribution of one or more divisions of the trigeminal nerve
- Pain is paroxysmal and very severe
- Trigger zones in the area
- Absence of objective sensory loss
- Absence of detectable organic cause

Acute sinusitis is the most common paranasal disease that causes facial pain but antral carcinoma is rare (Ch. 28).

Mumps is a common cause of pain from, and swelling of, the parotid glands. In children the diagnosis is usually quickly made on clinical grounds. In adults the diagnosis may not be immediately suspected and, occasionally, these patients think they have dental disease.

Suppurative parotitis is uncommon but may be a complication of dry mouth. Acute parotitis may therefore be seen as a complication of Sjögren's syndrome or irradiation damage to the glands. Sjögren's syndrome itself can occasionally cause parotid pain and swelling of the glands.

Swelling rather than pain is usually the first symptom of malignant tumours of salivary glands. Parotid gland tumours can also cause facial palsy and, finally, ulceration and fungation.

Myocardial infarction usually causes constricting or crushing pain substernally, but pain may radiate down the inside of the left arm or up into the neck or jaw. Rarely, cardiac pain is felt in the jaw alone. There is even a case on record where a dentist recognised the cardiac cause of jaw pain, to the dismay of his patient who was a cardiologist. This pain can come on at any time, at rest or during exercise. The clinical picture is variable, but in typical cases the patient is obviously anxious, pale and sweating with a rapid pulse and low blood pressure.

Intracranial and psychological disorders

Trigeminal neuralgia is one of the most important of these conditions (Table 34.8).

Trigeminal neuralgia

Typical features are summarised in Table 34.9. Elderly patients are affected, and though the pain is excruciatingly severe, there is complete or almost complete, relief between spasms. During an attack the patient's face is often distorted with anguish, while between attacks the patient may appear apprehensive at the thought of recurrence. The severity of the pain may also make the patient depressed. The pain is paroxysmal, i.e. severe, sharp and stabbing in character but lasts only seconds or min-

utes and may be described as like lightning. However, attacks may sometimes be quickly recurrent at short intervals. Stimuli to an area (trigger zone) within the distribution of the trigeminal nerve can provoke an attack. Common stimuli are touching, draughts of cold air, or toothbrushing. Occasionally, masticatory effort induces the pain.

There are no objective signs. Either the second or third division of the trigeminal nerve is usually first affected, but pain soon involves both. The first division is rarely affected and pain does not spread to the opposite side. Less typical features of trigeminal neuralgia, which make diagnosis difficult, are more continuous, long-lasting, burning or aching pain, absence of trigger zones, and extension of the pain beyond the margins of the trigeminal area, though not to the opposite side.

Typically, the disease undergoes spontaneous remissions, with freedom from pain for weeks or months. These remissions may make it difficult to decide whether treatment has been effective.

Diagnosis

In typical cases the diagnosis should be readily made from the features described. In young patients multiple sclerosis should be excluded. A careful search should be made for diseased teeth, though pain of this severity is unlikely to be due to dental disease. An inflamed pulp can cause stabs of severe pain in its early stages, but the pain changes in character and soon becomes more prolonged. Pulpitis can usually also be identified as toothache by most patients and is felt to be different in character from pain in the face due to neuralgia. Any diseased teeth should of course be treated, though this does not affect the neuralgia. In the absence of disease, teeth should not be arbitrarily extracted, as this only adds to the patient's misfortunes.

Pulp stones in particular, seen on a radiograph, are not a reason for extracting teeth.

Treatment

The most effective drugs are anticonvulsants, particularly carbamazepine and to a lesser extent phenytoin. Carbamazepine, with or without phenytoin, will usually relieve the pain, at least for a time. The action seems specific and other types of pain are not relieved. Abolition of the pain of trigeminal neuralgia by giving an anticonvulsant, such as carbamazepine, also helps to confirm the diagnosis. Carbamazepine (100 mg/day but gradually raised if necessary to 800 mg/day) must be given long-term (essentially prophylactically) to reduce the frequency and severity of attacks. If a patient has trigeminal neuralgia which appears unresponsive to carbamazepine it sometimes transpires that instructions about continuous use have either not been given or not understood, so that the drug has been used as if it were an analgesic. Up to 80% of patients are relieved of pain partly or completely by carbamazepine, but minor side-effects are common. Drowsiness, dryness of the mouth, giddiness, diarrhoea and nausea are all to some extent dose-related. A small initial dose should therefore be given and gradually raised as necessary. In some patients tolerance to the side-effects may develop. Leukopenia is a rare toxic effect.

Surgical treatment. A few patients are unresponsive to carbamazepine or cannot tolerate the side-effects. If drug treatment fails, the final resort is surgery. The simplest option is cryotherapy to the trigeminal nerve or, if this fails, cryotherapy at the base of the skull. If these fail, microvascular decompression of the trigeminal ganglion may be required. This operation requires great skill and a mortality of 1% has been noted in some studies. In a series of over 1000 patients treated in this way in the USA, the mortality was 0.2%, 30% had recurrences of pain and 11% underwent a second operation. Overall it was claimed that 70% of the patients were pain-free without medication 10 years postoperatively.

Glossopharyngeal neuralgia

This rare condition is characterised by pain similar to that of trigeminal neuralgia but affects the base of the tongue and fauces on one side. It may also radiate deeply into the ear. The pain, which is sharp, lancinating and transient, is typically triggered by swallowing, chewing or coughing. It may be so severe that patients may be terrified to swallow their saliva and try to keep the mouth and tongue as completely immobile as possible. Glossopharyngeal neuralgia sometimes responds to carbamazepine, but less often than trigeminal neuralgia. Once an organic cause has been excluded, surgical treatment may be needed. However, like trigeminal neuralgia, there can be spontaneous remissions, sometimes for years.

Postherpetic neuralgia

Up to 10% of patients who have had trigeminal herpes zoster,

particularly if elderly, may develop persistent neuralgia. The pain is more variable in character and severity than trigeminal neuralgia. It is typically persistent rather than paroxysmal. The diagnosis is straightforward if there is a history of facial zoster or if scars from the rash are present.

Unfortunately, postherpetic neuralgia is remarkably resistant to treatment. Nerve or root section are ineffective and the response to drugs of any type, including carbamazepine, is poor. When pain is severe, large doses of analgesics can be given, and may give relief. Application of transcutaneous electrical stimulation to the affected area by the patient him- or herself is sometimes effective. The instrument is applied hourly for 5–10 minutes every day, and persistent bombardment of the sensory pathways by the stimulator may prevent perception of pain centrally.

Multiple sclerosis

A minority of patients with multiple sclerosis have pain indistinguishable from trigeminal neuralgia, usually as a late symptom. Between 2% and 3% of patients with 'classical' symptoms of trigeminal neuralgia may have multiple sclerosis, but younger persons (under 50) are typically affected. In about 30%, pain, unlike trigeminal neuralgia, may be persistent and lack trigger zones, or may spread beyond the trigeminal area. Disturbances of sensation are capriciously distributed according to the sites of lesions in the brain. The lip may be affected and symptoms may range from paraesthesia to extreme hypersensitivity whereby the patient will literally jump or scream with pain if the lip is touched.

The diagnosis usually depends on the presence of multiple deficits, particularly defects of vision, weakness of the limbs, and sensory losses. Disturbed sensation in the trigeminal area is likely only to be seen in patients with advanced disease and multiple paralyses. There is unlikely to be any doubt about the diagnosis as a consequence.

Carbamazepine is sometimes effective for trigeminal neuralgia-like pain, otherwise surgical treatment as for trigeminal neuralgia may be required.

Migrainous neuralgia (cluster headache)

Migrainous neuralgia is caused by vascular changes at the base of the skull and may occasionally be mistaken for trigeminal neuralgia. It is rarely seen in dental practice. Migrainous neuralgia has many features in common with classical migraine (hemicrania) and is due to oedema and dilatation of the wall of the internal carotid and probably also the external carotid arteries.

Cluster headache mainly affects men, usually young adults but up to the age of 50. Attacks may be precipitated by alcohol or vasodilators or come on spontaneously 1–3 times a day. Attacks sometimes recur at precisely the same time each day or may disturb sleep. Pain is localised to the region of the orbit, temple or maxilla. The duration is 0.5–2 hours. Obvious vascular changes in the affected side of the face typically accompany the pain. The eye may become suffused and water, the nostrils may be blocked, the skin over the cheek may become red and there may be sweating on that side. After one to several months there is usually sudden and spontaneous complete remission and the patient remains completely free from pain for months, or even years. An uncommon variant of cluster headache is a chronic variety with attacks confined to the cheek or lower jaw, known as *lower half headache*.

Unlike migraine, there are neither visual symptoms nor nausea or vomiting. Cluster headache may respond to simple analgesics or to ergotamine. Ergotamine should be given an hour before the expected attack and is most effective by subcutaneous injection or by suppository. Alternatively, ergotamine powder can be inhaled from a spinhaler. Success depends on an accurate idea of the timing of the attacks, and two or three doses a day for the duration of the cluster of attacks may be necessary. Treatment should preferably be stopped for one day each week to see whether there has been spontaneous remission. Sumatriptan or indomethacin may be more effective.

In a double blind trial, intranasal lignocaine (4%) has been shown to provide rapid relief from the headache of classical migraine in approximately 55% of patients. The effectiveness of this treatment for migrainous neuralgia is not known but it is simple and safe, and worth a trial.

Intracranial tumours

Pain resembling trigeminal neuralgia can rarely be caused by intracranial tumours. Features suggesting an intracranial lesion are associated sensory loss, especially if associated with cranial nerve palsies. Frequently, anatomically related nerves (especially III, IV and VI, causing disordered oculomotor function) are affected.

Bell's palsy

As discussed later, facial paralysis is the predominant and most troublesome feature. In about 50% of cases, pain, usually in or near the ear but sometimes spreading down the jaw, either precedes or develops at the same time as the facial palsy. Rarely a patient with early Bell's palsy seeks a dental opinion for the pain felt in the jaw, since this may precede paralysis by several days.

Psychogenic (atypical) facial pain

Pain is not a simple sensation, but has been described as the unpleasant experience felt 'when hurt in body or mind'. The psychological aspects of pain are often overwhelmingly important, and the patient's reaction is affected by such factors as mood, emotional characteristics, personality and cultural background. At one extreme a footballer may receive a relatively severe injury in the middle of a game without feeling it. At the other extreme there are patients who complain bitterly and per-

sistently about trivial lesions. Pain causes emotional disturbance, and prolonged severe pain, as in rheumatoid arthritis, can cause depression. There are also many patients whose facial pain is psychogenic rather than organic in nature.

It must be emphasised that the diagnosis of psychogenic facial pain is a diagnosis by exclusion, but it is important to try to recognise the condition, however limited diagnostic methods may be. The symptoms (Table 34.10) cause real enough suffering to the patient and should if possible be relieved. It is also important to avoid unnecessary surgery.

Table 34.10   Features suggestive of psychogenic (atypical) facial pain

- Women of middle age or older mainly affected
- Absence of organic signs
- Pain often poorly localised
- Description of pain may be bizarre
- Delusional symptoms occasionally associated
- Lack of response to analgesics
- Unchanging pain persisting for many years
- Lack of any triggering factors
- Sometimes good response to antidepressive treatment

A common site for the pain is the maxillary region or in relation to the upper teeth, but localisation may not be precise or in a recognisable anatomical pattern. The pain may be described as vague, bizarre ('drawing' or 'gripping') or exaggerated ('unbearable') but without obvious effect on the patient's health. It is often described as having been continuous, even unremittant, and unchanging for several years.

Pain is usually not provoked by any recognisable stimulus, such as hot or cold foods, or by mastication. Despite the fact that the pain may be said to be continuous and unbearable, the patient's sleeping or even eating may be unaffected. Analgesics are often said to be completely ineffective, but some patients have not even tried them, despite the stated severity of the pain. Objective signs of disease are absent. Although teeth have often been extracted and diseased teeth may be present, none of these can be related to the pain. As a consequence, treatment of diseased teeth does not relieve the symptoms.

Other signs of emotional disturbance are highly variable. Some patients are more or less obviously depressed; some of them mention, in passing, difficulties they have had, for instance at work with their colleagues. Others may complain how miserable the pain makes them. Others may complain of bizarre (delusional) symptoms such as 'slime' in the mouth or 'powder' coming out of the jaw.

Pain can be a symptom of depression. Since mental illness, even now, carries with it a stigma, patients frequently suppress the overt misery of depression. The patient may also fear (often rightly) that doctors or dentists are intolerant of what is regarded as their weakness in being unable to cope with their life situation.

This pain can be regarded as their cry for help. This is occasionally strikingly evident in a patient who appears emotionally in control but who, when given a chance to describe the complaint at length, suddenly loses control and starts to weep uncontrollably. At the other extreme, there are patients who so aggressively reject the idea of mental illness that they insist from the start that the pain is not 'due to their nerves' and typically refuse psychiatric help.

Occasionally, anxiety such as cancerophobia can give rise to atypical facial pain and may respond to reassurance.

Management

The first essential is to exclude organic disease by a careful search for all possible sources of pain. Any potential sources of pain must be dealt with, but there should not be too much expectation of benefit. If no organic cause can be found and if sympathetic discussion suggests psychogenic factors, then it may help to explain to the patient in simple terms that depression and other emotional disturbances are just as much illnesses and cause as much suffering as physical diseases. It is also important to explain that emotional disturbances affect almost everyone to some degree. It may also help to point out that more common symptoms, particularly headache, are rarely due to organic disease. Patients should also be reassured that there is no dangerous disease and that frightening possibilities such as cancer can be confidently excluded. Such reassurance is sometimes remarkably effective.

While it is obviously reasonable gently to recommend psychiatric help, patients are often resentful of the idea and it is more tactful to refer to the psychiatrist as a 'pain expert'. Sometimes, antidepressant treatment with dothiepin, or one of the newer generation, antidepressive drugs, is strikingly effective.

Unfortunately, there is a hard core of patients who complain of persistent facial pain, have gone the round of specialists (including psychiatrists), have been treated with a wide range of drugs, but still continue to complain of severe pain. This problem may be a reflection of the limited range of treatment available, or perhaps such patients 'need' their pain for obscure emotional reasons.

It is essential also to appreciate that a few patients thought to have atypical facial pain are found later to have some disease, such as an occult adenoid cystic carcinoma infiltrating nerve fibres.

Psychogenic dental pain (atypical odontalgia)

This is a less common variant of atypical facial pain. Pain is often precisely localised in one tooth or in a row of teeth, which are said either to ache or to be exquisitely sensitive to heat, cold or pressure. If dental disease is found, treatment has no effect, or if as a last resort the tooth is removed, the pain moves to an adjacent tooth. Again, if no organic cause can be found and treatment is ineffective, psychiatric assessment is needed. Early diagnosis is essential to avoid overtreatment and serious dental morbidity.

PARAESTHESIA AND ANAESTHESIA OF THE LIP

Paraesthesia of the lip can be caused by osteomyelitis or fracture of the jaw. Very occasionally it results from neurological disease. The main causes of anaesthesia or paraesthesia of the lip are summarised in Table 34.11.

Table 34.11   Important causes of paraesthesia or anaesthesia of the lip

- Inferior dental blocks
- Trauma (fracture or operative damage)
- Acute osteomyelitis
- Malignant tumours of the mandible
- Exposed mental foramen
- Herpes zoster
- Multiple sclerosis
- Tetany

Prolonged anaesthesia or paraesthesia of the lip can occasionally follow *inferior dental blocks*, possibly as a result of damage to the nerve by the needle. Spontaneous recovery usually takes place.

Paraesthesia of the lip can be a complication of *fractures of the mandible* where the nerve has become stretched, particularly over the sharp edge of the canal. The effect is temporary but complete recovery may take some months. The inferior dental nerve may occasionally be damaged in *operations on the mandible* and there may be anaesthesia or paraesthesia lasting for many months. Complete loss of sensation is unusual but recovery may take a year or more.

The inferior dental nerve is rarely involved in *osteomyelitis* but, with effective treatment, recovery is the rule. Alternatively it may be compressed by a *neoplasm* or a tumour may infiltrate the nerve sheath. A jaw tumour causing pain or paraesthesia strongly suggests malignancy. In such cases the prognosis is poor, either because the tumour may be a secondary carcinoma or a primary but highly malignant tumour, such as an osteosarcoma.

The mental foramen can become exposed by *excessive resorption of mandibular bone* in an edentulous patient. The denture can then press upon the nerve as it leaves the foramen. Though these changes are common, they rarely cause paraesthesia of the lip.

Herpes zoster affecting the trigeminal nerve can leave residual disturbances of sensation. The most severe and troublesome is postherpetic neuralgia, but in other patients there may be persistent paraesthesia of the lip.

Disturbances of sensation of the face and other regions can be caused by *multiple sclerosis*, as discussed earlier.

Tetany is the result of hypocalcaemic states and causes heightened neuromuscular excitability together with minor disorders of sensation such as paraesthesia of the lip. A significant cause of tetany is overbreathing, usually due to anxiety (*hyperventilation syndrome*).

FACIAL PALSY

Important causes of facial palsy, which include both upper and lower motor neurone lesions, are summarised in Table 34.12.

Table 34.12 Causes of facial palsy

- Extracranial causes
   Bell's palsy
   Malignant parotid neoplasms
   Parotid surgery
   Sarcoidosis (Heerfordt's syndrome)
   Misplaced local anaesthetic
   Melkersson–Rosenthal syndrome
- Intracranial causes
   Strokes
   Cerebral tumours and other neurological diseases
   Multiple sclerosis
   HIV infection
   Lyme disease
   Ramsay Hunt syndrome
   Trauma to the base of the skull

Bell's palsy

Bell's palsy is a common cause of facial paralysis. It probably results from compression of the facial nerve in its canal as a result of inflammation and swelling. A viral infection, particularly *Herpes simplex*, is suspected as the cause. Either sex may be affected, usually between the ages of 20 and 50. As mentioned earlier, pain in the jaw sometimes precedes the paralysis or there may be numbness in the side of the tongue. Though this disease is uncommon in dental practice, its recognition is important as early treatment may prevent permanent disability and disfigurement.

Function of the facial nerve is tested by asking the patient to perform facial movements. When asked to close the eyes, the lids on the affected side cannot be brought together but the eyeball rolls up normally, as the oculomotor nerves are unaffected. When the patient is asked to smile, the corner of the mouth on the affected side is not pulled upwards and the normal lines of expression are absent (Fig. 34.1). The wrinkling round the eyes which accompanies smiling is also not seen on the affected side and the eyes remains staring.

The majority of patients recover fully or partially without treatment; at least 10% of patients with Bell's palsy are unhap-

Fig. 34.1 Bell's palsy (a). When trying to shut the eyes, that on the affected (right) side fails to close completely but the eyeball rolls up normally (b). When trying to smile, the mouth fails to move on the affected side, which remains expressionless, having lost all natural skin folds. The difference is made more striking by covering each side of the picture in turn. This patient, incidentally, complained primarily of facial pain, though increasingly aware of the facial disability. The severely disfiguring effect of this disorder and the need for early treatment is obvious. In this case response was complete. (By kind permission of the patient.)

py about the final outcome because of permanent disfigurement or other complications. A guide to the need for treatment is the severity of the paralysis when first seen. Full recovery is usual in patients with an incomplete palsy seen within a week of onset, but more than half of those with a complete lesion fail to recover completely. Electromyography and other electrodiagnostic techniques can be used to measure the degree of functional impairment as a guide to the need for treatment. Prednisolone, by mouth (20 mg four times a day), may be given for 5–10 days and then tapered off over the following 4 days, and may be effective if given within 24 hours of the onset. The addition of acyclovir appears to produce more reliable results and also suggests a role for a herpes virus.

If treatment fails or is not given, persistent facial weakness is disfiguring. The affected part of the face sometimes also contracts involuntarily in association with movement of another part. There may, for example, be twitching of the mouth when the patient blinks. More uncommon is unilateral lacrimation (crocodile tears) when eating. The majority of patients with persistent denervation have contracture of the affected side of the face. Watering of the eye (epiphora) due to impaired drainage of tears, or occasionally to excessive and erratic lacrimal secretion, may remain particularly troublesome. Sagging of the affected side of the face may be limited by an intraoral prosthesis.

Melkersson–Rosenthal syndrome

Melkersson–Rosenthal syndrome in its rare complete form comprises unilateral recurrent facial paralysis, which may become permanent, labial or facial swelling and fissured tongue. Recurrent, soft, painless facial swelling is more common, but may become persistent due to progressive fibrosis. The buccal mucosa may have a cobble-stone pattern like that in Crohn's disease and, histologically, granulomas are found. Facial palsy is troublesome and disfiguring but there is no specific treatment.

Other causes of facial palsy

Cerebrovascular accidents (thrombosis or haemorrhage) are a common complication of hypertension in the elderly. Unilateral paralysis (hemiplegia) and often loss of speech (aphasia) are frequent in survivors of the acute episode. Unilateral facial palsy is common but differs from Bell's palsy in that the lower part of the face is mainly affected and spontaneous emotional facial reactions may be retained. As in the case of persistent paralysis in Bell's palsy, an intraoral prosthesis may limit sag-ging of the face. A stroke is occasionally the cause of an emergency in the dental surgery (Ch. 36).

Facial palsy is an uncommon but characteristic manifestation of a *malignant parotid tumour*. Alternatively, a facial nerve may have been sacrificed during resection of a malignant tumour, or is accidentally damaged during a parotidectomy. The variable course of the facial nerve within the parotid gland makes it particularly vulnerable to surgical injury and great skill is needed to trace its course.

Ramsay Hunt syndrome is severe facial palsy with pain, usually felt in the throat. Vesicles of herpes zoster may be seen in the external auditory meatus or throat.

Lyme disease is caused by *Borrelia burgdorferi* and transmitted by animal ticks. It is common in the USA but now seen in many other countries. Facial palsy or cervical lymphadenopathy are sometimes prominent but arthritis is the chief effect.

Heerfordt's syndrome is the rare combination of facial palsy, uveitis and parotid swelling caused by sarcoidosis of cranial nerves and salivary glands.

SUGGESTED FURTHER READING

Adour K K, Rubioyianes J M, von Doerstein P G et al 1996 Bell's palsy treatment with acyclovir and prednisone compared with prednisone alone: a double-blind, randomized, controlled trial. Ann Otol Rhinol Laryngol 105:371–378

Baringer J R 1996 Herpes simplex virus and Bell's palsy. Ann Intern Med 124:63–65

Barker F G, Jannetta P J, Bissonette D J et al 1996 The long-term outcome of microvascular decompression for trigeminal neuralgia. N Engl J Med 334:1077–1083

Bergdahl J, Anneroth G, Perris H 1995 Cognitive therapy in the treatment of patients with resistant burning mouth syndrome: a controlled study. J Oral Pathol Med 24:213–215

Devlen J 1994 Anxiety and depression in migraine. J R Soc Med 87:338–341

Fields H L 1996 Treatment of trigeminal neuralgia (editorial). N Engl J Med 334:1125–1126

Huong W, Rothe M J, Grant-Kels J M 1996 The burning mouth syndrome. J Am Acad Dermatol 34:91–98

Kost R G, Straus S E 1996 Postherpetic neuralgia — pathogenesis, treatment and prevention. N Engl J Med 335:32–42

Maizels M, Scott B, Cohen W, Chen W 1996 Intranasal lidocaine for treatment of migraine. JAMA 276:319–321

Morgan M, Nathwain D 1992 Facial palsy and infection: the unfolding story. Clin Infect Dis 14:263–271

Shafshak T S, Essa A Y, Bakey F A 1994 The possible contributing factors for the success of steroid therapy in Bell's palsy: a clinical and electrophysiological study. J Laryngol Otol 108:940–943

Whitley R J, Weiss H, Gnann J W 1996 Acyclovir with and without prednisone for the treatment of herpes zoster. A randomized, placebo-controlled trial. Ann Intern Med 125:376–383

Zakrzewska J M 1996 Assessment of a patient with orofacial pain. Primary Dent Care 3:57–60

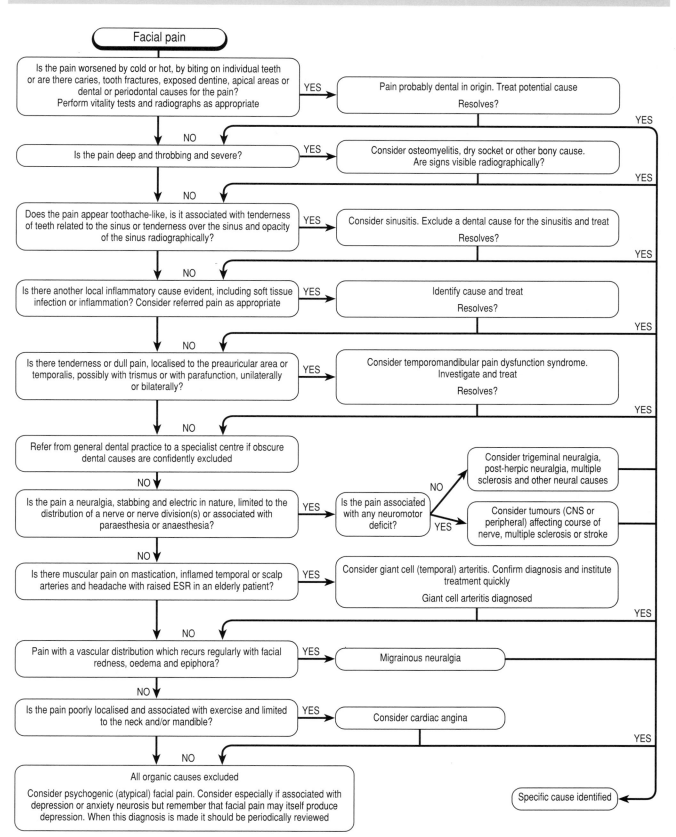

Summary 34.1   Steps in the diagnosis of important causes of facial pain.

Complications of systemic drug treatment

About 10% of ambulant outpatients may be having systemic drug treatment. Though not a common source of difficulties, some drugs can complicate dental management, occasionally catastrophically. Drug addicts are also a growing clinical problem. The effects of systemically administered drugs on dental management are varied (Table 35.1).

Table 35.1   Significance of drug treatment to dental management

- Drugs may complicate dental treatment itself (Table 35.2)
- Drugs given for medical purposes may react with drugs given for dentistry
- Drugs may cause stomatitis or have other oral effects (Table 35.2)

Table 35.2   Examples of drugs having dentally-relevant adverse effects

Type of drug	Dentally-relevant adverse effects
Antibiotics	Superinfection (usually candidosis)
	Allergy (mainly penicillin) (Figs 35.1 and 35.2)
Anticoagulants	Risk of postoperative haemorrhage
Antihypertensives	Severe hypotension in general anaesthesia
Calcium channel blocker antihypertensives (e.g. nifedipine) and diltiazem (an antidysrhythmic)	Gingival hyperplasia
Phenytoin	Gingival hyperplasia
	Lymphadenopathy occasionally
	Folate deficiency occasionally
Aspirin	Potentiation of any haemorrhagic tendencies
	Avoid in children because of risk of Reye's syndrome
Other non-steroidal anti-inflammatory analgesics	Oral lichenoid reactions rarely
Hypnotics and sedatives*	Potentiation of general anaesthetics and other sedating drugs
Barbiturates	Risk of bullous erythema multiforme
Phenothiazine antipsychotics ('major tranquillisers')	Dry mouth
	Tardive dyskinesia (uncontrollable facial movements)
	Parkinsonian tremor
	Postural hypotension
	Oral mucosal pigmentation

Table 35.2   (cont'd)

Metoclopramide	Clenching of jaw muscles
Tricyclic antidepressants (e.g. amitriptyline)†	Dry mouth
Monoamine oxidase inhibitors†	Dry mouth
	Dangerous interactions with opioids, particularly pethidine
Insulin	Risk of hypoglycaemic coma
Antistamines	Dry mouth
	Drowsiness
	Potentiate sedatives
Corticosteroids	Opportunistic infections
	Risk of circulatory collapse (see also Table 31.8)
Other immunosuppressive and cytotoxic drugs	Oral ulceration (especially methotrexate)
	Opportunistic infections
	Cisplatin can cause grey gingival line
	Vincristine can cause jaw pain and weakness of the facial muscles
Cyclosporin	Gingival hyperplasia

*Benzodiazepines ('minor tranquillisers') have few adverse effects apart from sedation, additive effects with other CNS depressants, and slight respiratory depression which is not significant in normal persons. However they are addictive.
† Do *not* cause significant interactions with adrenaline in local anaesthetics.

Oral reactions to drugs

Many drugs can occasionally cause oral reactions. They are varied in character but frequently lichenoid or ulcerative (Figs 35.3 and 35.4).

The mechanisms of reactions to drugs are often obscure but the important types are shown in Table 35.3.

Local reactions to drugs

Chemical burns.   The best-known example is that of aspirin tablets held against the mucosa close to an aching tooth. This causes superficial necrosis and a white patch. When the irritant is removed, dead epithelium is shed and the mucosa heals. Other irritant chemicals are chromic acid or phenol dropped on the mucosa.

Fig. 35.1   Collapse caused by type I hypersensitivity to penicillin.

Fig. 35.2   Hypersensitivity to penicillin. There is a generalised slight oedema of the face, pallor and a macular rash.

Fig. 35.3   Lichenoid reaction to captopril. In this milder reaction there are several small ulcers, but the main effect is the production of striae covering the whole ventral surface of the tongue.

ceptible patients, use of a topical antibiotic may precipitate candidal infection within 48 hours.

Systemically-mediated reactions

Depression of marrow function.   Few drugs significantly depress red cell production alone, though any drug which causes anaemia might give rise to oral signs. The main example is prolonged use of phenytoin (for epilepsy) which, in susceptible patients, can occasionally cause folate deficiency and macrocytic anaemia. This in turn can cause severe aphthous stomatitis. Response promptly follows administration of folate.

White cell production is depressed by a variety of drugs. Leukopenia may be severe enough to produce the clinical picture of agranulocytosis, with necrotising ulceration of the gingivae and throat. This can go on to a severe prostrating illness

Interference with the oral flora: superinfection.   Prolonged topical use of antibiotics (particularly tetracycline) in the mouth kills off sensitive organisms and allows resistant ones, particularly *Candida albicans*, to proliferate, causing thrush. In sus-

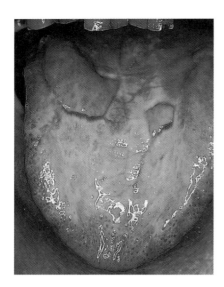

Fig. 35.4 Lichenoid reaction to gold treatment for rheumatoid arthritis. There is extensive ulceration of the dorsal tongue, atrophy and keratosis. Biopsy showed changes very similar to lichen planus.

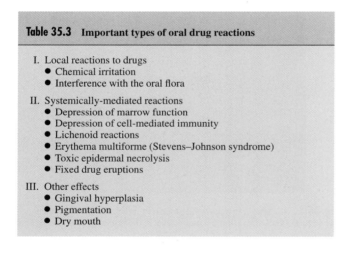

Table 35.3   Important types of oral drug reactions

I. Local reactions to drugs
   ● Chemical irritation
   ● Interference with the oral flora
II. Systemically-mediated reactions
   ● Depression of marrow function
   ● Depression of cell-mediated immunity
   ● Lichenoid reactions
   ● Erythema multiforme (Stevens–Johnson syndrome)
   ● Toxic epidermal necrolysis
   ● Fixed drug eruptions
III. Other effects
   ● Gingival hyperplasia
   ● Pigmentation
   ● Dry mouth

and septicaemia if untreated. Drugs which may have this effect include antibacterials, (particularly co-trimoxazole and chloramphenicol), analgesics (particularly amidopyrine, but obsolete in the UK), phenothiazines and antithyroid agents. When the main effect is on granulocytes, low-grade oral pathogens, particularly of the gingival margins, are able to overcome local resistance and produce necrotising ulceration.

Other drugs may affect haemostasis and cause oral purpura (Ch. 23). Drug-induced purpura is often also an early sign of aplastic anaemia caused by drugs such as chloramphenicol, which depress marrow function, as indicated above. Purpura can cause severe spontaneous gingival bleeding or blood blisters and widespread submucosal ecchymoses.

Depression of cell-mediated immunity. Immunosuppression by such drugs as corticosteroids and cytotoxics is induced in patients having organ transplants (Ch. 24) or with immuno-

logically-mediated diseases (Ch. 25). Viral and fungal infections of the mouth are common in transplant patients and can be severe. Recurrences of childhood viral infections such as measles and chickenpox are also seen.

Lichenoid reactions. Several drugs, notably gold and antimalarials (both used in the treatment of rheumatoid arthritis or other collagen diseases) and the antihypertensive agent methyldopa can cause disease indistinguishable from lichen planus, both clinically and histologically. The mechanism of such reactions is unknown.

Acute erythema multiforme. As discussed earlier, sulphonamides, barbiturates or other drugs are occasionally implicated, but the mechanisms are unknown and more frequently there is no evidence of a drug reaction.

Toxic epidermal necrolysis. This, which probably represents the extreme end of the spectrum of erythema multiforme, is one of the most dangerous and severe types of drug reaction. Mucosal involvement is common and causes widespread erosions due to epithelial destruction. Oral ulceration may precede the dermal changes, and cause the patient to seek treatment for the extreme soreness of the mouth. Early diagnosis and treatment is important as the reaction can be lethal. Metals such as gold salts are important causes but phenylbutazone, barbiturates and other drugs have also been implicated. Healing of oral lesions may leave a pattern of lichen planus.

Fixed drug eruptions. These consist of sharply circumscribed skin lesions recurring in the same site or sites each time the drug is given. Many drugs are capable of causing this reaction, but phenolphthalein, a widely used component of purgatives, is one of the more common causes. Involvement of the oral mucous membrane has been described but is exceedingly rare.

Other drug effects

Gingival hyperplasia. Phenytoin and other drugs (Table 35.2 and Ch. 5), can cause fibrous hyperplasia, particularly concentrated at the interdental papillae.

Oral pigmentation. Heavy metals such as mercury, bismuth and lead can cause black or brown deposits in the gingival sulcus by interaction with bacterial products to form sulphides. The blue lead line may be particularly sharply defined and indicate the level of the floor of the pocket. These effects are rarely seen now that mercury and bismuth are no longer used in medicine and lead is no longer a major industrial hazard. However, cisplatin, a cytotoxic drug, can cause a blue line. Topical antibiotics and antiseptics may cause dark pigmentation, particularly of the dorsum of the tongue, due to overgrowth of pigment-forming bacteria.

Dry mouth is a relatively common side-effect of drugs, particularly those with antimuscarinic (atropine-like) actions, such as the tricyclic antidepressants, which are widely used (Ch. 18).

Management considerations

Oral reactions to drugs are not common on the whole; nevertheless, they may be important as an early sign of a dangerous or lethal reaction.

However, a drug being taken by a patient is not necessarily the cause of any oral symptoms. Coincidence is often difficult to exclude, particularly with common oral diseases such as lichen planus. The problem is made more difficult by multiple drug treatment. It is essential to get a detailed history of drug treatment as this may affect other aspects of dental treatment.

Precautions

Though drugs only occasionally cause clinical difficulties, patients must always be asked whether they are under medical treatment. In such enquiries the word 'drugs' should be avoided as inevitably leading to misinterpretation. Patients should be asked whether they are taking 'medicines, tablets, injections or any sort of medical treatment for *any* purpose', or have received any of medications recently, or whether they have been given any sort of hospital card.

DRUG DEPENDENCE

Drug dependence, particularly addiction to intravenous drugs, is a major social problem, particularly in large cities. However, alcohol remains the most widely abused drug. There are few direct oral effects of drug dependence, apart from maxillofacial injuries secondary to alcohol abuse particularly, but difficulties in management are more common (Table 35.4).

Addicts may manipulate dentists into prescribing drugs, particularly opioids, by complaining of pain. Multiple drug abuse is also common, and attempts may be made to obtain any drugs such as benzodiazepines or antihistamines which are mood-altering or sedative. Benzodiazepines can also cause dependence and should only be prescribed for short periods.

Liver function damaged by alcoholism or hepatitis impairs

Table 35.4   Implications of drug dependence for dental management

- Stealing prescription pads
- Attempting to manipulate dentists into prescribing drugs
- Carriage of hepatitis viruses or HIV by intravenous addicts
- Maxillofacial injuries, particularly among alcoholics
- Impaired liver function secondary to alcoholism or hepatitis
- Lymphadenopathy secondary to drug injection in unusual sites
- Infective endocarditis secondary to dirty injections
- Severe infections such as osteomyelitis among alcoholics
- Increased risks from general anaesthesia
- Gross oral neglect and sometimes enhanced sensitivity to pain
- Rarely, ulceration of the palate secondary to cocaine-induced ischaemia of the nasal cavity
- Occasionally, parotid swelling in alcoholics
- Interactions with other drugs

drug metabolism. This makes general anaesthesia, in particular, hazardous, as does respiratory disease or covert use of the drug of abuse preoperatively. Once infective endocarditis has resulted from dirty injections, the damaged heart becomes vulnerable to endocarditis after some types of dental procedures (Ch. 27).

SUGGESTED FURTHER READING

Cawson R A, Spector R G, Skelly A M 1995 Basic pharmacology, and clinical drug use in dentistry, 6th edn. Churchill Livingstone, Edinburgh
Passeri L A, Ellis E, Sinn D P 1993 Relationship of substance abuse to complications with mandibular fractures. J Oral Maxillofac Surg 51:22–25
Robb N D, Smith B G N 1996 Chronic alcoholism: an important condition in the dentist–patient relationship. J Dent 24:17–24
Strang J 1995 Substance abuse: the size of the problem. Medicine Int 23:41–44
Vale A 1995 Alcohol intoxication and alcohol–drug interactions. Medicine Int 23:51–53

Emergencies in dental practice

Dentists must know how to recognise and manage medical emergencies, rare though they may be. Their professional skill and equipment should enable them occasionally to save patients' lives. Patients suffering life-threatening emergencies should be quickly transferred to hospital, but city traffic and the load on ambulance services are so heavy that the delay can be considerable. Under such circumstances, measures taken by the dentist may be critical.

Dentists are also required to ensure that all members of their staff are able to provide practical assistance in these circumstances.

Many types of emergencies may have to be faced (Table 36.1).

Table 36.1   Emergencies that may arise during dental procedures

Sudden loss of consciousness (Collapse)
1. Fainting
2. Acute hypoglycaemia
3. Circulatory collapse secondary to corticosteroid therapy
4. Myocardial infarction
5. Anaphylactic shock
6. Cardiac arrest
7. Strokes

Acute chest pain
1. Angina
2. Myocardial infarction

Difficulty in breathing
1. Asthma
2. Anaphylactic shock

Convulsions
1. Epilepsy
2. Any other cause of loss of consciousness, including fainting

Other Emergencies
1. Haemorrhage
2. Drug reactions and interactions
3. Major maxillofacial injuries

SUDDEN LOSS OF CONSCIOUSNESS

Fainting

Fainting, caused by transient hypotension and cerebral ischaemia, is the most common cause of sudden loss of consciousness in the dental surgery. There are several predisposing factors (Table 36.2), but some patients are particularly prone to faint and frequently do so. Signs and symptoms are usually readily recognisable (Table 36.3).

Table 36.2   Factors predisposing to fainting

- Anxiety
- Pain
- Injections
- Fatigue
- Hunger

Table 36.3   Signs and symptoms of fainting

- Premonitory dizziness, weakness or nausea
- Pale, cold moist skin
- Initially slow and weak pulse becoming full and bounding
- Loss of consciousness

Sometimes consciousness is lost almost instantaneously. Minor convulsions or incontinence are occasionally associated. Principles of management are summarised in Table 36.4.

Table 36.4   Management of a fainting attack

- Lower the head, preferably by laying the patient flat*
- Loosen any tight clothing round the neck
- Give a sweetened drink when consciousness has been recovered
- If no recovery within a few minutes, consider other causes of loss of consciousness

*To keep the patient upright worsens cerebral hypoxia and is harmful.

Prevention

Regular fainters are frequently helped by an anxiolytic, such as temazepam 5 mg orally, on the night before and again an hour before treatment, if there is a responsible accompanying adult.

Acute hypoglycaemia

Hypoglycaemia affects diabetic patients after an overdose of insulin or if prevented from eating at the expected time by dental treatment. Signs and symptoms are summarised in Table 36.5.

Table 36.5 Signs and symptoms of acute hypoglycaemia
• Premonitory signs are similar to those of a faint, but little response to laying the patient flat • Unconsciousness steadily deepens

Management of hypoglycaemia is important (Table 36.6). If there is any doubt about the cause of loss of consciousness, insulin must never be given as it can be fatal to a hypoglycaemic patient.

Table 36.6 Management of hypoglycaemia
• Patients often aware of what is happening and able to warn the dentist • Before consciousness is lost, give glucose tablets or powder, or sugar (at least four lumps) as a sweetened drink, repeated if symptoms not completely relieved • If consciousness is lost, give subcutaneous glucagon (1 mg), then give sugar by mouth during brief recovery period. • Alternatively, give sterile intravenous glucose (up to 50 ml of a 50% solution) • *Hypostop*, a gel containing glucose, may provide sufficient glucose absorbed through the oral mucosa to combat declining consciousness

Circulatory collapse in patients on corticosteroid treatment

The response of patients on long-term corticosteroid treatment to surgery is unpredictable, but near-fatal circulatory collapse can follow minor dental extractions under anaesthesia in a patient taking as little as 5 mg of prednisone a day. All patients who are taking or have been taking systemic corticosteroids are at risk. Adrenocortical function may possibly take up to 2 years to recover. Corticosteroid skin preparations used liberally, particularly for widespread eczema, can also lead to stress-related collapse.

Since large doses of corticosteroids given for a short period are safe and can be life-saving, management should lean towards being overprotective. Prevention is all important.

Causes and clinical features of corticosteroid-related collapse

General anaesthesia, surgical or other trauma, infections or other stress are the main causes. Signs and management of corticosteroid-related collapse are summarised in Table 36.7.

Table 36.7 Signs and management of corticosteroid-related collapse
Signs • Pallor • Rapid, weak or impalpable pulse • Loss of consciousness • Rapidly falling blood pressure *Management* • Lay the patient flat and raise the legs • Give at least 200 mg hydrocortisone sodium succinate intravenously* • Call an ambulance for immediate transfer to hospital • Give oxygen and, if necessary, artificial ventilation • Consider other possible reasons for loss of consciousness
*The intramuscular route can be used if a vein cannot be found but absorption is slower.

Myocardial infarction

A patient typically has severe chest pain, but may suddenly lose consciousness as a result of a myocardial infarct (see below).

Anaphylactic reactions

Penicillin is the most common cause of these type I hypersensitivity reactions. Similar reactions due to direct histamine release by morphine or intravenous barbiturate anaesthetics are rare. Anaphylactic reactions can also be precipitated by insect stings, foods (nuts or shellfish particularly) and exceptionally rarely by aspirin.

In general, the quicker the onset the more severe the reaction. A severe reaction to penicillin may start within a minute of an injection, but immediate loss of consciousness is more likely to be due to fainting. A reaction starting 30 minutes after an injection is unlikely to be dangerous. Acute reactions to oral penicillins are rare but can develop after half an hour or more because of slower absorption from the gut.

Collapse is due to widespread vasodilatation and increased capillary permeability causing potentially fatal hypotension.

Signs and symptoms

The clinical picture is variable (Table 36.8).

Table 36.8 Acute anaphylaxis — typical features
• Initial facial flushing, itching, paraesthesiae or cold extremities • Facial oedema or urticaria • Bronchospasm (wheezing) sometimes prominent • Loss of consciousness • Pallor going on to cyanosis • Cold clammy skin • Rapid weak or impalpable pulse • Deep fall in blood pressure • Death if treatment is delayed or inappropriate

Management

Adrenaline is the mainstay of treatment (Table 36.9). It raises cardiac output, combats excessive capillary permeability and bronchospasm, and also inhibits release of mediators from mast cells.

Table 36.9   **Management of anaphylactic collapse**

- Lay the patient flat. Raise the legs to improve cerebral blood flow
- Give 0.5–1 ml of 1:1000 adrenaline by intramuscular injection
  Repeat every 15 minutes if necessary, until the patient responds
- Give 10–20 mg chlorpheniramine (diluted in the syringe with 10 ml of blood) slowly intravenously
- Give 200 mg of hydrocortisone sodium succinate intravenously
- Give oxygen and, if necessary, assisted ventilation
- Call an ambulance

Circulatory collapse is probably largely due to histamine release which is combated by parenteral chlorpheniramine. Hydrocortisone is slow to take effect but maintains the blood pressure for some hours and combats the continued effect of the antigen–antibody reaction.

Rapid transfer to hospital is necessary to provide circulatory support by intravenous fluids and other measures. The patient must also be given a card, warning against the use of the causative drug.

Minor anaphylactic reactions such as urticaria can be treated with oral or intramuscular chlorpheniramine.

Cardiac arrest

Cardiac arrest can follow myocardial infarction or the acute hypotension of an anaphylactic reaction or of corticosteroid insufficiency. Otherwise, it may be the result of an anaesthetic accident and due to hypoxia, anaesthetic overdose or severe hypotension.

Dentists should be aware of, and alert to, the possibility of cardiac arrest and be able to recognise it (Table 36.10) when it happens. Speed of response is essential and there is a legal obligation that the dental team should be trained in cardiopulmonary resuscitation and be able to carry it out immediately.

Table 36.10   **Signs and symptoms of cardiac arrest**

- Sudden loss of consciousness
- Absence of arterial pulses (the carotid artery, anterior to sternomastoid, should be felt)

Respiratory arrest and eventual cyanosis, pupil dilatation and loss of reaction to light, and absence of measurable blood pressure are other signs but resuscitation must be started before they develop.

Principles of management of cardiac arrest are summarised in Table 36.11.

Table 36.11   **Management of cardiac arrest**

- Summon help. Telephone for an ambulance and state that there has been a cardiac arrest
- Put the patient on a firm flat surface, i.e. the floor, if possible*
- Clear the airway and keep it clear by extending the neck and holding the jaw forward
- Start external cardiac compression immediately. Kneel (or stand) beside the patient and put one hand over the other on the patient's lower sternum. Forcefully depress the sternum about 1.5–2 inches (4–5 cm) at about 80 times a minute
- The assistant should inflate the lungs between each five compressions of the sternum, either as a mouth-to-mouth procedure or with a self-inflating bag with oxygen supplementation, as described below†
- Persist until expert help arrives or there are signs of restoration of blood pressure with disappearance of facial pallor, and a good spontaneous pulse. Other signs of success are contraction of the pupils, return of reflex activity, such as the blink reflex and reaction of the pupils to light, lightening of unconsciousness and purposeful spontaneous movements — not twitching or convulsions
- Transfer the patient to hospital for advanced life support

*If the patient is too heavy to lift out of a dental chair but can be laid supine there, resuscitation can be carried out by the operator and assistant standing beside the chair. An operator's stool can be placed under the headrest to stabilise the chair.
† If there is no assistant, the ratio of chest compressions to lung inflations should be 15:4.

The optimal pressure for chest compression is about 40 or 50 kg (the weight of the upper part of the body applied through stiffly extended arms). External cardiac massage is tiring and another person should preferably take over as soon as the first operator becomes fatigued. If no signs of life appear within 15 minutes (timed by the clock) recovery is unlikely.

Unless the operator is skilled in its use, time should not be wasted in trying to pass an endotracheal tube. However, a self-inflating bag with an oxygen supply should be available to provide positive pressure ventilation. A plastic airway should be put in the patient's mouth and the mask applied firmly over the nose and mouth with the resuscitation bag attached. The patient's lungs should be inflated with oxygen by squeezing the bag, so that the chest is visibly expanded at each respiration. Passive recoil of the chest wall causes spontaneous expiration as soon as the pressure is removed.

If a self-inflating bag is not available, mouth-to-mouth ventilation can be given, preferably with an intervening Laerdal pocket mask.

During artificial ventilation the patient's nose must be closed. Deep inflations are given by the operator and time allowed for passive recoil of the chest. If there is no airway adjunct available, direct mouth-to-mouth resuscitation, with the nose occluded, must be given. Causes of failure are summarised in Table 36.12.

> **Table 36.12** Causes of failure of cardiopulmonary resuscitation
>
> - Giving external cardiac compression without artificial ventilation
> - Giving artificial ventilation without cardiac compression
> - Failing to clear the airway or to keep it open by failing to hyperextend the head adequately
> - Failing to close the nose during mouth-to-mouth ventilation
> - Failing to fit the mask closely on to the patient's face when using an inflating bag
> - Failing to make sure that ventilation is adequate, as shown by movement of the chest
> - Timidity in applying external cardiac compression, and using insufficient force to compress the heart. The risk of cracking a rib should be disregarded
> - Failing to release pressure on the chest completely between compressions and thus preventing cardiac filling
> - Compressing the chest too rapidly to allow the heart to fill between compressions
> - Putting the hands in incorrect positions
> - Failing to act sufficiently quickly and fretting about details rather than getting on with the essentials of external cardiac compression and artificial ventilation

Strokes

Patients are usually hypertensive and middle-aged or elderly.

The clinical picture varies with the size and site of brain damage. Subarachnoid haemorrhage from a ruptured berry aneurysm on the circle of Willis is the main cause of stroke in a younger person. It typically causes intense headache followed by coma without localizing signs. Signs and management of a stroke are summarised in Table 36.13.

> **Table 36.13** Signs and management of a stroke
>
> *Signs*
> - Loss of consciousness
> - Weakness of an arm and leg on one side
> - Drooping of the side of the face
> - Often stertorous breathing
>
> *Management*
> - Maintain the airway
> - Call an ambulance for transfer to hospital

CHEST PAIN

Angina pectoris

A patient with coronary atheroma might have a first anginal attack as a consequence of an emotional response to dental treatment. However, most patients have already had attacks and carry medication. Acute chest pain due to myocardial ischaemia is the only symptom. Principles of management are summarised in Table 36.14.

> **Table 36.14** Management of angina
>
> - Give the patient his antianginal drug (usually 0.5 mg of glyceryl trinitrate sublingually) OR
> - Glyceryl trinitrate spray (400 mg)* gives rapid relief
> - If there is no relief within 3 minutes the patient has probably had a myocardial infarct (see below)
>
> *Glyceryl trinitrate spray has a better shelf-life for the emergency kit.

Myocardial infarction

Myocardial infarction is a common cause of death and must be recognised, as the patient's fate may be decided by the first few minutes' treatment. Typical signs and symptoms are summarised in Table 36.15. Several aspects of dentistry, particularly apprehension, pain or the effect of drugs, might contribute to make this accident more likely in a susceptible patient.

Some patients die within a few minutes after the start of the attack and it is rash to try overambitious treatment. Drugs, apart from those described below, should not be used, as without continuous monitoring they may do more harm than good.

> **Table 36.15** Typical signs and symptoms of myocardial infarction
>
> - Severe crushing retrosternal pain
> - Shallow breathing
> - Vomiting
> - Weak or irregular pulse

Pain can radiate to the left shoulder or down the left arm but very occasionally is felt only in the left jaw. Vomiting is common and there is sometimes shock or loss of consciousness.

Principles of management are summarised in Table 36.16. Aspirin is a valuable antiplatelet drug but it is only feasible to give a fibrinolytic drug such as streptokinase in hospital where lignocaine or other antidysrhythmic drugs can be given, as appropriate.

> **Table 36.16** Management of myocardial infarction
>
> - Put the patient in a comfortable position that allows easy breathing.
> - Do not lay flat if there is left ventricular failure and pulmonary oedema
> - Send an assistant to telephone for an intensive care ambulance
> - Give 50/50 nitrous oxide and oxygen from a general anaesthetic or relative analgesia machine, to relieve pain and anxiety
> - Constantly reassure the patient
> - Give oxygen if necessary
> - Give aspirin 150 mg by mouth as soon as more urgent measures have been carried out
> - Check for possible cardiac arrest

There is concern about dentists giving aspirin under these circumstances in case there has been a misdiagnosis and the pain is due to a perforated peptic ulcer or dissecting aneurysm. However, the danger of giving a single tablet of aspirin in such conditions is unlikely to be significant.

DYSPNOEA

Status asthmaticus

Causes

Loss of, or forgetting to bring, a salbutamol inhaler, anxiety, infection or exposure to a specific allergen are possible causes.

Important signs and management are summarised in Table 36.17.

Table 36.17 Signs and management of status asthmaticus

Signs
- Breathlessness
- Inability to talk
- Expiratory wheezing (may be disguised as shallow breathing).
- Rapid pulse (usually over 110 per minute). Progress to bradycardia is a danger sign
- Accessory muscles of respiration start to come into action
- Cyanosis

Management
- Reassure the patient
- Do NOT lay the patient flat
- Give normally-used anti-asthmatic drugs (such as salbutamol) by inhaler or, better, by nebuliser
- Give hydrocortisone sodium succinate 200 mg intravenously
- Give oxygen
- If no response within 2–3 minutes, ideally give salbutamol 250 μg by slow i.v. injection
- If i.v. salbutamol not available and patient continues to deteriorate, give adrenaline, as for anaphylaxis
- Call an ambulance for transfer to hospital

CONVULSIONS

Epilepsy

Hunger, menstruation and some drugs such as methohexitone, tricyclic antidepressants, alcohol or frequently flashing lights (*not* merely turning the operating lamp on and off) may sometimes precipitate a fit.

Important signs and management are summarised in Table 36.18.

Status epilepticus

If convulsions do not stop within 15 minutes, or are rapidly repeated, the patient is in status epilepticus and can die from anoxia. Principles of management are summarised in Table 36.19.

Table 36.18 Signs and management of a tonic-clonic epileptic attack

Signs
- Sometimes a brief warning cry as the chest muscles contract and air is forced through a closed larynx
- Consciousness lost immediately
- The body becomes rigid (tonic phase) and cyanosis appears
- Widespread jerking movements start (clonic phase)
- Sometimes incontinence or frothing of the mouth
- Flaccidity sometimes follows after a few minutes
- Consciousness regained after a variable period. Confusion or drowsiness may persist

Management
- Put the patient prone in the coma ('recovery') position as soon as possible
- Prevent patients from injuring themselves
- Do not try to put anything in the mouth in the attempt to prevent the patient biting the tongue
- Make sure the airway is clear after convulsions have subsided
- Do not give any medication but await recovery
- Reassure patients as soon as consciousness returns
- Only allow patients to return home when fully recovered and accompanied by a responsible adult

---

Table 36.19 Management of status epilepticus

- Give 10 mg intravenous diazepam to an adult patient
- If venous access cannot be obtained give 5 mg of intramuscular midazolam* (absorption of intramuscular diazepam is slow and erratic)
- Repeat diazepam or midazolam if no recovery within 5 minutes
- Maintain the airway and give oxygen
- Call an ambulance and transfer to hospital

*Not officially approved for this purpose but may be life-saving.

OTHER EMERGENCIES

Haemorrhage

Prolonged bleeding is usually due to traumatic extractions. A major vessel is unlikely to be opened during dental surgery and patients are unlikely to lose any dangerous amount of blood if promptly managed. Postextraction bleeding is usually only an emergency in the sense that the dentist may be woken up at 3 o'clock in the morning by a frightened patient.

Occasionally bleeding is due to unsuspected haemophilia or other haemorrhagic disorders. Principles of management are summarised in Table 36.20.

Drug reactions and interactions

Apart from anaphylactic reactions discussed earlier, very few other drug reactions or interactions endangering life are likely to be seen in the dental surgery.

Table 36.20   Management of prolonged dental haemorrhage

- Reassure the patient
- Usher excited relatives out of the surgery
- Clean the mouth with swabs and locate the source of bleeding
- Give adrenaline-containing local anaesthetic, remove ragged tissue, squeeze up the socket edges and suture it
- When bleeding has been controlled, ask about the history and especially any family history of prolonged bleeding
- If bleeding continues despite suturing or if the patient is obviously anaemic or debilitated, transfer to hospital for investigation and management of any haemorrhagic defect
- Meanwhile, limit bleeding as much as possible with a pressure pad over the socket and by supporting the patient's jaw with a firm barrel bandage
- Ideally, tranexamic acid (500 mg, by slow intravenous injection) should be given and may be effective in a mild haemophilic while awaiting transfer to hospital

Local anaesthetics with vasoconstrictors

Noradrenaline (1:20 000), used as a vasoconstrictor in local anaesthetic solutions, has caused deaths from acute hypertension or cerebral haemorrage. Such reactions can be combated by an α-blocker such as phentolamine. Quite apart from its dangers, noradrenaline has no advantages and is no longer available.

Adrenaline. There is no clinical evidence of hypertensive reactions to adrenaline used in normal concentration and quantity.

Interactions with β-blockers. Adrenaline, in *large* doses, can interact with drugs such as propranolol to raise the blood pressure. Adrenaline causes constriction of skin and visceral vessels (α effect), but dilatation of muscle arterioles (β effect).

Dilatation of muscle vessels by adrenaline is opposed by the β-blocker but adrenaline's α effect on skin and visceral vessels is unopposed. The consequent constriction of both muscle and skin vessels raises the peripheral resistance and blood pressure.

Clinically, occasional cases of hypertensive interactions between adrenaline and propranolol have been reported in patients receiving large amounts of adrenaline in local analgesics for plastic surgery. In 1995, a dentist was convicted of manslaughter after causing the death of a patient on β-blockers by giving her 16 cartridges of lignocaine with adrenaline, though it appears overdose of lignocaine was the cause. Though healthy adults can tolerate large amounts of lignocaine with adrenaline, the dose should be limited to five cartridges given over the space of an hour.

Otherwise, in all three deaths associated with dental local anaesthetics in the 10 year period 1980–1989, prilocaine had been given.

Monoamine oxidase inhibitors

These can cause severe reactions with opioids. The onset can be very sudden and, with pethidine, can be fatal. Monoamine oxidase inhibitors also interact with indirectly-acting sympathomimetic drugs (such as ephedrine used as a nasal decongestant) to cause acute severe hypertension. The treatment is to give an α-blocker such as phentolamine. Adrenaline or noradrenaline in local anaesthetics do not cause hypertensive reactions with monoamine oxidase inhibitors.

General anaesthetics

These, particularly intravenous barbiturates, have been the main cause of fatalities in the dental surgery.

Corticosteroids

As already described, patients on long-term corticosteroid treatment when exposed to stress can suffer circulatory collapse as a result of adrenal suppression.

SUGGESTED FURTHER READING

Cawson R A, Spector R G, Skelly A M 1995 Basic pharmacology and clinical drug use in dentistry, 6th edn. Churchill Livingstone, Edinburgh

Edmondson H D, Frame J W, Malins A F 1989 Medical emergencies in dental practice: an update on drugs and the management of acute airway obstruction. Dent Update August: 254–256

European Rescuscitation Council Basic Life Support Working Group 1993 Guidelines for basic life support. BMJ 306:1587–1589

European Rescuscitation Council Working Party 1993 Adult advanced cardiac life support: the European Rescuscitation Council guidelines 1992 (abridged). BMJ 306:1589–1593

Fisher M 1992 Treating anaphylaxis with sympathomimetic drugs. In severe anaphylaxis adrenaline by any route is better than none (editorial). BMJ 305:1107–1108

Gallagher E J, Lombardi G, Gennis P 1995 Effectiveness of bystander cardiopulmonary rescuscitation and survival following out-of-hospital cardiac arrest. JAMA 274:1922–1925

Pennycook A, Makower R, Brewer A et al 1993 The management of dental problems presenting to an accident and emergency department. J R Soc Med 86:702–703

Sanders B J, Weddell J A, Dodge N N 1995 Managing patients who have seizure disorders: dental and medical issues. J Am Dent Assoc 126:1641–1647

Index